SOCIAL ASPECTS OF DRUG DISCOVERY, DEVELOPMENT AND COMMERCIALIZATION

SOCIAL ASPECTS OF DRUG DISCOVERY, DEVELOPMENT AND COMMERCIALIZATION

ODILIA OSAKWE, MS, PhD
Industrial BioDevelopment Laboratory, UHN-MaRS Centre
Toronto Medical Discovery Tower and Ryerson University,
Toronto, Canada

**SYED A. A. RIZVI, MSc, MBA, MS, PhD (Pharm),
PhD (Chem), MRSC**
Department of Pharmaceutical Sciences,
Nova Southeastern University, Fort Lauderdale, FL, USA

Amsterdam • Boston • Heidelberg • London
New York • Oxford • Paris • San Diego
San Francisco • Singapore • Sydney • Tokyo

Academic Press is an imprint of Elsevier

Academic Press is an imprint of Elsevier
125 London Wall, London EC2Y 5AS, UK
525 B Street, Suite 1800, San Diego, CA 92101-4495, USA
50 Hampshire Street, 5th Floor, Cambridge, MA 02139, USA
The Boulevard, Langford Lane, Kidlington, Oxford OX5 1GB, UK

British Library Cataloguing-in-Publication Data
A catalogue record for this book is available from the British Library

Library of Congress Cataloging-in-Publication Data
A catalog record for this book is available from the Library of Congress

ISBN: 978-0-12-802220-7

For information on all Academic Press publications
visit our website at http://store.elsevier.com/

Typeset by Thomson Digital

Publisher: Mica Haley
Acquisition Editor: Kristine Jones
Editorial Project Manager: Molly McLaughlin
Production Project Manager: Lucía Pérez
Designer: Vicky Pearson

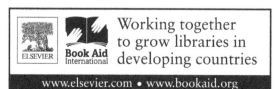

To

Philomena and Chioma

CONTENTS

Preface   *xiii*
Introduction   *xvii*

SECTION I: PHARMACEUTICAL INDUSTRY, SOCIETY, AND GOVERNANCE
1. Pharmaceutical Regulation: The Role of Government
in the Business of Drug Discovery   **3**
Odilia Osakwe

    1.1. Introduction   4
    1.2. The legal instruments   5
    1.3. The National Regulatory Authorities and Administration   6
    1.4. Analytical framework for regulatory approval: Benefit–risk assessment   11
    1.5. The pharmaceutical product life cycle   13
    1.6. The global pharmaceutical industry: Harmonization and partnerships   18
    1.7. Modernization of the global pharmaceutical systems: Regulatory strategies,
        roadmap initiatives, and partnerships   22
    References   26

2. Trends in Innovation and the Business of Drug Discovery   **29**
Odilia Osakwe

    2.1. Introduction   30
    2.2. Evolutionary trends in pharmaceutical innovation   32
    2.3. Advances in pharmaceutical innovation technology   36
    2.4. Select medical milestones of 2014   37
    2.5. Factors contributing to pharmaceutical innovation setback   38
    2.6. Case: Challenges in antimicrobial drug discovery   45
    2.7. Consequence of innovation setback   46
    2.8. Strategies and approaches to addressing innovation failure   47
    2.9. Concluding remarks   52
    References   52

3. Cash Flow Valley of Death: A Pitfall in Drug Discovery   **57**
Odilia Osakwe

    3.1. Introduction   58
    3.2. Product valuation as an investment decision-making tool   59
    3.3. Challenges associated with the valley of death   60
    3.4. Firms involved in the pharmaceutical value chain   66

3.5. Strategies for bridging the Valley of Death and innovation failure   67
3.6. Funding models   74
3.7. Nongovernmental funding models   76
3.8. Other financial concepts   77
3.9. Private–public sector groups   78
References   79

SECTION II: DRUG DISCOVERY CYCLE I: DISCOVERY AND PRECLINICAL
DRUG DEVELOPMENT
4. Prediscovery Research: Challenges and Opportunities   85
Odilia Osakwe

4.1. Introduction   85
4.2. Models of human disease biology   88
4.3. Diseases considered in biopharmaceutical research and development   91
4.4. Modern trends in drug discovery   91
4.5. Current challenges in early drug discovery   101
References   105

5. The Significance of Discovery Screening and Structure
Optimization Studies   109
Odilia Osakwe

5.1. Introduction   109
5.2. Screening tools in drug discovery   110
5.3. *In silico* models in drug discovery and design   114
5.4. From hit to lead: Summary of compound optimization in drug discovery   123
References   126

6. Preclinical *In Vitro* Studies: Development and Applicability   129
Odilia Osakwe

6.1. Introduction   129
6.2. Predictability of preclinical disease models   130
6.3. Trends in preclinical drug development   132
6.4. Relevance of ADME/PK studies   133
6.5. Experimental tools used in preclinical development   135
6.6. Drug eliminating agents and mechanisms   139
6.7. Application of zebrafish as a model whole organism: A landmark
in preclinical development   144
References   145

7.   **Animal Utilization in Drug Development: Clinical, Legal,**
      and Ethical Dimensions   **149**
      Odilia Osakwe

      7.1. Introduction   150
      7.2. The scientific value of animal studies: Pharmacology objectives   150
      7.3. Laboratory animals model in the frontiers of drug discovery   151
      7.4. Relationships in animal taxonomy and implications in pharmaceutical
            research and development   152
      7.5. The effect of species differences on study results   154
      7.6. How reliable is the animal toxicity information generated across
            the animal species?   157
      7.7. Landmarks in preclinical development: Species selection and rationale   158
      7.8. Animal models in the development of biopharmaceuticals:
            The exceptional use of nonhuman primates   161
      7.9. Legal accommodations on the use of animals in pharmaceutical research
            and development   161
      7.10. Animal alternatives in drug development: Replacing, reducing,
            and refinement of animals   163
      References   165

8.   **Pharmaceutical Formulation and Manufacturing Development:**
      Strategies and Issues   **169**
      Odilia Osakwe

      8.1. Introduction   169
      8.2. Regulatory aspects of pharmaceutical development   171
      8.3. Formulation and manufacturing in pharmaceutical development   173
      8.4. Clinical trials materials   175
      8.5. Concepts used in pharmaceutical development   177
      8.6. Drug shortages   179
      8.7. Manufacturing problems leading to drug shortages   180
      8.8. Addressing drug shortages: strategies   184
      References   185

SECTION III: THE DRUG DISCOVERY CYCLE II: CLINICAL DEVELOPMENT
9.   **Clinical Development: Ethics and Realities**   **191**
      Odilia Osakwe

      Part I   192
      9.1. Introduction   192

Part II Clinical development of candidate drugs   194
    9.2. Clinical trial: principles and approach   194
    9.3. Evaluation tools in clinical trials, clinical outcomes, and relevance   199
    9.4. Selected topics in clinical trials   204
    9.5. Implications of inappropriate study design   205
Part III Clinical trial ethics   207
    9.6. Ethical conduct in clinical trials   207
    9.7. Informed consent   209
    9.8. Conflict of interest in clinical research   210
    9.9. Crucial cases in clinical trials with implications on society 211
    9.10. International clinical trials across the globe   213
    References   218

10. **Pharmacogenomics in Drug Discovery, Prospects
     and Clinical Applicability**   **221**
     Odilia Osakwe

     10.1. Introduction   222
     10.2. Genetic variations and implications in drug development   227
     10.3. The effectiveness of clinical implementation of pharmacogenomics   230
     10.4. Promising outcomes associated with clinical application
            pharmacogenomics: cases   233
     10.5. Economic and social implications of pharmacogenomics application   236
     10.6. National regulatory agencies on pharmacogenomics implementation   237
     References   239

**SECTION IV: THE DRUG DISCOVERY CYCLE III: AUTHORIZATION
              AND MARKETING**
11. **Patents, Exclusivities, and Evergreening Strategies**   **245**
     Syed A. A. Rizvi

     11.1. Introduction: Patents and exclusive marketing rights   245
     11.2. US Patent Law Amendments Act of 1984   246
     11.3. The interplay of patents and exclusivities during the product lifecycle   248
     11.4. Patents in the global pharmaceutical market place   249
     11.5. Evergreening   250
     11.6. Conclusions   252
     References   253

12. Drug Pricing and Control for Pharmaceutical Drugs   **255**

Odilia Osakwe

12.1. Introduction   255
12.2. Drug assessment and pricing in various geographical locations   256
12.3. Pharmaceutical drug pricing and ethics   263
References   264

13. Direct-to-Consumer Advertising   **267**

Odilia Osakwe

13.1. Introduction   267
13.2. Ethics and relevance of pharmaceutical advertising   268
13.3. Pharmaceutical advertising and government control   272
13.4. Prescription medicine advertising codes   276
13.5. Conclusions   278
References   278

Index   **281**

PREFACE

A considerable number of textbooks have delivered substantial information on the scientific and technological aspects of drug discovery and development, but very few have touched upon the social aspects. The idea of writing this book was stimulated by this necessity along with an emergent notion, which grew out of my experience as a lecturer on this subject, in Ryerson University.

The *Social Aspects of Drug Discovery, Development and Commercialization* presents a holistic overview of the entire drug discovery process, as it transitions from inception, to a pill in the hands of the patient. It explains the importance for it to be addressed comprehensively, to include all areas that interact with the society. This will enable a proper understanding of the workings of the pharmaceutical enterprise, from which springs forth the medical products that are supplied to the wide public. This will serve as a knowledge base to streamline ideas and perspectives about how drugs are created and distributed; for a regular citizen, an investor in the pharmaceutical business, or students or professionals who need to be updated on pharmaceutical affairs. In other words, this information helps the reader in decision making on the proper approach to healthcare and its products; and provides for the scholar or professional, a strong grounding in this subject area.

One outstanding characteristic of this textbook is that, it provides definitions and explanations of the relevant background information to serve as a framework for understanding the social aspects, making it a user-friendly resource for a wide range of readers. It details the key participants, relationships, and processes involved in the full drug discovery programs that span the pharmaceutical product lifecycle that are necessary for creating the medical solutions delivered to the public, as represented in the pharmaceutical ecosystems. Analysis of the paths of pharmaceutical innovation is within the context of the pharmaceutical ecosystem. For example, pharmaceutical policy and laws have emanated from extensive debate by a hierarchy of government-appointed groups, agencies, social groups, such as patient representative groups, representatives of charities and consumer associations, pharmaceutical and allied professionals, and other groups from various strata of the healthcare systems who are the voice of command in these decision making activities. Pharmaceutical ecosystems embrace the stakeholders, the processes, and technologies whose cross-interactions strengthen the drug discovery programs.

What type of knowledge is gained by the readers of this book?

The introductory chapter gives a general overview of the whole process, which serves as a foundation for the rest of the 13 chapters. Every chapter sequentially builds from the previous and all of which represent a progressive pathway in the discovery of an investigational drug molecule as it morphs into a full drug product that is accessed by the public.

This book attempts to answer certain exemplary questions. Chapter 1: What is the origin, meaning, and relevance of the pharmaceutical laws and regulations? Chapter 2: What is the pharmaceutical productivity landscape? Is pharmaceutical innovation sustainable? What is the technological flow, applicability, and effectiveness? What is the economic landscape for emerging pharmaceutical firms? What are the prospects and trend over the years? Chapter 3: What is responsible for hiatus or demise of the drug discovery pipeline in the initial stages of the drug discovery events? What are the relationships between the emerging and the big pharmaceutical companies? Chapters 4-6: How is the drug discovery pipeline advancing toward providing the needed medical solutions to diseases, especially the deadly ones? What are the hopes of families that have to grapple with life-threatening diseases? What is new in finding disease pathways and new drug molecules? Chapter 7: The animals chosen for testing of drug candidates, does this decision directly correlate with therapy pursued or are animals over utilized? How do the different species differ in pharmacological response? Chapters 8 and 9: Are drugs manufactured to precision? What is the reason for drug recalls? Chapter 9: Are clinical trials conducted to reflect specific public interests? What are the patients' rights as participants in clinical trials? What are the opportunities and setbacks in multinational clinical trials? Chapter 10: Why are certain drugs more compatible with certain individuals and the experienced adverse events in only certain individuals? What is the applicability of individualized or precision medicine? Chapter 11: How does patents alter drug accessibility? What are the legal factors that affect patents and emergence of generics? How fast could generics be reached? Chapter 12: How does drug marketing benefit the end user? Chapter 13: What is the flow of drug pricing around the globe?

This book could serve as a training tool or reference guide for students and professionals in most of health science and allied disciplines; pharmacy, pharmaceutical sciences, pharmacology, clinical and translational research, medicine, nursing, and more. This also applies to those in pharmaceutical law and policy, health policy and management, and pharmacoeconomics. It can also be a useful information base for students and professionals in regulatory affairs, who are expected to be thorough in the knowledge of drug discovery.

The text is delivered in a concise, direct, and soft language to stimulate interest and enliven your readership.

I would like to extend my personal gratitude to Dr Syed A.A. Rizvi for his valued contribution to this work. Most and foremost, my hearty thanks goes to He who is the pillar of my life and who supplied the knowledge, courage, and strength that carried me throughout this process.

Introduction

1 TRENDS IN DRUG DISCOVERY

The pharmaceutical industry is of tremendous value to society, mainly because of the active discovery and development of pharmaceuticals, which have increased quality of life through both ameliorating pain and suffering, and the treatment of diseases.

Major landmarks in drug discovery that preceded the thalidomide tragedy in the 1950s have led to a total overhaul of regulatory systems. Extensive federal governance has been deemed necessary to address the unsatisfactory efficacy and safety standards that characterized earlier drug manufacturing systems, which underlie the high standards imposed on companies that manufacture and distribute drugs to the public. Since then, increasingly innovative breakthroughs have contributed immensely to the changing pharmaceutical landscape.

The first major historical accomplishment was the innovation boon of the 1990s, a period marked by a rise in the production of blockbuster drugs that has contributed to more than one-third of the total pharmaceutical revenues, totaling US$149 billion [1]. Market growth rate skyrocketed due to expansion of the number of high selling drugs, which lifted the position of the pharmaceutical industry in the global economy [2]. Products from the leading five pharmaceutical companies – Pfizer, Roche, AstraZeneca, Merck & Co., and Novartis – topped the list of the best-selling drugs, such as Prozac, an antidepressant drug; Lipitor® (atorvastatin), which is used to treat blood cholesterol; and Plavix® (clopidogrel), which inhibits the formation of blood clots following myocardial infarction. Many of these drugs attract interest, particularly because they target chronic diseases. Large financial returns generated from just a handful of these drugs sustain the research and development (R&D) for emerging drugs. However, this business model is no longer very promising because patents are expiring. Diversification to niche market drugs is increasingly being expected so as to shift focus from the blockbuster drugs market to those drugs that target other diseases in demand of medical therapy. Thus, today's R&D is largely driven by new medical discoveries associated with a high probability of economic and technical risk. These types of diseases require discovery of difficult targets that limit innovation speed and cash flow with a high price of unpredictability. For example, the emergence of HIV/AIDS points to the need to expect a therapy that has hitherto been a distant reality.

Incremental shifts in the configuration of the industry over time culminated in the technological breakthroughs of the early twentieth century when interpretation and understanding of molecular biology changed drastically. Groundbreaking biological techniques like proteomics and genomics emerged along with more sophisticated techniques that utilize advanced statistical and mathematical platforms coupled with computer-based strategies in biology and chemistry. Most of these are molecular modeling, simulations, combinatorial chemistry, high-throughput technology, and high-performance computing. Dynamic models created a framework to integrate the knowledge base within the functional areas and, most importantly, the high technology applications further facilitated a better handling of the rapidly growing volume of "big data" to scale down the complicated R&D processes for a better workflow and output. The "omics" revolution represents an advancement in molecular science that improved understanding of the molecular linkage of cause and function of diseases to enable the finding of the networks of pathways and, ultimately, the disease targets [3–5]. A model mechanism of drug action enables the drug discovery and development team to understand how drugs act in whole body systems, organs, and at a subcellular level. There is a growing technical competence in targeting smaller patient populations to narrower therapeutic areas for personalized medicine – a greater selectivity offered by genomics.

The Orphan Drug Act was intended to advance treatments for rare disease. This is increasingly leading to new drugs that are effective on smaller defined patient populations that fall into the "orphans" category, with a foreknowledge furnished by an increased understanding of the causes of the diseases. This presents an opportunity for companies to specialize in particular aspects of the drug development process, which is a more promising pathway to innovation success.

These revolutionary scientific and technological discoveries have brought changes that underscore a dynamic society undergoing major transformation – a change encompassing all the varied levels of the complex processes. This dynamic society requires an integrated framework to bring together all the processes within and across all aspects of the pre- and post-drug launch of candidate drugs. A robust pharmaceutical innovation system that would promote effective cooperation and communication among the stakeholders is highly desirable.

2 THE PHARMACEUTICAL ECOSYSTEM

The pharmaceutical ecosystem refers to the interdependent relationships among levels of interacting stakeholder networks in connection with processes, tools, and infrastructures that are controlled by policies, laws, and opinions. The stakeholder groups are the discovery and development team, academia, physicians, healthcare providers, payers, patients, advocacy groups, consumers groups, and the public or civic society. All these players have unique perspectives about the pharmaceutical industry in connection with the needs, values, and preferences of the area of the public they represent. The infrastructure is the technological platform and core facilities used to drive the drug product from concept to access. The strategic issues – regulatory structures and reform, local and national cultures, politics, federal laws, economic and reimbursement policies, intellectual property and patent policies, product factors, and marketing dynamics – are also the tools for streamlining the utility of medicines during the pre- and postmarketing stages. This is the pivot upon which the pharmaceutical industry rotates. That is to say, all the R&D operations that are the core aspect of drug discovery and development are extensively affected and controlled by these social values. The definition mentioned earlier implies that all aspects of the ecosystem contribute toward most or all of that which translates into a new medical product. A functional ecosystem is characterized by uniform interdependent relationships, which is critical for the continuation of the system. Thus, a pharmaceutical industry that exhibits a functional ecosystem will be more efficient in satisfying its anticipated intended purpose. Figure 1 shows the relatedness of all the players in the pharmaceutical value chain leading to a functional pharmaceutical ecosystem with inference to the drug product.

The pharmaceutical value chain is the totality of functions that are performed within big pharmaceutical companies until product phase-out.

There are networks of multichannel interactions at various levels around the development of a pharmaceutical product. This explains the enormous complexity of pharmaceutical innovation. Meaningful cooperation among all the elements offers the promise of high-performance collaboration, processes, and utility of tools and infrastructure [6].

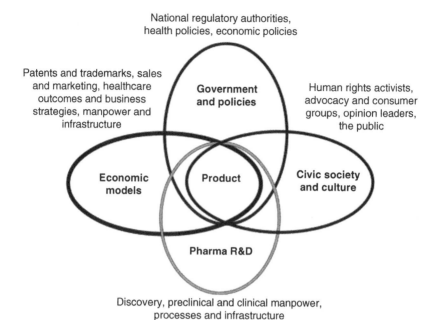

Figure 1 *Cross-Functional Interactions in the Pharmaceutical Ecosystem.*

The pharmaceutical ecosystem could be defined as the convergence of networks of cross-interacting subsystems across the drug product pipeline, which has a stake in the efficiency of the drug development and access to the marketed drug.

3 ASPECTS OF THE PHARMACEUTICAL SYSTEMS AND THE STAKEHOLDERS

3.1 Government and Policies

The government provides revolutionary policies that improve the entire pharmaceutical environment, such as federal laws, economic/reimbursement policies, intellectual property and patent policies, and health policies. The major national regulatory authorities are the Food and Drug Administration (FDA) for United States, the European Medicines Authority (EMA) for Europe, and the Pharmaceuticals and Medical Devices Agency (PMDA, KIKO) for Japan.

3.2 Drug Discovery Research and Development

Target identification through the optimization stage involves biochemists, pharmacologists, systems biologists, cell biologists, immunologists, and bioinformaticians, as well as synthetic, medicinal, analytical, and computational chemists, biotechnologists, and therapeutic area specialists. The preclinical R&D stage involves quality assurance professionals, assay development scientists, safety pharmacologists, and toxicologists. Those that study pharmacokinetics (PK) are the drug metabolism and PK scientists. Formulation and pharmaceutical scientists are involved in pharmaceutical development. Clinical R&D involves clinical research associates, pharmacologists, biostatisticians, molecular biologists, pharmacovigilance professionals, and drug safety scientists.

3.3 Economics Models

Economics models attempt to address scarcity of resources by evaluating economic outcomes of pharmaceuticals and their impacts on people, organizations, and society. Economics modeling involves business experts that implement product strategies to further their corporate objectives. The sales and marketing department partakes in market research to provide information about consumers, including the sales and prescriptions for an indication. Marketing communications provide projections of the anticipated sales trajectory of the drugs under development. The health outcomes are concerned with analysis of causes and effects of diseases, pricing and reimbursement, and economic value. Epidemiologists and strategic pricing executives are also part of this process. Patents cases are overseen by the patent attorneys.

3.4 The Civic Society

Civic society refers to the social groups, patient advocacy groups, consumer groups, other functional groups, and the public.

3.5 The Processes

Processes refer to the utilization of infrastructure and tools that convert knowledge and ideas into tangible products, marketing, and patient access. These include technical skills, machinery and equipment purposed for product innovation, process and product strategies and planning, protocol development, analysis, reporting, and data management.

Cross-functional interactions and coordination enable the pharmaceutical company to leverage knowledge across the value chain stream to optimize product innovation.

4 THE MUTUAL EFFECT OF THE PHARMACEUTICAL SYSTEMS AND SOCIETY

4.1 Pharmaceutical Policy and Regulation

Pharmaceutical policy is concerned with processes by which medicines are developed, approved, manufactured, distributed, and consumed, as well as the innovation tools for pricing access.

Policy could be defined as a means of furthering the administrative objectives and responsibilities of the government.

The regulators employ stringent strategies in their regulatory mechanisms, so as to always satisfy favorable risk–benefit requirements for safety and quality. The public expect the regulators will continue to exercise this mandate seamlessly. For instance, the regulators are expected to recognize the mutual implication of trying to emphasize access to therapies over safety or vice versa. As discussed by Miller and Henderson [7], a policy that focuses more on access to drugs at the expense of safety would lead to exposing the patient to a health risk. However, if access is preferably emphasized, it could affect costs and the ability of the patient to have life-saving medical therapy. Thus, in exercising its statutory authority, the regulator is expected to seek those interests that would promote the utility of a drug that benefits society. Pharmaceutical R&D is structured around governmental regulatory control for a drug product that is manufactured and distributed to the public [8].

Federal government policies provide financial sponsorships and incentives in support of biomedical/pharmaceutical-related research. The relevant organizations receive enormous funding from government agencies such as the National Institutes of Health (NIH) in the United States and the Canadian Institutes of Health Research (CIHR) of Canada. The Small Business Innovation Research and Small Business Technology Transfer programs of the NIH are a major financial funding source for innovative small companies with early-stage capital to engage in biomedical R&D that has a strong potential for commercialization. Over US$750 million was invested in 2014 alone (http://sbir.nih.gov/). About C$11.5 billion were issued between 2000 and 2014 by CIHR (http://www.cihr-irsc.gc.ca/).

A recent demonstration of interdependence among the social sectors of the pharmaceutical ecosystems in advancing drug discovery (Source: p. 24 CEN.ACS.ORG February 2, 2015).

4.1.1 Patent Linkage

Patents render exclusive permissions allowing the pioneering drug manufacturers monopoly of over sales of their drugs (preventing others from selling the drug) that have successfully passed through the drug approval cycles. Federal laws provide for linkages between the drug approval process and the registration of patents in most of North America and other countries spread over the globe. The prices of patented drugs are set by federal legislation that mandates the regulatory authority to the control of prices such that they are not excessive. There is a direct connection between drug prices and availability of generics in the sense that entry of a generic drug into the market accompanies a decrease in drug prices. Nevertheless, patent linkage is not a thriving strategy for the generic companies. The reason is because the lengthy procedure involved in drug approval was not considered when a generic company is permitted to initiate the application process only toward the end of the brand drug's lifetime. This introduces delay in a drug entering the generic market and, as such, will also limit the low pricing effect [9].

4.1.2 Political Interests
Political activists, lobbyists, and special interests groups impress upon the government a need to accommodate their own interests in decision making. These could lead to controversy and uncertainties. If the applicable laws are not implemented, private interests surge and escalate leading to calls for action. This kind of social movement has dire consequences for the pharmaceutical industry [10–14].

4.2 Access to Drugs
Pharmaceuticals are expected to be readily available, effective, safe, and accessible. The drug discovery process is very complex, costing up to $1 billion with extensive development time of up to 15 years, and has been blamed on scientific, economic, and regulatory uncertainties. Efficiencies in drug discovery R&D are strictly dependent on the ability to provide a confirmatory evidence of robust experimental outcomes that satisfy the efficacy, safety, and quality mandate. But sometimes unforeseen biological activities undermine the clinical utility of the developmental drug. Such an encounter is not uncommon because it has often led to innovation failure, to the detriment of both the drug maker and the public. For example, a drug molecule might exhibit toxic off-target activities that were not determined in the early discovery research and during clinical development. This underlying toxicity might only manifest during the postmarketing period leading to drug recalls and revenue loss for the pharmaceutical company. In such a situation, there has been a tendency to resort to proceeds from other

thriving pipeline drugs to sustain its R&D, and which translates into high prices for the drugs intended for the public.

Access to pharmaceuticals can be defined as the timely availability, subject to economic and physical conditions, of quality, safe, and effective medicines to those patients who need them. Many intertwined factors determine the level of access to quality medicines, such as the availability of financial resources, government policies, infrastructure conditions, private and public sector insurance programs, appropriate use, supply management, and manufacturing capacity[1].

4.3 Drug Pricing and Payment

The ability to receive discounted drugs and adequate coverage is a top priority. But commercialization goals need to be met, which more often have been pursued through established pricing mechanisms for cost recovery – the high cost of prescription drugs has been blamed on these huge pipeline expenditures. Revenue generated by the pharmaceutical company is partly dependent on what the third party is willing to pay. However, third party payers would want to reduce costs by excluding sales of highly costly drugs that are listed in the formularies and permit therapeutic substitution. Highly priced prescription drugs are largely unattractive especially those that are extensions of already marketed products that offer only marginal improvement in therapeutic value. To the lawmaker, the need for unrestricted access would sometimes necessitate the industry to compromise its high profitability intentions and operate like a not-for-profit business. Yet, the firm's owner's ultimate desire is to maximize wealth. In general, increasing the cost of drugs affects access to drugs, screening off those who are unable to afford pricey drugs and consequently jeopardizing their quality of health.

4.4 Communication

Communicating crucial information, risks, costs, and complexities to the public enables an understanding of all the hurdles of drug development risks and prices. Intuitively, the public relies on the drug firms to decide what data to disclose [15–17]. As such, common interests need to be communicated seamlessly. Trudo Lemmens in his publication "Pharmaceutical knowledge governance: a human rights perspective" expressed a growing concern over the extent of industry control of pharmaceutical data that it produces and how it impacts the therapeutic quality of the approved drug and public health. The report emphasized how dissemination of promotion,

---

[1]For further information, go to http://www.ifpma.org/global-health/access/about-access.html.

prescription, and consumption of pharmaceuticals and medical devices, and the adverse reporting system information, should take into consideration the protection and promotion of public health [18]. Advances in technology innovation drives the discovery of new drugs and these trends need to be communicated among the advisory bodies and regulatory authorities, investment and funding agencies, public health officials, medical societies, health professionals, public and private payers, and the general public. The purpose is to communicate values, opportunities, and challenges that will help transform the future of public health worldwide. Media influence arises when reports emphasize excessive profits and unethical behavior or promotional information, knowing that favorable remarks will not attract public attention.

4.4.1 Direct-to-Consumer Advertising/Gift Giving

The act of advertising is meant to help the consumer achieve positive health outcomes, to increase awareness of available options, and to build trust in the industry's marketed products. The societal norms of "right to health" relates to the right to receive all the information that is crucial to health and freedom of expression. The drug company is expected to dispense candid information during an advertisement without commercial preference or deception. Advertising for marketing gains is a noncompliant gesture, which draws complaints and misgivings from the public. Quite often, elaborate funding has been invested toward advertising at the expense of the end user who indirectly pays for these practices through the purchase of drugs with built-in advertisement expenditures on price tags [19]. Funding of patient advocacy organizations has resulted in the protection of the interest of the funding partners. This sometimes overshadows its own objectives, leading to conflicts of interest and loss of confidence from the patients they represent [20]. The European Medicines Agency (EMA)'s Patients' and Consumers' Working Party is the platform for interaction of patients and with EMA. A group of representatives from patients' and consumers' organizations provide recommendations to the Agency and its human scientific committees on issues that align with the patient's medical needs.

4.5 Drug Repositioning or Repurposing

Drug repositioning or repurposing is intended to find alternative uses for a pioneering drug or a drug that is made by another innovator. It mostly involves developing approved or failed compounds. Drug repositioning is expanding in the area of rare and neglected diseases. It is a new way of approaching drug compounds and targets that have been "derisked" during the development stages, which accelerates the process and thus saves money, because the drug could be produced with less effort and marketed with a huge profit margin. Drug repositioning has helped to mitigate failures in drug discovery and has been associated with therapeutic breakthroughs. For example, the thalidomide medicine that had deleterious effects in the past has found a new indication. This is a growth opportunity that brings value to society. However, there are divided interests over the choice of the repurposed drug and the objective of such an endeavor [21].

4.6 Stratified/Personalized Medicine

Stratified/personalized medicine holds the promise of a more precise and effective standard of care when medications are targeted to the responsive patient population who show fewer adverse reactions.

5 CYCLICAL INTERACTIONS IN THE PHARMACEUTICAL ECOSYSTEM

Cyclical interactions within the pharmaceutical ecosystem are due to cross-relationships among the various aspects of the pharmaceutical ecosystems as detailed in Figure 1. Networks of interactions across the subsystems emphasize the interdependence of the industry and society (Figure 2). The cyclical interactions are as follows:

Government/Industry

Consultation: In the initial stages of the drug development program, the drug regulatory authority, such as FDA, issues guidance that defines the content of the drug product development plan to ascertain that it does not deviate from its intended purpose. Thus, communication between the sponsor/drug maker and the regulatory body is necessary at the initial stage. The agenda for such a meeting would be patient driven because it incorporates discussions that promote well-informed decisions for clinical trial design and the preclinical development program in support of the intended clinical trial design and therapeutic application [22,23].

Industry/Public Community

Consultation: The drug development program is often initiated in consultation with the stakeholders: physicians, patients, and payers to enable a well-informed clinical trial design. The obtained information is essential in identifying the product characteristics that promotes its commercial suitability [24,25].

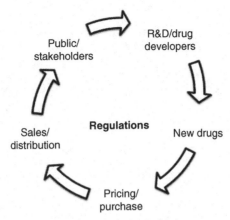

Figure 2 *Cyclical Interactions of the Pharmaceutical Subsystems.*

Decisions made by one subsystem affect the other in a feedforward and feedback fashion. For example, patient/public values predispose the scientific or medical rationale to R&D portfolio prioritization or which projects take the lead. These could include unmet medical needs (type of indications to address), target patient population, and propensity to boost sales and market competitiveness (the purchasing power of the target population). Drug development projects and drug attributes influence a drug's cost effectiveness and accessibility. As mentioned earlier, access to drugs and drug pricing affect the extent of market access, whereas for the company, low demand would drop profit margins. Consequently, this would reflect in the extent of future financial projections that drive R&D and limit the number of new drug entrants to the market. Decrease in innovation rates is a major concern considering those members of the public in need of medical therapy. In the same vein, communications, personalized medicine technology, and patents as explained in section 4 are aspects of the pharmaceutical systems that affect the practical value of medicines.

6 THE PHARMACEUTICAL PRODUCT LIFECYCLE

The pharmaceutical drug product is a "cross-technology" product that emerges through a combination of core pharmaceutical R&D processes and strategic/social issues across a wide range of disciplines (Figure 3) within the realm of a drug discovery program. The drug discovery and development continuum represents a sequence of efforts that combine the strength of basic and applied scientific knowledge in bringing a new drug product

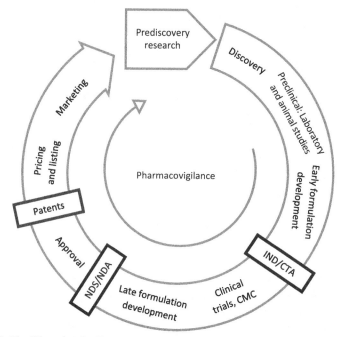

Figure 3 *The Lifecycle of a Pharmaceutical Product.*

to the marketplace. It is a collaborative function of pharmaceutical companies, start-up, small-to medium companies, governmental agencies, and the academic sector. The drug discovery process is complex, needing iterative efforts and exhaustive dedication, which is instrumental in bringing lasting and measurable improvements in performance toward the intended objective. Basic R&D relies on classical scientific methods and computations, which are applied through the entire discovery and development stage. Well-coordinated efforts at various levels, within and across the discrete functional units, foster information complementarity and efficiencies, which are crucial to the performance and success of drug development processes. These activities are expected to be interpreted in a way that maintains transparency and accountability with government and the public, and integrity within the healthcare industry.

As shown in Figure 3, the concentric circular scheme represents the entire bio/pharmaceutical R&D projects.

The business of pharmaceutical or bio/pharmaceutical R&D requires keeping a portfolio of R&D projects. Bio/pharmaceutical R&D has been used interchangeably with drug discovery and development. The term "Project" refers to related tasks that focus on a common goal for the drug product.

The core processes (inner circle) and the strategic/social issues (outer circle) bridge the drug discovery processes with society. The social aspects of drug development encompass the social tools used to analyze the theories, themes, attitudes, and opinions of the government and the general public in response to these underlying factors through which this "cross-technology product" emerges. These social factors are considered in all stages of the drug product lifecycle, discovery and development, clinical research, authorization, marketing, patient access, monitoring of drug access, and outcomes. Therefore, social aspects of drug discovery and development are the public tools or aspects of public life within the pharmaceutical ecosystem that have a mutual impact on drug discovery and development concerning drug quality, efficacy, and safety. The goal of this book is to communicate these strategic issues, regarded as the social aspect of drug discovery and development to shed light on the mutual impact of drug discovery and society.

7 CONCLUSIONS

The overall framework used to describe, evaluate, and judge the pharmaceutical industry is in terms of the medical quality of drugs and the social value to society. All aspects of human culture, law, and philosophy have a mutual relationship with drug discovery and development, and thus the latter cannot exist independently of the social system and its organizational characteristics. Thus, the ecosystem of the pharmaceutical industry must transform within itself and leverage new opportunities that enrich the global landscape. It is conceivable that in the near future, understanding the social aspects of drug development and discovery will lead to a culture of change in our attitude, which is based on how we focus on and interrogate the regulated pharmaceutical industry.

REFERENCES

[1] Debnath B, Al-Mawsawi LQ, Neamati N. Are we living in the end of the blockbuster drug era? Drug News Perspect 2010;23(10):670–84.
[2] Grabowski HG, Vernon J. The distribution of sales revenues from pharmaceutical innovation. Pharmacoeconomics 2000;18(S1):21–32.
[3] Sleno L, Emili A. Proteomic methods for drug target discovery. Curr Opin Chem Biol 2008;12:1–9.
[4] Niwayama S. Proteomics in medicinal chemistry. Mini Rev Med Chem 2006;6:241–6.
[5] Ahn NG, Wang AHJ. Proteomics and genomics: perspectives on drug and target discovery. Curr Opin Chem Biol 2008;12:1–3.
[6] Patel AC, Coyle AJ. Building a new biomedical ecosystem. Clinical Pharmacology & Therapeutics; 2013 May. Pfizer's Centers for Therapeutic Innovation.

[7] Miller HI, Henderson DI. Governmental influences on drug development: striking a better balance. Nat Rev Drug Discov 2007;6:532–9.

[8] Liberti L, McAuslane JN, Walker S. Standardizing the benefit-risk assessment of new medicines: practical applications of frameworks for the pharmaceutical healthcare professional. Pharm Med 2011;25(3):139–46.

[9] Brief: European Commission orders Italy to drop patent linkage delaying generics. Intellectual Property Watch 2012 Jan; European Commission – Press release. Available from: http://europa.eu/rapid/press-release_IP-12-48_en.htm?locale=en

[10] Lessig L. Republic Lost: How Money Corrupts Congress – and a Plan to Stop It. New York: Twelve; 2011.

[11] Thompson DF. Ethics in Congress: From Individual to Institutional Corruption. Washington, DC: The Brookings Institution; 1995.

[12] Thompson DF. Two Concepts of Corruption: Making Campaigns Safe for Democracy. George Washington Law Rev 12 2005;73(5):1036–69.

[13] Safra EJ. Center for ethics. Available from: http://www.ethics.harvard.edu/lab

[14] Jorgensen PD. Pharmaceuticals, political money, and public policy: a theoretical and empirical agenda. J Law Med Ethics 2013;41(3):553–5.

[15] Sismondo S, Nicholson SH. Publication Planning 101: a report. J Pharm Pharmaceut Sci 2009;12(3):273–9. Available from: www.cspsCanada.org.

[16] Healy D, Cattell D. Interface between authorship, industry and science in the domain of therapeutics. Brit J Psychiat 2003;183:22–7.

[17] Matheson A. Corporate science and the husbandry of scientific and medical knowledge by the pharmaceutical industry. BioSocieties 2008;3:355–82.

[18] Sismondo S. Ghost management: how much of the medical literature is shaped behind the scenes by the pharmaceutical industry? PLoS Med 2007;4(9):e286.

[19] Podolsky SH, Greene JA. A historical perspective of pharmaceutical promotion and physician education. JAMA 2008;300:831–3. IFPMA Code of Pharmaceutical Marketing Practices 2012 Revision Appendix 1. Available from: http://www.ifpma.org/fileadmin/content/Publication/2012/IFPMA_Code_of_Practice_2012_new_logo.pdf.

[20] Rose SL. Patient advocacy organizations: institutional conflicts of interest, trust, and trustworthiness. J Law Med Ethics 2013;41(3):680–7.

[21] Moynihan R. Doctors' education: the invisible influence of drug company sponsorship. BMJ 2008;336:416–7.

[22] Tebbey PW. Target product profile: a renaissance for its definition and use. J Med Market 2009;9(4):301–7.

[23] Don R. Target product profile: starting with patients in mind. DNDI Newsletter 2005;12. Available from: http://www.dndi.org.

[24] Gagnon MA. Corruption of pharmaceutical markets: addressing the misalignment of financial incentives and public health. J Law Med Ethics 2013;41(3):571–80.

[25] Prahalad CK, Krishnan MS. The New Age of Innovation: Driving Cocreated Value through Global Networks. McGraw-Hill; 2008.

SECTION I

Pharmaceutical Industry, Society, and Governance

1. Pharmaceutical Regulation: The Role of Government in the Business of Drug Discovery   3
2. Trends in Innovation and the Business of Drug Discovery   29
3. Cash Flow Valley of Death: A Pitfall in Drug Discovery   57

CHAPTER 1

Pharmaceutical Regulation: The Role of Government in the Business of Drug Discovery

Odilia Osakwe

Contents

1.1 Introduction   4
    1.1.1 Evolution of the Pharmaceutical Regulatory System   4
1.2 The Legal Instruments   5
    1.2.1 The Act/Enabling Act   5
    1.2.2 Regulations   5
    1.2.3 Guidelines   6
1.3 The National Regulatory Authorities and Administration   6
    1.3.1 The Food and Drug Administration   7
    1.3.2 Health Canada   8
    1.3.3 European Medicines Agency   9
    1.3.4 Pharmaceuticals and Medical Devices Agency of Japan   10
1.4 Analytical Framework for Regulatory Approval: Benefit–Risk Assessment   11
1.5 The Pharmaceutical Product Life Cycle   13
    1.5.1 Modules for Drug Regulatory Assessment: The Decision Points   13
    1.5.2 Patents   16
    1.5.3 Labeling   17
1.6 The Global Pharmaceutical Industry: Harmonization and Partnerships   18
    1.6.1 International Conference on Harmonisation of Technical Requirements
        for Registration of Pharmaceuticals for Human Use   19
    1.6.2 Government Regulations: Prospects for Multinational Clinical Trials   21
1.7 Modernization of the Global Pharmaceutical Systems: Regulatory Strategies,
    Roadmap Initiatives, and Partnerships   22
    1.7.1 The Critical Path Initiative   22
    1.7.2 The European Medicines Agency's Roadmap to 2015   23
    1.7.3 The Progressive Licensing Model of Health Canada   24
    1.7.4 Global Initiatives   24
    1.7.5 World Health Partnerships   25
References   26

Social Aspects of Drug Discovery, Development and Commercialization   Copyright © 2016 Elsevier Inc.
http://dx.doi.org/10.1016/B978-0-12-802220-7.00001-6   All rights reserved.

1.1 INTRODUCTION

1.1.1 Evolution of the Pharmaceutical Regulatory System

The initial restructuring of the federal regulation of drugs in the United States took place around 1902 when Harvey Wiley, a chemist with the Department of Agriculture, scrutinized drug ingredients through the Drug Laboratory Program. In 1906, the Federal Food and Drugs Act was enacted, which prevented the trade of misbranded or adulterated foods and drugs. It required evidence of active ingredient purity for every marketed drug as outlined in the United States Pharmacopeia compendium. The 1906 Act was not actively enforced, leaving ambiguities in the pharmaceutical regulatory system. During this period, manufacturers could make false claims on drug efficacy to promote sales. The Shirley Amendments were passed in 1912 to prohibit labeling medicines with false therapeutic claims that defrauded the purchase [1].

In 1937, tragic ethylene glycol poisoning associated with the use of sulfanilamide solvent in a drug formulation claimed over 100 lives. This laid the foundation for the enactment of the Federal Food, Drug, and Cosmetic Act (FD&C Act) in 1938 following a 5-year debate process. As a consequence, major revisions were made to the 1906 legislation [2].

Decades later, the unprecedented thalidomide-induced disaster that took place around 1959 affected several countries and attracted global attention. Thalidomide (racemic mixture) was prescribed to pregnant women to treat the symptoms associated with morning sickness. Unfortunately, it led to serious health impairment in thousands of babies – most of who were born with various forms of congenital malformations. The drug was later withdrawn from public access. During much of that period, pharmaceutical regulation was not well-established for postmarketing monitoring.

These laws fundamentally changed the legal standards for marketing new products. In the United Kingdom, the regulatory system received a total facelift and prompted the setting up of the Committee on Safety of Drugs in 1963. Subsequently, a voluntary adverse drug reaction reporting system emerged in 1964. In the United States, the thalidomide aftermath brought a quick call to action leading to the passage of the 1962 Kefauver–Harris Amendment [3,4]. The Drug Amendments Act of 1962 implemented the Kefauver–Harris recommendations, which demanded that drug manufacturers specifically show proof of efficacy and safety as well as compliance with current good manufacturing practices (GMP) in order to receive approval for new drug applications (NDA). GMP guidelines mostly outline the requirements for drug manufacturing facility operations. In Canada, this ushered a new requirement demanding manufacturers to submit evidence of efficacy to obtain a Notice of Compliance for the sale of drugs. In some countries, such as, Belgium, Brazil, Canada, Italy, and Japan, thalidomide sales persisted for several months after withdrawal from the West German and British markets. In Japan, where thalidomide was finally withdrawn in September 1962, incidences of birth deformity heightened while those in West Germany declined. In countries like the Netherlands, Sweden, Ireland, Italy, and the United Kingdom there was a correlation between the amount of thalidomide sales and birth deformities over time.

Today, pharmaceutical regulations have advanced tremendously through a series of additions that support continual improvement in pipeline activities. The introduction of the "pharmaceutical quality systems" is a means of enriching the circumstances to promote a strong connection within the pharmaceutical development processes for continual improvement across the entire product life cycle and to sustain an appropriate level of oversight for medical products.

1.2 THE LEGAL INSTRUMENTS

These legal instruments are legal statutes and other types of documents used to communicate the legal requirements for conducting a controlled activity. The following are typical legal instruments.

1.2.1 The Act/Enabling Act

The Act/Enabling Act is a statute with the force of law, made by delegated bodies appointed by the executive legislative authorities. The Act grants a dependent entity, the legitimacy of power to enforce the laws. It explicitly defines the legal requirements necessary for the agency to certify a drug product that has sufficiently and convincingly been found to be effective, based on well-conducted development program and controlled clinical studies. Examples are the FD&C Act of the United States, the Food and Drug Act of Canada, and the Pharmaceutical Affairs Act (PAA) of Japan.

1.2.2 Regulations

Regulations are most often defined as complex systems of interrelated principles, rules, or laws. They are made under the authority of the Act, by the body to whom the authority to make regulations has been delegated. They are sometimes referred to as subordinate legislation, which defines the application and enforcement of legislation. These regulations are continuously amended and supplemented. Examples are the Code of Federal Regulations (CFR) of the United States and the Food and Drug Regulations (FDR) of Canada.

A framework is composed of several complementary elements or concepts in support of something larger. A regulatory framework can be defined as the macro-level steps that regulators must complete in order to bring forward regulations.

1.2.3 Guidelines

Guidelines are departmental documents that are derived from legislation; their purpose is to instruct in simplistic terms. The guidance documents communicate regulations in such a way as to promote uniformity and consistency in their application. They do not possess the force of law but allow a proper and effective regulatory compliance. The national regulatory authority adapts the guidelines within the context of the manufacturer's specific goals and objectives. Examples are GMP and the International Conference on Harmonization (ICH) guidelines.

1.3 THE NATIONAL REGULATORY AUTHORITIES AND ADMINISTRATION

Every country concerned with the manufacture of drugs and sales establishes a strong national regulatory authority (NRA) to ensure that the manufacture, trade, and use of medicines are properly regulated with the ultimate goal of satisfying the overall public health needs and necessities. The NRA mostly reviews all applications for marketing approval and controls the distribution of pharmaceuticals and related products, such as drug product quality and efficacy, labeling, reporting, surveillance, drug safety studies, risk management, information dissemination, off-label use, and direct-to-consumer advertising and patents. Drug discovery follows set regulatory standards as published in the websites. Examples are the US Food and Drug Administration (FDA) (www.fda.gov), Health Canada (http://www.hc-sc.gc.ca/index-eng.php), and the European Union (EU) (http://www.ema.europa.eu/ema/). In Japan, details of the Ministry of Health, Labour, and Welfare (MHLW) are available from: http://www.mhlw.go.jp/english/ or http://www.pmda.go.jp/english. In this section, the prominent NRAs will be discussed. These are the FDA, the European Medicines

Agency (EMA), Health Canada, and the Pharmaceutical and Medical Devices Agency (PMDA).

1.3.1 The Food and Drug Administration

FDA is the NRA for the United States and has administrative authority over the manufacture of pharmaceuticals for distribution to the public. The most referenced centers for pharmaceuticals are the Centre for Drug Evaluation and Research (CDER) and Centre for Biologics Evaluation and Research (CBER). These centers are responsible for the licensure and monitoring of therapeutic products throughout the product life cycle. CDER regulates the pharmaceutical drugs and all marketing approval applications are completed by this subsection of the FDA. CBER regulates the biological products: vaccine, blood or blood component, allergenic, somatic cell, gene therapy, tissue, recombinant therapeutic protein, or living cells that are used as therapeutics to treat diseases. Other centers are, the Center for Devices and Radiological Health (CDRH) and the Office of Regulatory Affairs (ORA) (http://www.fda.gov, www.fda.gov/cder/index.html).

1.3.1.1 Federal Food, Drug, and Cosmetic Act

FD&C Act is a set of laws passed by Congress in 1938 giving authority to the FDA to oversee the safety of food, drugs, and cosmetics. The United States is the largest market for prescription medicines and thus FDA regulatory processes became the benchmark for the global pharmaceutical and biotechnology industry. FD&C Act was passed under the Kefauver–Harris amendments in 1962. It provides the statutory basis for drug approval in the United States. The Act empowers the FDA to the licensing of drugs based on sound evidence of safety and efficacy and requires a premarket authorization for new drugs that were marketed in the United States. The FDA also regulates products other than drugs; biological products, medical devices, dietary supplements, foods, cosmetics, animal drugs, and tobacco products. In addition, these amendments also gave the FDA authority to regulate research in humans with investigational drugs; specifically, manufacturers could not transport drugs in interstate commerce without full market approval or the appropriate legal approval for the status of the drug.

The CFR is promulgated by the agencies of the federal government to carry out the provisions of the Act. It is subdivided into 50 sections. Section 21 of the CFR contains most regulations pertaining to food and drugs and, as such, documents all the activities that are required under the federal law. The Electronic Code of Federal Regulations (eCFR) is a current version of the CFR produced by the National Archives and Records Administration's Office of the Federal Register and the Government Printing Office (http://www.gpo.gov/fdsys/browse/collectionCfr. action?collectionCode=CFR).

Evolution of Drug Laws Under the FD&C Act

1983 – Orphan Drug Act, provided incentives for pharmaceutical manufacturers to develop drugs, biotechnology products, and medical devices for the treatment of rare diseases and conditions.

1984 – Hatch-Waxman Act, promoted the prescriptions for low-cost generic drugs by establishing a generic drug approval process for pioneer drugs first approved after 1962.

1992 – Prescription Drug User Fee Act (PDUFA), introduced user fees and performance goals for accelerated drug approvals.

1997 – FDA Modernization Act (FDAMA), created a mechanism designated as "Fast Track" for drugs that addressed serious or life-threatening conditions and met medical needs. This also eased access to experimental therapies with relaxed clinical testing requirements, and allowed an extension of 6 months of marketing protection on testing of pediatric drugs.

2002 – Public Health Security and Bioterrorism Preparedness and Response Act, reauthorized the FDAMA pediatric testing provision and granted an extension of the drug user fee law for 5 more years.

2003 – Pediatric Research Equity Act, required drug makers to include pediatric assessments in NDAs.

2007 – FDA Amendments Act, streamlined the regulatory processing by mandating the FDA authority to regulate drug safety.

1.3.2 Health Canada

Health Canada is the NRA for all foods and drugs sold in Canada. Its regulatory mandate is subject to the Food and Drugs Act (FDA) under which it administers its legislative framework through FDRs. The division of the Health Products and Food Branch of Health, Therapeutic Products Directorate (TPD), and the Biologic and Genetic Therapies Directorate (BGTD) are the three major subsidiaries of Health Canada, which specifically oversee adulteration of bio/pharmaceutical products and manufacturing compliance. Health Canada's TPD is the national authority that regulates, evaluates, and monitors therapeutic and diagnostic products available to Canadians. These products include drugs, medical devices, disinfectants, and sanitizers with disinfectant claims. Health Canada's BGTD is the Canadian federal authority that regulates biological drugs (products derived from living sources) and radiopharmaceuticals for human use in Canada, whether manufactured in Canada or elsewhere. In the same manner, the Natural Health Products, Directorate covers regulation of natural products.

1.3.2.1 Canadian Food and Drugs Act

The FDA is an act of the Parliament of Canada regarding the production, import, export, interprovincial commerce and sale of food, drugs, contraceptive devices, and cosmetics (including personal cleaning products such as soap and toothpaste). It was introduced in 1920 following the founding of a federal Department of Health in 1919. Regulations developed under the Act laid out the requirements for licensing drugs and a penalty for noncompliance. Also the thalidomide incident brought a fundamental change in the Canadian regulatory regime that marked the inception of a rebuilt regulation requiring manufacturers to submit evidence of efficacy in seeking a Notice of Compliance. The FDR is enforced under the authority of the FDA. It was recreated in 1947 and has undergone processes of incremental change, leading to the inclusion of a requirement for the filing of new drug submissions (NDS) prior to marketing authorizations (http://laws-lois.justice.gc.ca/eng/regulations/C.R.C.,_c._870/page-1.html, http://laws-lois.justice.gc.ca/eng/acts/F-27/index.html) and follows its regulatory mandate under the FDR (http://laws-lois.justice.gc.ca/eng/regulations/C.R.C.%2C_c._870/). C-51 is a bill for amendment of the FDA for current regulatory systems for health products in Canada (details for Health Canada are available from: http://www.hc-sc.gc.ca/dhp-mps/index-eng.php).

1.3.3 European Medicines Agency

In 1993, the EMA was founded primarily to render sound and enabling scientific evaluation for all applicable medicinal products, for the participating EU constituencies. The European Community (EC) system for the authorization of medicinal products was founded in 1995 to allow uniform distribution of marketed drugs within the EC countries through mutual recognition agreements (MRAs). The harmonization process centralized the regulatory procedure to foster smoother international trade processes, in parallel with the US model. Later, the EMA came into being in 1993 as a decentralized body of European Union, headquartered in London (http://www.hma.eu/). A drug product that has been approved by the European Commission follows a centralized authorization procedure. Thus, a product approval procedure generally follows either a centralized or a decentralized procedure. For the centralized procedure, a mutual recognition procedure (MRP) allows recognition of prior marketing authorization and covers a majority of conventional medicinal products for the MRA partners. The decentralized procedure requires that an application for the marketing authorization of a medicinal product be submitted. One out of these states serves as the "Reference Member State." This procedure is applicable to most of the medicinal products.

The Heads of Medicines Agencies is a network for the regulation of medicinal products for human and veterinary use in the European Economic Area. The Heads of Medicines Agencies cooperates with the EMA and the European Commission in the operation of the European Medicines Regulatory Network ("the Network") [5]. The European Medicines Evaluation Agency (EMEA) (http://www.emea.europa.eu/) and the FDA share information on new or changes to premarketing procedures, and postmarketing surveillance for pharmaceutical products under review. Department of Health and Medical Research Council guidance on compliance with provision of European Clinical Trials Directive is available from http://www.ct-toolkit.ac.uk/.

1.3.3.1 The European Drug Regulatory Legislation

The European Drug Regulatory Legislation (EudraLex) is a collection of rules and regulations governing medicinal products in the European Union and is comprised of 10 volumes. EudraLex – Volume 1 contains "pharmaceutical legislation medicinal products for human use." It complies with the body of EU legislation in the pharmaceutical sector for medicinal products for human use.

The legislations of the EudraLex are mostly the regulations and the directives. The regulations conform to the national law while the directives are general rules adapted into national law by the European member states. An example is Directive 2001/83/EC for medical products.

1.3.4 Pharmaceuticals and Medical Devices Agency of Japan

The Pharmaceuticals and Medical Devices Agency (PMDA, KIKO) is an independent agency founded on April 1, 2004, under the Pharmaceutical Affairs Law (PAL) or Pharmaceutical Affairs Act (PAA) (http://www.jpma.or.jp/

english/parj/1003.html). It was created through a combined effort of the Pharmaceuticals and Medical Devices Evaluation Center of the National Institute of Health Sciences, the Organization for Pharmaceutical Safety and Research, and part of the Japan Association for the Advancement of Medical Equipment. Its regulatory function is mostly for drug and medical devices. These functions have been classified under three major categories:

- Adverse drug reactions (ADR) relief work
- Review work, which involves premarket review and approval processes based on PAL
- Safety measures that focus on risk management, consultations pertaining to safety, and drug monitoring activities

The EMA and the European Commission have a confidentiality arrangement with the Japanese MHLW and the Japanese PMDA.

1.3.4.1 The Pharmaceutical Affairs Act of Japan

Pharmaceutical legislation found its roots in Japan when the regulations on handling and sales of medicines emerged in 1889 (http://www.jpma.or.jp/english/parj/pdf/2014_ch02.pdf). The Pharmaceutical Affairs Law was enacted in 1943 and was subject to series of revisions that cumulated in the modernized Pharmaceutical Affairs Act (PAA), initiated in 1960 [6]. The regulation of manufacturing, importation, and sale of drugs, and medical devices in Japan followed the PAA. Subsequently, the 2002 amendment was modeled after the European Union, Australia, Canada, and the United States. The amendment adopts a greater global cooperation and, in accordance with its legislative provisions, adopts the science- and risk-based approach in evaluations for marketed drugs. The June 2006 amendment to the law (Law No. 69 of 2006, with effective date of June 2009) changed the marketing of over-the-counter drugs for the first time in 46 years [6]. The amended law allowed the retail of certain over-the-counter drugs without prior consultation or prescription, and thus were readily available throughout the regular retail stores.

1.4 ANALYTICAL FRAMEWORK FOR REGULATORY APPROVAL: BENEFIT–RISK ASSESSMENT

The benefit–harm effect is a major consideration in evaluating drug safety and of whose potential benefits must clearly outweigh uncertainties regarding safety and efficacy. Benefit could be regarded as the intended positive effect and risk; the unintended effect that diminishes human health.

An important element of the benefit–risk assessment is ensuring that the baseline scenarios are properly defined. Baseline scenarios enable identification of the elements that are important factors in the decision-making. These elements, when identified and measured, could be systematically incorporated into the design process of regulatory actions. The FDA Benefit–Risk Assessment Framework is a product of extensive review and analysis of previous and ongoing regulatory decisions. For example, in the PDUFA V provisions, the Patient-Focused Drug Development program is a novel FDA-inspired initiative aimed at obtaining a patient's perspective on certain disease areas. This information is instrumental in the critical evaluation of disease severity previously treated and the current treatment options available over the period of PDUFA V (http://www.fda.gov/ForIndustry/UserFees/PrescriptionDrugUserFee/ucm326192.htm). It is this optimized baseline scenario that is used to determine the incremental benefits and associated risks over the life cycle of the pharmaceutical product. Thus, the PUDFA V strategy is a more systematic approach and a critical aspect of FDA's decision making as it establishes the context in which the regulatory decision is made.

PDUFA was enacted in 1992 and renewed in 1997 (PDUFA II), 2002 (PDUFA III), 2007 (PDUFA IV), and 2012 (PDUFA V). It authorizes the FDA to accept a fee or levy from companies to accelerate drug approval processes. The fee is also a form of initiative targeted to improve the drug review process.

The EMA Benefit–Risk Methodology Project is the development and testing of tools and processes for evaluating benefits and risks to inform science-based regulatory decisions about medicinal products (http://www.ema.europa.eu/ema/index.jsp?curl=pages/special_topics/document_listing/document_listing_000314.jsp). The benefit–risk assessment method for the EMA's benefit–risk methodology project involves a working group of the Committee for Medicinal Products for Human Use that published decision-making models in March 2008. Some of the simpler models, such as the Number Needed to Treat/Number Needed to Harm method, applied in clinical trials. Another method employed was quality-adjusted life years, which is a way of measuring both the quality and quantity of life lived, as an aid in quantifying the benefit of a medical intervention. Most of these are yet to be fully development and could be applicable only when successfully tested [7,8].

For Health Canada, the regulatory process follows a two-tier approach of which the first hinges on scientifically sound evidence; a second tier requires evidence of overall favorable benefit balance. This is based on satisfactory evidence that demonstrates compliance for marketing authorization. Canada's benefit–risk model is reflected in a life cycle approach to drug regulation that requires a continuous assessment of benefit–risk profile for the authorized conditions of use throughout the drug's life cycle (http:// www.hc-sc.gc.ca/dhp-mps/homologation-licensing/model/evaluation-eng.php).

In a wider scope, the higher level benefit–risk evaluation takes into consideration the societal, ethical, or constitutional influences such as vulnerability of children and the elderly to certain drug usage, mostly duration, indication, and dosing of a drug. Unexpected issues that might arise are severity of the disease and patterns of drug. Marketing-associated risks are the availability and performance of other therapies; domestic and international clinical practice environments; nontraditional patterns outside those originally established and studied in premarket trials; drug access issues to the drug in the premarket environment; type of clinical trials performed and ethical reasons; and risk or uncertainty acceptance by other regulatory authorities (outside the region). The postmarketing risks include duration; effect on real-world target populations at postmarketing stage; manageability of risks; impact of other uncertainties about the drug; severity of disease for the drug therapy; and the nature of the target population.

1.5 THE PHARMACEUTICAL PRODUCT LIFE CYCLE

The pharmaceutical product life cycle comprises all the pharmaceutical processes from drug discovery through launch to access. These activities are monitored closely by the regulators, who intercept at the strategic decision points as shown in Figure 1.1.

The decision-making process is an integral aspect of drug development and determines the fate of a drug in terms of progressing to the next stage in the pharmaceutical product life cycle. The modules of assessing a developmental drug will be discussed in the following section.

1.5.1 Modules for Drug Regulatory Assessment: The Decision Points

1.5.1.1 Decision Point I

At this stage, the product dossier submission is known as investigational new drug (IND) application/clinical trial application (CTA)/investigational medicinal product dossier (IMPD). In order to meet eligibility, the applicant or

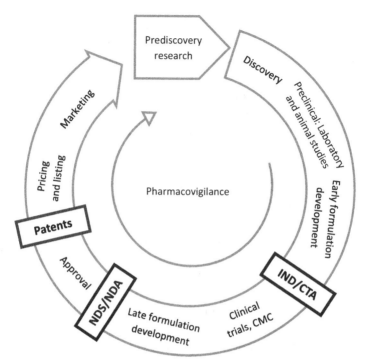

Figure 1.1 *The Pharmaceutical Product Life Cycle Showing Intersection of the Regulator at Different Points: IND/CTA, NDS/NDA, and Patents.*

drug sponsor is required to submit evidence of the effectiveness of the drug compound under investigation together with all the background technical data. Generally, these applications authorize the manufacturers to distribute or conduct clinical evaluations to obtain data about the safety and efficacy of that drug. The medical reviewer evaluates the clinical trial protocol to determine if the data confirms protection from unnecessary risks; if the study design would generate data to support safety and effectiveness of the drug. Phase I study is concerned with risk exposure and toxicity of the drug. Phases II and III must strictly demonstrate sound scientific evidence of all aspects of quality to support the licensing of the drug. Once the relevant health authorities have reviewed and approved an application, the drug advances to the clinical trials phase. The details can be obtained from the CDER Guidance – Content and Format of Investigational New Drug Applications (INDs) for Phase I Studies of Drugs. Submitting Application Archival Copies in Electronic Format, Drug Master. The guidance documents, laws, regulations, policies, procedures, and related resources pertaining to IND are

available from: http://www.fda.gov/drugs/developmentapprovalprocess/
howdrugsaredevelopedandapproved/approvalapplications/investigational-
newdrugindapplication/default.htm. The guidance index is available from:
http://www.fda.gov/Drugs/GuidanceComplianceRegulatoryInformati
on/Guidances/ucm121568.htm.

1.5.1.2 Decision Point II

The second decision point is essential for marketing authorization known
as New Drug Submission (NDS)/NDA/Marketing Authorization (MAA).
Upon the completion of Phase III clinical trials, the sponsor is required
to submit evidence of safety and effectiveness supported by the technical data on the series of studies performed according to the regulatory
requirement [9]. The decision made recommends the market worthi-
ness of the drug compound under investigation by the FDA [10] (http://
www.fda.gov/downloads/Drugs/GuidanceComplianceRegulatoryInfo
rmation/Guidances/ucm079748.pdf). Guidance for Industry: Management of Drug Submissions is available from: http://www.hc-sc.gc.ca/dhp-
mps/prodpharma/applic-demande/guide-ld/mgmt-gest/mands_gespd-
eng.php#a5.2). Priority Review of Drug Submissions Policy is available
from: http://www.hc-sc.gc.ca/dhp-mps/prodpharma/applic-demande/
pol/prds_tppd_pol-eng.php. For the European Commission see http://
ec.europa.eu/health/files/eudralex/vol-2/a/chap4rev200604_en.pdf
[11,12]. EMA preauthorisation procedural advice for users of the central-
ised procedure. A change to the label or dosage strength of the drug or
manufacturing requires Supplemental Abbreviated New Drug Submission.
The Abbreviated New Drug Application (ANDA) grants approval for a generic drug product – "Abbreviated" means that the processing and approval
precludes preclinical (animal) and clinical (human) but rather bioequivalence (similar function as the innovator drug) in establishing safety and
effectiveness.

1.5.1.3 NRA/Industry Meetings

Before any major regulatory approval, presubmission meetings are organized to initiate a discourse in the light of a new product in the pipeline
prior to the main submission. This enhances the preparedness of the manufacturer or sponsor. It also helps to identify potential flaws in the process.
Thus, communication is pivotal in promoting compliance standards and
efficiency in the process. Examples are pre-IND, End-of-Phase I, End of

Phase II, a pre-NDA, or Biologics License Application Conference. There are also other types not mentioned here. These meetings are not compulsory in the United States and Canada.

The Common Technical Document (CTD) is a common format for the organization of information in marketing authorization (registration) applications. This format is principally acceptable in the United States, Europe, and Japan. Content requirements are not fully harmonized and there are differences between the three regions. An example is module 1 of the ICH document (Figure 1.1). Prior to conducting the clinical trials, IND or its equivalent is filed with the respective NRA.

Typical considerations in an NDA review are as follows:
- Safety and effectiveness in its proposed use and benefit–risk balance (by how much do the benefits outweigh the risks)
- Content and suitability of the drug's proposed labeling (package insert)
- Competence of the methods for the drug manufacture in demonstrating the drug's identity, strength, quality, and purity [13]

In summary, given the variations in regulatory standards among different countries, certain guidelines are generally imposed and respected globally: NDA must contain evidence of nonclinical testing conducted according to the specified guidelines. It must accompany all the nonclinical and clinical testing and manufacturing that satisfies the regulatory requirements and also information related to pricing and reimbursement including postmarketing activities. All the information must have been thoroughly scrutinized and reviewed by the relevant NRA prior to granting a marketing authorization. The marketing authorization issued is valid throughout the patent period for brand-named products and obeys the law subject to the jurisdiction involved, which vary by country.

Following drug marketing, there is a constant monitoring of safety-related aspects of the drug. The marketing authorization holders are required to have a well-established pharmacovigilance system in place to ensure that the benefit–risk profile of the drug is fully reported in a timely fashion and reports on ADRs are expedited.

1.5.2 Patents

A patent for any innovative product is a property right granted by the government to the originator or inventor of the product. Depending on the country (mostly in the developed countries), property rights associated with a patent also grant the patent holder the monopoly of selling an invention. For an innovative therapeutic product, patent is granted for a period of

20 years from the date the patent is filed. Patents address extended regulatory lag periods and high costs of innovation [14,15]. The US Congress passed the Patent Act in 1790, which has been subject to several changes. In 1984, the Price Competition and Patent Term Restoration Act (Public Law 98-417), informally the Hatch–Waxman Act, stipulated the process for pharmaceutical manufacturers to file an ANDA for approval of a generic drug by the FDA. The pharmaceutical patents are legally tied to drug approval under provisions of the Act respecting drug-marketing authorization, the FD&C Act, or the FDA.

The North American Free Trade Agreement (NAFTA) and the World Trade Organization's Agreement on Trade Related Aspects of Intellectual Property Rights (TRIPS) lead to the implementation of regulations that allow generic manufacturers to depend on research and clinical studies conducted by brand manufacturers [16]. A free trade agreement, Canada and EU Comprehensive Economic and Trade Agreement (CETA), is an overarching trade initiative, far surpassing that of NAFTA. It presents Canadian firms with secure and unparalleled marketing opportunity with the EU's 28 member states and other flanking entities (http://international.gc.ca/trade-agreements-accords-commerciaux/agr-acc/ceta-aecg/understanding-comprendre/brief-bref.aspx?lang=eng).

The Canadian linkage regulations were modeled after the US Hatch-Waxman linkage regime with patent protection under the Patent Act (Patent Act, RSC 1985, c.P-4, s.44). Prior to 1993, patent protection and regulatory approval of pharmaceuticals were governed by different statutes with separate policy goals and objectives, which sometimes were confounding and contrasting. Variations in statutory schemes among different countries for pharmaceutical patent protection sometimes complicate generic market entry. The European Commission's regulatory authority denounces patent linkage as it is conceived as not promising for the generic product markets and that it could hinder innovation [17]. The United States, Malaysia, Vietnam, Australia, Peru, and Japan are in the process of building the patent-linkage system [17]. With these amendments, the intellectual property laws will continue to fulfill international intellectual property obligations and protect innovative medicines.

1.5.3 Labeling

Each statement proposed for drug labeling must be justified by data and results submitted in the NDA. In addition to demonstrating the drug's safety and effectiveness, the manufacturer is expected to obtain approval for the drug's labeling, which refers to all written material about the drug such as packaging, prescribing information for physicians, and patient brochures. Labels incorporate information on the available dosage forms to which the labeling applies.

1.6 THE GLOBAL PHARMACEUTICAL INDUSTRY: HARMONIZATION AND PARTNERSHIPS

Due to increasing international focus on manufacturing and clinical trial activities, globalization has become a matter of importance to the pharmaceutical industry. International regulators have increasingly recognized that international partnering enhances the pharmaceutical market and facilitates the regulation of health products in a sustainable way. The NRA has a shared global approach, as they align their initiatives to reduce limitations in actualizing this process. Globalization and harmonization have resulted in several initiatives. The following are some examples: the establishment of TRIPS and agreement of the World Trade Organization play prominent roles in international pharmaceutical regulation. TRIPS was formed in order to promote the intellectual property rights and to subject it to common international control. The Regulatory Cooperation Council unifies the Canada–United States regulatory systems for across the border operational gain and efficiencies in trade, eliminating unnecessary differences and repetitions to sustain appropriate levels of oversight of their products. A vehicle to harmonization, the MRA, enables pharmaceutical products that have been inspected and certified in a member nation to be recognized within the MRA countries. The MRA taps into the value of reciprocity allowing each sovereign nation to recognize standards within the other participating nations. MRA also promotes trade and market access within the European Union, the United States, Canada, Japan, Switzerland, Australia, New Zealand, and Israel. EMA supports the European Commission's collaboration with China, India, and Russia. This can be found at http://www.ema.europa.eu/ema/index. jsp?curl=pages/partners_and_networks/document_listing/document_ listing_000233.jsp&mid=WC0b01ac05801f0a04. A memorandum of understanding is a common agreement platform that promotes greater global cooperation. The International Organization for Standardization (ISO), the International Conference on Harmonisation of Technical Requirements for Registration of Pharmaceuticals for Human Use (ICH), and the International Cooperation on Harmonisation of Technical Requirements for Registration of Veterinary Medicinal Products (VICH) all contain regulatory guidelines that are collectively recognized internationally.

There is an increasing focus toward harmonization as it has been demonstrated to promote effective globalization of the pharmaceutical sector, which is the key aim of establishing the ICH documents.

1.6.1 International Conference on Harmonisation of Technical Requirements for Registration of Pharmaceuticals for Human Use

1.6.1.1 Scope

ICH is the harmonized format for drug registration applications for new pharmaceutical products, biologicals, the abbreviated (abridged) applications. ICH represents a point of convergence to straighten the uneven global regulatory landscape. Thus, it was created in an attempt to address the unilateral development of requirements and to reduce time and resources needed to compile applications and enhance reviews, communication, and exchange between regional countries.

The International Conference of Drug Regulatory Authorities (organized by the World Health Organization (WHO), attended by delegates from Japan, the European Union, and the United States and observers from WHO, the European Free Trade Association, and Canada, took place in 1989. Other participants were trade associations: European Federation of Pharmaceutical Industries Association, Pharmaceutical Research and Manufacturers of America, and Japan Pharmaceutical Manufacturers Association. A consensus was reached and it led to the launch of the International Conference on Harmonisation of Technical Requirements for the Registration of Pharmaceuticals for Human Use. Guidelines for active pharmaceutical ingredients (API), by the ICH, and GMPs now apply in the European Union, Japan, and the United States, and also in other countries (e.g., Australia, Canada, and Singapore), which adopt them for the manufacture and testing of active raw materials.

The United States, Europe, Japan, and Canada are the major trade groupings that are the signatories to ICH. Other regions are Asia Pacific, Latin America, Africa, Russia, Australia, and New Zealand. These nations incorporate the dossier requirements for quality, preclinical and clinical studies for developmental healthcare products and drug master file (Figure 1.2). According to Figure 1.2, module 1 is region specific while modules 2–5 are common to all the applicable regions.

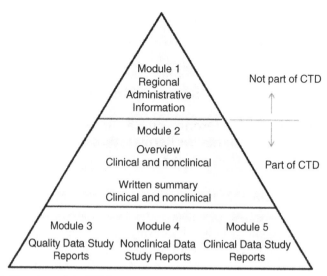

Figure 1.2 *Structure of the ICH Document.*

The ICH Global Cooperation Group comprises representatives from the regional harmonization initiatives, which are: Asia-Pacific Economic Cooperation, Association of the Southeast Asian Nations, Gulf Cooperation Council, Pan American Network for Drug Regulatory Harmonization, and Southern African Development Community. Certain non-ICH countries are now major contributors/consumers of the global pharmaceutical market. The regulators forum that started in 2008 includes representatives from Australia, Brazil, China, Taiwan, India, Russia, Singapore, and South Korea most of which are not part of harmonization initiatives and are focusing on the API, GMP, clinical trials, and pharmacovigilance. While promoting the efficiency and integrity of clinical trials, increasing reforms are bringing appreciable impact on globalization due to its widening scope and geographical coverage. The evolutionary changes and international harmonization endeavors are opening avenues for collaboration among the national regulators to facilitate faster "time to launch" while mitigating the regulatory burden. Continual cooperation among the NRAs is a priority and essential toward the moving forward of the regulatory agenda.

ICH terminology used in the Quality Safety and Efficacy Classification Systems:

ICH-Q: Quality. This pertains to pharmaceutical quality based on GMP risk management.

ICH-S: Safety. This pertains to risks like carcinogenicity, genotoxicity, and reprotoxicity.

ICH-E: Efficacy. This pertains to effective design, conduct, safety, and reporting of clinical trials and processes pivotal for demonstrating efficacy including the use of pharmacogenetics/pharmacogenomics.

ICH-M: Multidisciplinary. This pertains to topics outside the quality, safety, and efficacy categories. It includes the ICH medical terminology, the CTD, and the development of Electronic Standards for the Transfer of Regulatory Information.

1.6.2 Government Regulations: Prospects for Multinational Clinical Trials

Outsourcing some aspects of pharmaceutical research and development (R&D) has been a cost-saving mechanism for many international sponsors. For example, conducting international clinical trials in less industrialized or less developed countries usually brings less expenditure for the sponsor. But to the middle to low income country or geographical region that is indisposed to meet the legal standards, regulatory compliance has been a challenge. Continual regulatory reform is streamlining processes in multinational clinical trials to help bridge the gap and promote its effectiveness.

1.6.2.1 Pharmaceutical Regulations in Asia

Asia is a rapidly growing pharmaceutical market that attracts drug development projects and marketing opportunities. However, incremental regulatory demands and reformations tend to mitigate the success opportunities for the affected companies. Thus, modernization of the pharmaceutical regulatory systems that have taken into consideration these economic barriers has played a major role in shaping the effectual multinational pharmaceutical R&D operations. This strongly elicits the strengthening of the global pharmaceutical marketplace – a crucial need for the industry and human health.

In Japan, the adoption of the ICH "Guideline on Ethnic Factors in the Acceptability of Foreign Clinical Data" (E5) in 1998, and the approval of the new "Basic Concepts for International Joint Clinical Trials" in 2007 by Japan's PMDA, relaxed the regulations that now permit pharmaceutical companies to accept clinical data from outside Japan. This has reduced the lengthy timelines for projects resulting from limitations in clinical trial studies performed in Japan. Prior to the recent regulatory changes, approval for new drugs in Japan could take up to 4 years longer than in the United States or Europe because of the difficulty of conducting trials in Japan.

China's population explosion (over a billion people) is an advantage for pharmaceutical manufacturers, as it attracts clinical trials and markets for emerging therapies, but these trials often have longer timelines. With increasing investment in R&D by foreign companies, the regulatory demands for multinational clinical trials performed in China have made it difficult for foreign drug sponsors and multinational sponsors to proceed with clinical trials in the country. On December 2, 2011, China's State Food and Drug Administration (SFDA) issued the Guiding Principles for Administration on Phase I Clinical Trials on Drugs (for Trial Implementation), in order to streamline Phase I clinical trials in China that has now enhanced multinational clinical trials in the country. In drafting the previously mentioned principles, the SFDA referred to British Pharmaceutical Industry and EMA clinical trials guidelines. The guidelines are found in the Association of the British Pharmaceutical Industry's Guidelines for Phase I Clinical Trials. The EMA's Guideline on Strategies to Identify and Mitigate Risks for First-in-Human Clinical Trials with Investigational Medicinal Products. EMA's Guideline for Good Clinical Practice. China Issues New Guidelines on Phase I Trials [18].

One significant regulatory change is that Certificates of Analysis (COA) must be issued locally for the ingredients in drugs to be tested in China. The COA requirement may now be waived for chemical-based products not registered for sale in China. This further widens the scope of multinational trials, providing a better opportunity for Chinese patients seeking new medicines. In October 2007, China's SFDA issued new timetable guidelines that have reduced the pharmaceutical review time by 1–2 months [19,20].

1.7 MODERNIZATION OF THE GLOBAL PHARMACEUTICAL SYSTEMS: REGULATORY STRATEGIES, ROADMAP INITIATIVES, AND PARTNERSHIPS

Modernized frameworks support evolving regulatory tools that incorporate adjustments to eliminate regulatory redundancies at various levels of pharmaceutical processes. They help to create robust systems customized to the growing needs of modern populations. Increasing challenges of product development and globalization demanded modernization and advancement in the regulatory systems that promote a prospering pharmaceutical R&D environment and the utility of its drug products.

1.7.1 The Critical Path Initiative

The Critical Path Initiative (CPI) was launched in the United States in March 2004. The FDA, like any other federal drug regulation authority, has a dual obligation in meeting its mandate of public wellness and safety. It is involved with both regulation of drug development procedures through implementing policies that ensure that the benefits of new products are sustained with minimal risks and promoting pharmaceutical innovations that can improve health. There is increasing public demand on the regulator and on the drug maker about drug development outcomes. However, these demands seem to coincide with a declining pharmaceutical innovation and, consequently, lapses in the ability of the healthcare industry to meet all the public medical needs. These social necessities and the challenges associated with this dual obligation to public health compelled the emergence of the CPI.

CPI is a roadmap initiative focused on modernizing the various aspects of biomedical and drug discovery science, from concept to launch, and on facilitating scientific breakthroughs that translate to increasing pharmaceutical introductions to the clinic. CPI is specifically focused on reforming the major dimensions of the drug discovery and development process, which are: safety, medical utility, and industrialization; and to improve the effectiveness, productivity, and approval rates of emerging therapies. One of the major goals is to promote innovation and effective utilization of technologies for clinical trials and pharmaceutical manufacturing, toxicity testing such as nephrotoxicity, neurotoxicity, adenovirus toxicity, and vaccine adjuvant therapies. CPI is aimed at developing an enhanced information database for postmarket safety monitoring, personal genomic information, and utility in product development. Its goals include development of new diagnostics and treatments, enhancement of testing technologies, and improved investigation of contamination outbreaks. The CPI has accomplished much in helping to qualify biomarkers and providing *in vitro* diagnostic tools to improve the effectiveness of clinical trials and manufacturing operations. It does so by leveraging the technology available to bring more safety, efficacy, and quality to the overall pharmaceutical manufacturing and testing process. Further information can be found in the Critical Path Initiative – Report on Key Achievements in 2009. Building on the milestones of the CPI, the Advancing Regulatory Science Initiative (ARS) was launched on February 24, 2010. ARS is concerned with developing innovative standards and tools for evaluating the safety, efficacy, and quality of all FDA-regulated products.

1.7.2 The European Medicines Agency's Roadmap to 2015

The EMA's Roadmap published "A Strategy for the Heads of Medicines Agencies 2011–15" toward improving the operational efficiency of medicines. This was authorized by the decentralized procedure and MRP, and it mirrors the FDA's CPI (http://www.hma.eu/fileadmin/dateien/ HMA_joint/02-_HMA_Strategy_Annual_Reports/02-HMA_Strategy_ Paper/2010_12_HMA_StrategyPaperII.pdf). The goal of the EMA's Road-map to 2015 is to address the diminishing efficiency in drug developments. It aims to improve pharmacovigilance and safety monitoring by provid-ing a regulatory framework to track the risks and benefits throughout a drug product's life cycle. It also strengthens R&D through its legislative reform that promotes patient safety – with special consideration for the aging population and the medical needs of elderly people. The novel dis-coveries in science and technology that are applicable to drug discovery are mostly nanotechnology, based on advanced cell and gene therapy, and tissue engineering, which needs further adaptation to accommodate the new trends. Personalized medicine is being considered for integration into medical practice, and is gradually becoming a standard of care but has not been fully attained.

EMA has launched the Trans-Atlantic Task Force on Antimicrobial Re-sistance in an attempt to resolve lack of development of antibiotics and an-timicrobial resistance. ECDC/EMEA Joint Technical Report: The bacterial challenge: time to react. There has been a call to narrow the gap between multidrug-resistant bacteria in the European Union and development of new antibacterial agents [21].

1.7.3 The Progressive Licensing Model of Health Canada

Health Canada uses the Progressive Licensing Model (PLM) to manage pharmaceutical regulation, which takes into consideration the stages or points of intersection with government authorities to ensure efficiency and effectiveness at each stage. Regulatory activities cover every stage of devel-opment through the postmarketing period. These activities are focused on managing increasing knowledge as the drug is developed and help to orga-nize information across the entire process. The aim of the PLM is to enhance business performance and regulatory confidence in the interest of cost and time. Government regulatory measures intersect with business processes at key functional areas to ensure accurate monitoring through the pipeline.

1.7.4 Global Initiatives

The International Federation of Red Cross and Red Crescent Societies and the International Federation of Pharmaceutical Manufacturers & Associa-tions proposed to launch a "4 Healthy Habits" global initiative. This was intended to reduce the rise of noncommunicable diseases (NCDs), which are, cardiovascular diseases, cancer, chronic respiratory diseases, and diabetes; and to promote healthy lifestyles in communities around the globe. The four main NCDs share four main behavioral risk factors: tobacco use, harmful use of alcohol, insufficient physical activity, and unhealthy diet/obesity, which contribute to the low-average life expectancy in many low- and middle-income countries according to the report [22].

1.7.5 World Health Partnerships

The largest world health partnerships are addressing the areas of availability of treatments through differential pricing, financial support, product donations, surgery, and technology transfer. The building of health care systems, infrastructure of small to medium income countries through development of physical infrastructure, outreach and medical services, provision of insecticide nets, salt fortification capacity, and training also strengthens healthcare delivery, access and awareness (http://partnerships.ifpma.org/pages/healthpartnerships/5/35/Global-mobilization-aimed-at-saving-lives-of-millions-of-women-and-children). Certain developments of innovative tools and approaches (http://partnerships.ifpma.org/partnership/glaxosmithkline-using-mobile-phones-to-tackle-counterfeiting-in-nigeria) have been made possible through world health partnerships. These initiatives have been brought forward in order to refine scientific knowledge in developing countries and facilitate discovery of new medicines. Prevention/awareness/outreach addresses areas of malnutrition, neglected and tropical diseases (NTDs), bridging cancer care, and delivering hope. In the areas of R&D there are increasing development endeavors for treatment of NTDs, such as, HIV, tuberculosis, and malaria. There has been pediatric R&D, promotion of innovating funding mechanisms, and expanding research capacity. The details and the participating companies can be found in http://partnerships.ifpma.org/partnerships/by-type.

A multilateral agreement among governments, inter- and nongovernmental organizations, private sector companies, universities, and foundations was intended to improve the therapeutic response to HIV/AIDS, malaria, TB, NCDs, NTDs, and those pertaining to women and children's health.

Case Report: Combating NTDs in Africa

The low- and middle-income countries have been tackling the highest burden of poverty-related neglected infectious diseases worldwide, along with incompetent biomedical and medical research originating from these regions. Some of the reasons have been attributed to lack of public funding for health systems. The feeble and substandard health systems currently underpin the debilitating West Africa-wide Ebola outbreak mayhem that has defiled the limited infrastructure and medical tools employed in combating this societal catastrophe.

There has been a considerable influx of funding for clinical research. For example, European and Developing Countries Clinical Trials Partnership (EDCTP) was established by EU member states and Norway under Article 169 Joint Programme of Activities [23]. The collaboration led to a €400 million investment in research funds for the advancement of clinical trials conducted in the developing countries. The major aim of the EDCTP was to expedite the development of promising therapies against the NTDs – HIV/AIDS, malaria, and TB – in developing countries, with a major interest in sub-Saharan Africa, and to promote effectual and promising medical research directed toward these disease areas with a focus on Phase II and III clinical trials in sub-Saharan Africa.

A recent report stated that certain limitations are the barriers to creating research capacity in sub-Saharan Africa – mostly lack of understanding of the policy makers and lack of infrastructure. EDCTP intends to offer a window of opportunity toward filling this pharmaceutical gap through international collaboration between African partners, Europe, and the United States, and regional collaboration between African research institutes (http://www.rand.org/randeurope/research/projects/health-research-sub-saharan-africa.html; http://www.edctp.org/media-centre/news/announcement/current-state-of-health-research-on-poverty-related-diseases-in-sub-saharan-africa/).

REFERENCES

[1] Swann JP. How chemists pushed for consumer protection. The Food and Drugs Act of 1906. U.S. Food and Drug Administration. Available from: http://www.fda.gov/AboutFDA/WhatWeDo/History/CentennialofFDA/Chemistsandthe1906Act/ucm126648.htm

[2] Moore SW. An overview of drug development in the United States and current challenges. South Med J 2003;96(12):1244–55.

[3] Borchers AT, Hagie F, Keen CL, Gershwin ME. The history and contemporary challenges of the U.S. Food and Drug Administration. Clin Ther 2007;29(1):1–16.

[4] Mossinghoff GJ. Overview of the Hatch-Waxman Act and its impact on the drug development process. Food Drug Law J 1999;54(2):187–94. Available from: http://www.oblon.com/files/news/107.pdf.

[5] Richards D. Drug development and regulation. Medicine 2008;36(7):369–76.

[6] Matsuo D. Effect of Amendment to Japan's Pharmaceutical Affairs Law. Nomura Research Institute Papers. Dec. 2009; No. 149.

[7] Hughes DA, Bayoumi AM, Pirmohamed M. Current assessment of risk-benefit by regulators: is it time to introduce decision analyses? Clin Pharmacol Ther 2007;82:123–7.

[8] Honig P. Benefit and risk assessment in drug development and utilization: a role for clinical pharmacology. Clin Pharmacol Ther 2007;82:109–12.

[9] Grignolo A. Meeting with the FDA. In: Pisano DJ, Mantus DS, editors. FDA regulatory affairs: a guide for prescription drugs, medical devices, and biologics. 2nd ed. New York: Informa Healthcare; 2008. p. 109–23.

[10] Office of New Drugs (US). Guidance for Review Staff and Industry. Good Review Management Principles and Practices for PDUFA Products. 2013 Apr. MAPP 6030.9.

[11] Notice to applicants. Volume 2A. Procedures for marketing authorisation. Mutual recognition. 2007 Feb. Available from: http://ec.europa.eu/health/files/eudralex/vol-2/a/vol2a_chap2_2007-02_en.pdf. European Commission [chapter 2].

[12] Notice to applicants. Volume 2A. Procedures for marketing authorisation. Centralized procedure. 2006 April. Available from: http://www.ema.europa.eu/docs/en_GB/document_library/Regulatory_and_procedural_guideline/2009/10/WC500004069.pdf [accessed 30.10.2014] [chapter 4].

[13] FDA (US). New Drug Application (NDA): Introduction. Available from: http://www.fda.gov/Drugs/DevelopmentApprovalProcess/HowDrugsareDevelopedandApproved/ApprovalApplications/NewDrugApplicationNDA/default.htm

[14] Boldrin M, Levine DK. Against intellectual monopoly. Cambridge University Press; 2008 [chapters 8 and 9].

[15] Macdonald S. When means become ends: considering the impact of patent strategy on innovation. Inform Econ Policy 2004;16:135–58. Available from: http://www.stuart-macdonald.org.uk/pdfs/Macdonald.pdf.

[16] North American Free Trade Agreement, U.S.-Can.-Mex., Dec. 17, 1992, T.S. No. 2 (1994).

[17] Asia IP magazine. 2012 Apr. 4(4), 50.

[18] Will it speed up approvals. Pharm Asia News: Drugs-Biologics-Devices 2012.

[19] SFDA, Regulations for Implementation of the Drug Administration Law of the People's Republic of China, Art. 30.2002. Available from: http://former.sfda.gov.cn/cmsweb/webportal/W45649038/A48335997.html

[20] SFDA. Regulations for the Supervision and Administration of Medical Devices, Art. 7. 2000. Available from: http://former.sfda.gov.cn

[21] ECDC/EFSA/EMEA/SCENHIR Joint Report on Antimicrobial Resistance (AMR) Focused on Zoonotic Infections. EFSA J 2009;7(11):1372. Question No. EFSA-Q-2008-781. doi:10.2903/j.efsa.2009.1372. European Medicines Agency Reference EMEA/CVMP/447259/2009.

[22] The Joint IFRC-IFPMA Reception on the occasion of the 67th World Health Assembly 2014 May 19; Geneva, Switzerland.

[23] European and Developing Countries Clinical Trial Partnership, Joint Programme of the Action, Part A, Technical content and the overall work plan for the entire period of the Action, Annex I, Part A, Final draft, Nov. 13, 2003.

CHAPTER 2

Trends in Innovation and the Business of Drug Discovery

Odilia Osakwe

Contents

2.1 Introduction	30
2.1.1 Pharmaceutical Innovation	30
2.1.2 The Global Pharmaceutical Business	30
2.2 Evolutionary Trends in Pharmaceutical Innovation	32
2.2.1 The Global Pharmaceutical Discoveries of the Twentieth Century	32
2.3 Advances in Pharmaceutical Innovation Technology	36
2.4 Select Medical Milestones of 2014	37
2.5 Factors Contributing to Pharmaceutical Innovation Setback	38
2.5.1 Research and Development Productivity	38
2.5.2 Complex Biological Systems	39
2.5.3 The Challenge of Adverse Drug Reactions	39
2.5.4 Economic Strategies	40
2.5.5 Between Risk and Return: The "Valley of Death"	41
2.5.6 Poor Product Strategies	42
2.5.7 Patent Protection	43
2.5.8 Clinical Development Challenges	43
2.5.9 Regulatory Burden	45
2.6 Case: Challenges in Antimicrobial Drug Discovery	45
2.7 Consequence of Innovation Setback	46
2.8 Strategies and Approaches to Addressing Innovation Failure	47
2.8.1 Regulatory Approach	47
2.8.2 Mergers, Acquisitions, and Outsourcing	48
2.8.3 Pharmaceutical Research and Development	50
2.8.4 New Avenues of Personalized Medicine: Application of Pharmacogenomics Technology in Drug Development	51
2.8.5 Drug Repositioning/Repurposing	52
2.8.6 Building the Pharmaceutical Ecosystem	52
2.9 Concluding Remarks	52
References	52

Social Aspects of Drug Discovery, Development and Commercialization
http://dx.doi.org/10.1016/B978-0-12-802220-7.00002-8

2.1 INTRODUCTION

2.1.1 Pharmaceutical Innovation

Pharmaceutical innovation or medical discovery is necessitated by the need to address a medical condition or disease and brings about efforts to identify a therapy. It is not only concerned with medical breakthroughs but also breakthrough tools for developing new treatments, creating the most desired performance standards and predictive tools needed to satisfy the overall public health needs and necessities [1]. In the twenty-first century, a time when basic biomedical knowledge is increasing exponentially, medical discovery tools build on knowledge delivered by recent advances in science, such as bioinformatics, genomics, imagining technologies, and materials science. According to Fredric J. Cohen [2], innovation involves scientific, technical, and market research; product, process, or service development and manufacturing; and marketing that supports dissemination and application of the invention. Moreover, the previously mentioned are the major aspects of the value chain [3–5]. The pharmaceutical innovation cycle is only complete when scientific ideas are duly translated into effective therapy and economic success (Figure 2.1).

2.1.2 The Global Pharmaceutical Business

The global pharmaceutical business (GPB) is the cornerstone of the knowledge-based economy (KBE) due to an astonishing increase in revenue over the last thirty decades. Evolution of technology contributes to its knowledge base and the largest drug companies (big pharmas) are the strongholds of the GPB. The pharmaceutical industry owns a 20–25% stake worldwide. The overall global pharmaceuticals market is worth US$300 billion a year of which over one-third is controlled by the big pharmas [6].

The United States is the world's largest market for pharmaceuticals and the world leader in biopharmaceutical research. US firms conduct 80% of the world's research and development (R&D) in biotechnology and hold

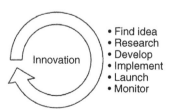

Figure 2.1 *The Innovation Cycle.*

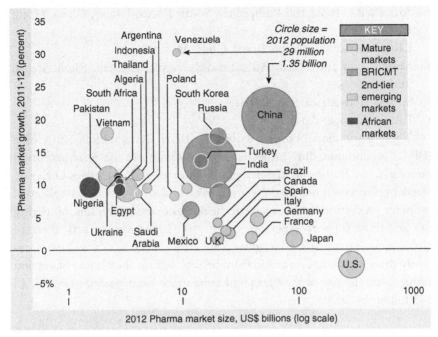

Figure 2.2 *The Global Pharmaceutical Market, 2012.*

the intellectual property rights to most new medicines [7,8]. President Obama reaffirmed the US commitment to an Open Investment Policy in 2011. The top six the pharmaceutical industries are based in the United States and four in Europe. These are regarded as the developed world, whose economies grant access to markets, attracting a multitude of multinational pharmaceutical developments, which are already settled in these regions [9]. The largest pharmaceutical companies are the multinational companies, headquartered in the United States and Western Europe. Revenue-based ranking in the United States follows the order Pfizer, Merck, Johnson & Johnson, Eli Lilly, Bristol-Myers Squibb, Abbott Labs, and Amgen, while in Europe the ranking is Novartis and Roche, (Switzerland), Sanofi-Aventis (France), GlaxoSmithKline and AstraZeneca (UK), Bayer and Boehringer Ingelheim (Germany), and Novo Nordisk (Denmark). In the rest of the world Teva (Israel) and Takeda, Astellas, Daiichi Sankyo (Japan) are ranked the highest. It was predicted that North and South America, Europe, and Japan will continue to account for a full 85% of the global pharmaceuticals market well into the twenty-first century [9] (Figure 2.2). More than 70% of the world's population (Asia Pacific and emerging markets) contribute most to the global pharmaceutical market:

- Asia Pacific: India, the Philippines, South Korea, Taiwan, China, Hong Kong
- Latin America: Argentina, Brazil, Chile, Mexico
- Middle East and North Africa: mostly Egypt, Pakistan, Saudi Arabia, Turkey
- Sub-Saharan Africa: South Africa
- Eastern Europe: Russia

There is substantial growth within the Brazil, Russia, India, and China (BRIC) economies, duly projected as an extension of the pharmaceutical business from Europe to these regions. Most of the challenges currently faced by the emerging markets are weak regulatory controls, intellectual property protection, and inadequate health insurance programs, hindering the ability to support expensive drugs [10]. Emerging markets' share of global spending is expected to grow from 20% (2011) to 30% in 2016. Currently, drug spending downsized from 58% to 48% in the United States and Europe, and the size of the African pharma market is expected to double to $45 billion by 2020.

2.2 EVOLUTIONARY TRENDS IN PHARMACEUTICAL INNOVATION

2.2.1 The Global Pharmaceutical Discoveries of the Twentieth Century (Table 2.1)

2.2.1.1 The Changing Pharmaceutical Productivity

Over the last decade, there has been a continual rise in pharmaceutical R&D spending. Drugs approvals by the US Food and Drug Administration (FDA) steadily declined by 40%, despite the growth in cost in R&D of drugs accessed by the public. A study report by Oliver Wyman [17] examined drugs approved between 1996 and 2010 by the FDA. He referred the "Era of Abundance" as a period when the number of approvals of new molecular entities (NMEs) reached 36, which was between 1996 and 2004, and the "Era of Scarcity" as a period when the number dropped to 22, between 2005 and 2010 (Figure 2.3); these periods were characterized as boom or failure, respectively, and with a defining separation marked by Vioxx withdrawal in 2004. Scannell et al. [18] also indicated that the proposed Eroom's law theory – "the number of new drugs approved per billion US dollars spent on R&D has halved roughly every nine years since 1950" – agrees with the proposal of Oliver Wyman. A total of $128 billion was spent yearly on R&D from 2009 through 2011,

Table 2.1 The global pharmaceutical discoveries of the twentieth century

1900–1929
1900 US life expectancy is 45
1908 Tuberculosis vaccine
1920 and on
   Launch of the first vaccines, diphtheria, pertussis, and tetanus
1922 Insulin for diabetes
1924 Tetanus vaccine
1928 Discovery of penicillin
1930s and 1940s
1932 Launch antibiotic (sulfa drugs)
1935 Discovery of cortisone
1938 Launch epilepsy therapy
1940 Launch penicillin
1944 Launch kidney dialysis
1945 Launch flu vaccine
1948 Launch chemotherapy drug

1950s
1950 Discovery of prednisone
1951 Chlorpromazine (thorazine) for schizophrenia
1953 First leukemia Rx
1954 Polio vaccine
1953 Discovery of the structure of the DNA molecule
1957 L-Dopa developed
1958 First diuretic to treat high blood pressure
1960s and 1970s
1963 Measles vaccine
1967 Launch beta blocker
1967 Launch mumps vaccine; first human heart transplant
1968 Launch antirejection medicines for organ transplants
1972 Advances in anesthesia
1973 Engineered recombinant DNA technique
1977 Launch nonsurgical treatment for ulcers
1978 Launch biotech synthetic human insulin
1978 Launch production of human insulin
1978 Initial biotech application in drug development
1979 First synthesis of human growth hormone
1980 Smallpox cleared

1980s
1981 Launch ACE inhibitor to treat high blood pressure
1986 Launch monoclonal antibody treatment
1987 Launch new class of depression medicines
   Launch AIDS therapy
   Launch statins to treat cholesterol
1990s
1993 Launch Alzheimer's Rx
1994 New breast cancer Rx Polio cleared in the Americas
1994 Breast cancer gene discovery
1996 Parkinson's disease associated gene with new suggestions for neurological therapy
1995 Advance AIDS therapy (HAART)
1995 Launch oral drugs for diabetes
1997 Advance Parkinson's therapies
1998 Launch rotavirus vaccine
1990 Launch human genome initial experimental gene therapy treatment on a child

Source: Refs [10–16].

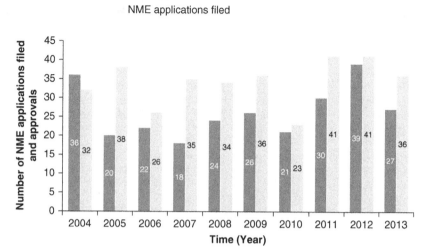

Figure 2.3 *A 10-year Comparison of new Drug Applications/Biologic License Applications/ new Molecular Entities Applications Received by CDER Through 2013.* Adapted *from January 2014 Novel New Drugs 2013 Summary. US Food and Drug Administration (FDA) Center for Drug Evaluation and Research [23].*

compared to only 60% spent per year from 2002 through 2004, and still there are fewer new entrants – only 29 new filings in 2011, compared to 32 in 2004. Some optimism reemerged in 2011, marked by the 30 NME approvals made by the FDA, the highest number recorded following the 36 NME approvals in 2004; this was the blockbuster era, a period when blockbuster drugs sales were leading the pharma market with high profit yields that prospered the innovator pharmaceutical companies [19]. Blockbuster markets are experiencing a diminishing revenue stream as the top 10 drugs that generated $15 billion in the United States in 2012 had lost their patents in 2013, and, as projected, could lose $8 billion by 2016; leading to a gradual rounding off of the "blockbuster era" for big pharma.

Patent expiry is regarded as the "patent cliff," which is gradually taking over the optimism that was the hallmark of the blockbuster era. It has been predicted that about $148 billion could be lost between 2012 and 2018 due to patent expiry. In addition, drug spending in developed markets will shrink by $127 billion between 2011 and 2016 due to an increasing focus on low-price generics. Between 2011 and 2016, global brand drug spending will grow by only 8%, compared to 80% growth in generic drug spending. Expenditures have been redirected to specialty drugs (biologics, orphan drugs) for cancer, HIV, hepatitis C, and rare diseases, which have recently picked up speed.

By 2011, Pfizer had gained profoundly due to its monopoly over the sale of Lipitor (while still on patent). About $115 billion in revenue has been reported since its release with 40% of total profits in 2005 alone [20]. Pfizer is currently facing a huge loss in profits due to loss of patent exclusivity over Lipitor. Also, the innovators of Plavix (clopidogrel) and Seroquel (quetiapine) are on the patent cliff with a revenue plunge totaling US $33 billion of sales in 2012 In addition to Lipitor, Plavix and Seroquel have suffered the steepest decline in revenue. In an attempt to minimize loses from patent expiration, a licensing agreement with the Indian pharmaceutical company Ranbaxy, was established [21,22]. Many of the mega-blockbuster drugs are now generic [23]. Other companies affected are Sanofi, Novartis, Roche Astra Zeneca and Eli Lilly.

The figure includes pending applications for 2013. The Center for Drug Evaluation and Research (CDER) approval averaged about 26 NME approvals per year excluding the 39 of 2012, an unusually high count above the rest within the decade.

One-third (33%) of the NMEs approved in 2013 (9 of 27) were identified by the FDA as first-in-class – with a new and unique mechanism of action for treating a disease. Orphan drugs, drugs that treat rare diseases (affecting around 200,000 Americans), comprise one-third (33%; 9 of 27) of the NMEs approved in 2013. This has been considered a significant accomplishment considering the prevailing paucity of orphan drugs due to low incidences of the diseases (see Tables 2.1 and 2.2).

NMEs or innovative new products are a new class of candidate drugs with therapeutic action against a disease that have not been licensed for marketing or clinical use. However, an NME may not therapeutically supersede existing therapies. First-in-class drugs are originator drugs with a novel action mechanism for treating a medical condition. Pharmaceutical companies essentially depend on incremental innovations to provide a revenue source that supports the development of the high risk, capital- and research-intensive drugs. Innovative new drugs increase manufacturer competition and lower drug prices. Me-too drugs differ slightly from others within the same class – drugs with similar chemical composition and which treat similar conditions. The slight difference enhances the ability of physicians to tailor drugs to the medical needs of a diverse patient population. Incremental improvements in the new classes of drugs tend to address the limits of the already existing ones. New drugs with adjusted formulations and dosing significantly increase patient compliance and therapeutic value.

Table 2.2 Select FDA drug approvals in 2013

Orphan – drugs and indications	First-in-class – drugs and indications
Imbruvica – Mantle cell lymphoma	Invokana – Type 2 diabetes glycemic
Gazyva – Chronic lymphocytic	control
leukemia	Kadcyla – HER2-positive late-stage
Kynamro – Homozygous familial	(metastatic) breast cancer
hypercholesterolemia	Sovald – Interferon-free oral treat-
Adempas – Pulmonary arterial	ment option for chronic hepatitis
hypertension	C
Opsumit – Pulmonary arterial	Mekinis – Metastatic melanoma
hypertension	
Gilotrif – Treat late stage (metastatic)	
nonsmall cell lung cancer	
Tafinlar – Forms of melanoma	
Tecfidera – Relapsing forms of	
multiple sclerosis	
Olysio – Chronic hepatitis C	

2.3 ADVANCES IN PHARMACEUTICAL INNOVATION TECHNOLOGY

In the 1980s, medical discovery was mostly by serendipity – a trial and error way of trying new compounds in model animals. These efforts did not consider the mechanism of a drug's action but assigned therapy based on attenuation of disease symptoms. Thus, research was focused on small molecules that were not probed in the biological systems. The discovery of the structure of DNA in the early 1950s led to the invention of genetic engineering in the 1970s.

This created a new path for pharmaceutical R&D – the field of biotechnology. The research techniques paved the way to understanding human systems, thus biology is an integral aspect of pharmaceutical R&D. The genome project that sequenced the whole human DNA revolutionized drug discovery and is the key to technological developments in fields such as gene therapy, cell therapy, tissue engineering, genomics, proteomics, and bioinformatics. These underpin the current innovative approaches in pharmaceutical developments leading to more sophisticated understanding of biological networks and pathogenic pathways, further fine-tuning discovery research leading to major therapeutic advancement in the cure or management of diseases.

Data mining and computation platforms complement the applied biological and chemical research. These have been duly utilized to address every possible drug target in terms of druggable characteristics. Using many of these tools collaboratively makes drug discovery more efficient [24]. PubChem, which provides information on the biological activities of small molecules, eMolecules, establishes and updates compound libraries to help accelerate discovery research. Collaborative drug discovery (CDD) allows the management and sharing of chemical and biological data and to collaborate with internal or external partners through the CDD vault interface. ChemSpider is a chemical structure database owned by the Royal Society of Chemistry. It permits fast access to compound structures, their properties, and associated information in the order of millions, enabling the discovery of freely available chemical data from a single online search. Assay Depot establishes a network with a wide range of service providers for speedy access to innovative tools for enhanced research [25]. The mining of real world data using electronic health records helps to identify comorbidities. Social media identifies patients' behavior in response to treatment and monitors applications that identify trends in lifestyle. Insurance claims data enable improvement in efficiency of delivery of drugs, tailored to patients at the right time. These and many more technological tools advance pharmaceutical innovations. Their application has created much value, contributing to years of economic growth and strong profits from novel drugs. Some positive outcomes are to be mentioned later.

2.4 SELECT MEDICAL MILESTONES OF 2014

The Pharmaceutical Research and Manufacturers of America (PhRMA) is comprised of prominent biopharmaceutical researchers and biotechnology companies in America. On account of improving medical solutions, the drug discovery and development pipeline has been termed the "Pipeline of Hope" [26]. A handful of medical accomplishments have been recorded by PhRMA, for example, new medical discoveries that have transformed the fatal HIV/AIDS disease to a manageable chronic disease [27]. Rheumatoid arthritis has been mechanistically addressed through targeting the physiological mechanism of action. This has increased the ability to target disease remission, which has been a bottleneck to therapy in the past. This was facilitated by growing knowledge built from technological advancement and which led to incremental breakthroughs while offering more hope for the future [28]. Available therapies now treat chronic myeloid leukemia, and recently its effectiveness in combating other devastating forms of leukemia, as well as gastrointestinal stromal tumors, has been identified. The historical account of higher survival rates (31–89%) is very promising; it renders hope for patients who depend on these therapies to extend their lifespans [29]. The eight Millennium Development Goals are to be enforced by 2015. The goals include cutting down on extreme poverty to meet the needs of the world's poorest and the spread of HIV/AIDS [30]. The National Institutes of Health (NIH), the largest US sponsor of biomedical research, has invested enormously in cancer research, contributing to the increasing amount of anticancer drugs in the market. In 1938, US funding in the area of cancer was through the National Cancer Institute and is estimated to be $100 billion and over $2000 billion worldwide [31,32]. The European Organization for Research and Treatment of Cancer (EORTC) was set up in October 2002 by the Translational Research Advisory Committee to support and provide expert advice on translational research projects conducted within EORTC [33].

2.5 FACTORS CONTRIBUTING TO PHARMACEUTICAL INNOVATION SETBACK

2.5.1 Research and Development Productivity

Despite historical advances in science and technology and concomitant improvement in the overall quality of care, pharmaceutical innovation versus capital expenditure balance has been more inclined to capital expenditure. The number of new drugs approved per billion US dollars spent on R&D decreased over time particularly as the current medical product development path has progressively been challenging, inefficient, and costly [34]. Recent innovations may not have proved significantly more effective or affordable, and according to the data in Figure 2.3, the average number of drugs produced over the past decade is running at a low average, designated as an "Era of Scarcity." Yearly new drug introduction has been very modest. Apart from 2004, the yearly average has been 22 with the highest being 26. This number, which rose to 30 in 2011 and more steeply to 39 in 2012, preceded a drop to 27 in 2013.

Recent tools and newly created technologies have not been harnessed productively to match technological advancement with pharmaceutical output. A disproportionate development of many new therapies for patients with only marginal improvement over the others has been considered a "pipeline problem." The principal reason for supplementing the already existing therapies is to avoid the huge R&D expenditures devoted to a high risk, low income results, and high attrition rates associated with drug development in new research areas. Another major problem is that the understanding of biological complexity in the inter- and intrahuman ecosystem is not yet absolute [35]. The changing demographics and disease profiles are a limitation that deters the ability to keep a balanced product pipeline.

2.5.2 Complex Biological Systems

The most challenging aspect of drug development is finding an approach that is commercially feasible to bring anticipated market value [36,37]. Numerous targets exist due to decades spent in research and suitable technologies that facilitate these findings. Estimates of the number of actual targets range from a few hundred to a few thousand. These need to be sifted through, requiring extensive labor and time investment in developing a therapeutically viable molecule. For example, the G-protein-coupled receptor is targeted by 30% of all marketed products but still uncharacterized ones are in the order of hundreds. The translating of this rudimentary arm of discovery to commercialization has been slowed by gaps in bringing definitive solutions to major diseases that afflict mankind, including cancer, cardiovascular disease, Alzheimer's disease, and diabetes. Intuitively, further development of a target depends on a number of factors. First among these is medical benefit. What benefit will a new drug bring to victims of the disease it is intended to treat? In the case of treatments for previously untreatable diseases the answer is obvious; that therapeutic outcomes of substantially improved tolerability, greater potency, or avoidance of side effects can justify the development of a new drug. The choice of a therapeutic target has been strategized as a means to address the risk involved. For example, the biomarkers (biological signatures) for diagnosis and the monitoring of progression of diseases have not been clearly delineated. Pharmaceutical R&D in these areas has not been "derisked" and is regarded as high risk and costly projects – the worst feared discovery issues.

2.5.3 The Challenge of Adverse Drug Reactions

Polypharmacology, which refers to off-target interactions that lead to adverse effects, is attributed to complicated biological pathways. Pharmacological profiling that identifies this attribute in a candidate drug requires adept abilities in scientific discovery and superior biological understanding [38]. The lack of fundamental knowledge has become a formidable barrier to understanding the underlying processes associated with disease development and maturity.

One of the aims of clinical development is to detect adverse drug reactions in a candidate drug prior to the marketing period. However, certain drug development methodologies do not exactly reflect the real world experience. Clinical development involves an average of 1500 patient exposures within a certain period of time or a few years. Thus, it might not provide a definitive estimate of the actual real world population. For example, Bromfenac (Durant), a nonsteroidal anti-inflammatory agent, was recalled in 1998, before its first year of introduction to the market, due to serious hepatotoxicity in a minority of the population taking the drug, which was about 1 in 20,000 patients over 10 years [39]. Thus, drugs that cause rare toxicity responses in humans might pass undetected during development but which could only be detected when exposed to a wider population within an extended period of time when taken by a wide range of patients while on the market. This exposes certain patient populations to safety risk. Market recalls could also be detrimental to the patient population that needed the drug. To the innovator pharmaceutical company, it means innovation failure and loss of revenue.

2.5.4 Economic Strategies

The ultimate goal of any pharmaceutical company is to create viable investment opportunities for robust yields, growth, and profits from proprietary drugs. The choice of a business model is informed by the particular therapeutic areas being pursued. This impresses on the pharmaceutical team a need to find a suitable innovation pathway that promotes the company's competitiveness. Expenditure and revenue generation follows cyclical feedback mechanism with revenue from product sales subsidizing the R&D of new drug compounds (Figure 2.4). In some cases, the path of market success could

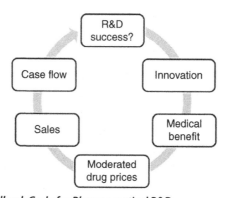

Figure 2.4 *The Feedback Cycle for Pharmaceutical R&D.*

be hampered by lack of sufficient revenue for R&D of new pipeline drugs, slowing down the entry of newer products to the market. Successful candidates based on a cumbersome process become costly. Product development programs have been dumped due to disproportionate investment of time and resources. Reports indicate that companies currently allocate a substantial portion of sales revenue to marketing their products. Previously, the cost of developing an NME has been increased from around $800 to up to $2 billion.

Failing R&D contributes to rising healthcare costs, with the burden of drug coverage costs and difficulties of medical product development contributing to stagnating innovation. Preferential use of generics and rising healthcare budgets in turn negatively impact financial performance for the innovator companies due to depleting revenue and failure in reinforcing pipelines through losses in the revenues as blockbusters come off patent. The result is a declining number of new drugs, raising doubts about the adequacy of biomedical revolution in addressing the public health burden. High drug pricing hinders drug accessibility especially for patients in the Third World where certain diseases are endemic while safety issues which has also further compounded the existing problems in part accounts for increased death rates. The one-size-fits-all paradigm to drug design and development, widely adopted by the drug developers, leaves the noncompliant patient population no option than to take drugs that are largely biologically nonconducive or unsafe.

2.5.5 Between Risk and Return: The "Valley of Death"

Most of the proposed research projects are based on speculative research ideas and are, consequently, high risk. The "Valley of Death" is a period of lack of funding and productivity in the drug development pipeline due to the paucity of business investors who are repelled by any high risk business with no clear indicators of future success. The "Valley of Death" is due to drug development projects based on complex pathologies markets, characterized as high risk and which have narrowed the probability of success [40,41]. Selection of a new research target is informed by the risk–return assessment, which is essential for the determination of the level of risk involved in developing a drug molecule and its costs. Recently, there has been a shift from the risk-adjusted, established project development processes to riskier alternatives. Success depends on the quality of the scientific hypothesis that established therapeutic efficacy of the drug and the technical effectiveness. Less validated new drug candidates are filling the pipelines due to the lessening of the number of well-validated options.

The outcome of a high risk venture with low prospects for financial success is due to difficulty in predicting the late stage success. This has resulted in the failure of important drugs developed at great expense due to unanticipated problems. The potential for a high financial return is not overruled, but depends on the therapeutic areas of interest, like cancer, inflammation, or cardiovascular disease. Speculative research targets and innovative improvements are major categories of consideration in target selection. A proof of biological efficacy would not be established for any candidate drug until the Phase II trial stage for the speculative research target, which is inherently at a greater risk. For the big pharmas, choice is narrowed to the most popular therapeutic areas, which are cardiovascular, central nervous system, cancer, and gastrointestinal, allergic, and metabolic diseases [42]. Sometimes the big biopharmaceutical companies reject certain high risk projects that are mostly taken over by smaller biotech companies with the hope of commercial success and growth if such a new area could be successfully developed and commercialized for company growth.

2.5.6 Poor Product Strategies

In the present competitive healthcare environment, translating innovation into medicines that are both approvable and commercially viable is difficult. Maintaining a competitive advantage depends on the scientific comprehension of the disease target. Drugs in development, especially first-in-class drug development (novel mechanisms), require an understanding of product strategies that would maximize the anticipated commercial performance. Product strategies are evaluated by disease areas that have not found pharmaceutical treatments due to limitation on basic scientific knowledge. Mostly, the underlying disease causes are not fully addressed, or that the developmental drug could never be optimized. It is also evaluated by patient or physician segmentation, which requires intensive search into the unmet medical needs. Understanding the physician preference by obtaining the information about how many patients are diagnosed, how many doctors are prescribing the drug, and how the treatment options could be complemented is essential. Other important aspects to consider are impact on regulatory environment, effect on pricing/reimbursement, and publication strategy. These are all predetermined to meet some fundamental objectives regarding performance in the market place.

The investigational drug could be well positioned in the competitive market place in collaboration with the marketing specialist. The marketing specialist collects, analyzes, and communicates information on the disease indication market place and, collecting information from the hospital situations (doctor–patient responses) pricing, acquires all the important facts related to the disease in a market place. The health outcomes personnel give information about patient segments. Commercial evaluations consist of an expected sales profile of the drug compound, which considers volume of sales, speed with which the drug compound reaches its maximum revenue potential, and possible decline from sales. The strategic and planning process incurs huge expenses in order to understand all conceivable risks and forms of success. Thus, not adequately incorporating these commercial assessments could lead to prioritizing a drug compound of limited potential over one of high potential. Failing to strategize the drug compound effectively and failing to maximize the compound's potential and returns would lead to innovation failure. This further leads to limiting possible revenue streams that could cover costs of failed compounds.

2.5.7 Patent Protection

Intellectual property is the proprietary knowledge that underlies the development of the marketed drug and could be seen as intangible capital that is secured through patent protection. Patent protection is a legal right that allows exclusive entitlement to the sale of an innovator drug for an allotted period of time. It is used as a tool by the innovator company to recoup the R&D investments expended in developing the drug. When patents expire, the so-called patent cliff results in depleting revenue streams, which impacts pharmaceutical innovation.

2.5.8 Clinical Development Challenges

In the drug development cycle, all the stages are important and contribute to product progression to marketing (Figure 2.3). A well-executed preclinical development contributes to effective clinical development and product success. A major concern in the preclinical drug development is the *in vitro* and *in vivo* models. Sometimes, the data generated using *in vitro* screening techniques do not recapitulate the systemic biology of the cell, organ, or whole organism, and cellular bioactivity. For example, the issue of animal models that do not exactly replicate the human pathophysiology and time to disease progression is not taken into consideration in experimental designs. This could lead to errors in presented data, which affect the integrity of generated clinical data. Thus, identification of candidates with a high probability of effectiveness remains a challenge [43]. Response to a drug tested in several healthy adults sometimes deviates from that in the target population manifesting the disease for the tested drug. In addition, adverse drug reactions (ADRs) might surface many years later. This rare type of ADR is called idiosyncrasy. It brings an abnormal trend in in new drug investigation.

New technologies require methods of evaluation that might be more complex than traditional methods, suggesting further validation steps, and time and money investment for complete utilization. Problems in the design, characterization, and manufacturing programs are other examples. Drug companies keep trying to reinvent themselves, or at least their research labs, with varying degrees of success and failure. Using study protocols in clinical trials that are poorly validated and targeting the wrong population in trials using poorly validated biomarkers to assign clinical endpoints are limitations in clinical development. More than 70% lack of success in Phase II trials have often been blamed on the market landscape and unmet medical needs. Additionally, recent large-scale Phase III failures, for example, Axitinib, Figitumumab, and Torcetrapib owned by Pfizer; Elesclomol and Syntha owned by GSK; AS404 and Antisoma owned by Novartis; Iniparib and BiPar owned by Sanofi; and Vandetanib owned by AstraZeneca have been attributed to scarcity of late-stage assets [44].

Bristol-Myers Squibb's candidate drug for hepatitis C is a nucleotide polymerase (NS5B) inhibitor. In 2012, drug administration in a Phase IIb study was suspended due to a heart failure response in a patient who had the highest daily dose, 200 mg, in combination with Bristol-Myers Squibb's daclatasvir, another hepatitis C drug candidate. Zaltrap (aflibercept) is an angiogenesis inhibitor for prostate cancer developed by Sanofi and Regeneron Pharmaceuticals. In 2012, the pipeline project was terminated as it failed to meet the threshold for primary endpoint of improvement in overall survival when administered intravenously as a first-line treatment. The treatment was for metastatic androgen–independent prostate cancer in combination with docetaxel and prednisone, in a VENICE Phase III study [45].

The dose–response evaluation is very critical and the methods need to be well established. The effectiveness of the use of clinical safety biomarkers in evaluating a disease condition has been questioned. This is why clinical pharmacology needs to be integrated into the multidisciplinary teams in this situation. Bioinformatics has led to a better understanding of human disease although it is not optimal. The filters are robotic and not based on the rational scientific judgment capability of humans.

2.5.9 Regulatory Burden

Drug companies undergo rigorous, heavily restricted and regulated discovery, applied research, and development processes, which on average, span 5 years of laboratory research and 8–10 years of clinical studies. Effectiveness must incorporate the regulatory-imposed elements in order for the appropriate legal and scientific standards to be met for drug licensing. Thus, the pharmaceutical company has to comply with standards strictly for business continuation and integrity. Novel compounds are produced under heavy regulatory guidance and the huge financial investment makes it a huge challenge [46]. Stringent regulatory standards are increasingly adding more filters that tend to constrict all the gateways to drug licensing.

2.6 CASE: CHALLENGES IN ANTIMICROBIAL DRUG DISCOVERY

Infections caused by antibiotic-resistant bacteria, especially the "ESKAPE" pathogens (*Enterococcus faecium*, *Staphylococcus aureus*, *Klebsiella pneumoniae*, *Acinetobacter baumannii*, *Pseudomonas aeruginosa*, and *Enterobacter* species), cause significant morbidity and mortality [47,48]. The ESKAPE pathogens are hard to eradicate being resistant to a vast majority of antibiotics in stock, accounting for a vast majority of intensive care unit patients. Increasing numbers of mortalities from infectious diseases across the world have been attributed to pharmaceutical limitations leading to the paucity in antibacterial drugs to combat infections.

Finding a small drug molecule to bind the features of the bacteria to neutralize its activity is difficult especially when there are only negligible differences between species. The breadth of evolution with microbial growth is huge when compared to that of mammals, making it more difficult to find the molecule with species-specific characteristics. The antibacterial drug development process has been failing to cross Phase II clinical trials [49].

The tumbling landscape of antibacterial discovery stimulated the emergence of the Infectious Diseases Society of America (IDSA) "10 × '20 Initiative" in 2010 [50, 51]. Beginning in 2002, the IDSA has been facilitating the search for novel therapeutics that treat multidrug-resistant infections, including those caused by Gram-negative bacteria. It was establish to support the rebuilding of the antibiotic pipeline by seeking development and regulatory approval of 10 effective and systematically administered antibiotics by 2020. IDSA continues to work with Congress, the FDA, NIH,

Centers for Disease Control and Prevention (CDC), and others who have joined hands to spur these ongoing efforts towards accomplishing its goals.

2.7 CONSEQUENCE OF INNOVATION SETBACK

R&D is capital intensive and relies on profits from pipeline drugs that it generates for developing the pipeline drugs (Figure 2.4). It could take as much as $800 million and a time span of 12–15 years to bring a new idea to a marketable drug and recoup investments. Thus, drug companies have been focusing on products with potentially high market return, directing their efforts to blockbuster drugs (for popular diseases) or those based on market value leading to gaps in addressing crucial medical needs. Global healthcare needs include the geographically stratified diseases such as the prevalent Third World diseases, rare diseases, pediatric use, prevention indications, and the debilitating diseases that have not found adequate therapy or individualized therapy. Some examples are HIV, tuberculosis, malaria, Alzheimer's disease, Parkinson's disease, schizophrenia, and bipolar disease. These diseases demand complex R&D efforts. When patented drugs expire, the resultant effect is reducing funds for future investment in R&D. For certain popular disease areas (such as hypertension), there is quite a handful of these medicines already in the market. Thus due to this high number, there is a narrowing of the propensity for economic success and public accommodation with continual market introduction of these me-too drugs, thereby requiring diversification to new research areas of increasingly complex science. The value of pharmaceutical innovation lies in the path towards new opportunities.

The Third World and low-income countries have been subjected to population reduction due to medical indications that have not found a well-defined therapeutic solution [52]. For the neglected diseases, therapies directed to these areas are in high demand in the undeveloped nations, requiring incentives that promote pharmaceutical innovation directed to these concerns. For example, the human immunodeficiency virus/acquired immunodeficiency syndrome (HIV/AIDS) has contributed to a decimated population and poor life expectancy in these countries. However, the development of a vaccine to combat HIV/AIDS is proving to be difficult and requires a solution.

Increasing evolution in population structure is due to the rapidly aging population and the baby boomers. This is leading to a wider population with elderly diseases. The most common and high burden diseases are osteoarthritis and Alzheimer's disease, which more often afflict the elderly; the disease progressions have not been effectively reversed. Chronic diseases are more widespread regardless of income or geography. Diseases such as diabetes, cardiovascular disease, depression, and cancers are mostly managed and not cured, requiring more therapeutic advances for people in countries throughout the world.

2.8 STRATEGIES AND APPROACHES TO ADDRESSING INNOVATION FAILURE

2.8.1 Regulatory Approach

The importance of facilitating a better access to medicines has been emphasized and efforts are addressing the productivity gap while streamlining regulatory consultations and information acquisition to harmonize these efforts. Continuous regulatory reform has led to roadmap initiatives that stimulate pharmaceutical productivity. Modernization incentives increase time to approval especially for the innovator drugs. For example, the FDA issued the Prescription Drug User Fee Act (PDUFA) 1992 requiring drug manufacturers to pay fees to speed up new drug and biologic drug applications reviewing to reduce the time to approval. A guideline document "A revised guideline on current Good Manufacturing Practices (cGMP) for the 21st century" recommends the effective application of new technological advances by the pharmaceutical industry and modern quality management techniques. National and international initiatives are introducing strategies that bring innovative medical solutions to the public. Some examples are Innovation and Stagnation: Challenge and Opportunity on the Critical Path to New Medical Products (United States), Innovative Medicines Initiative (Europe), New Safe Medicines Faster Project (Europe), and the Priority Medicines for Europe and the World Project "A Public Health Approach to Innovation" by the World Health Organization. They propose strategies for providing an enabling environment that fosters the steady integration of new and emerging science into modern medicine that builds on the lessons learnt previously to improve on their preparedness to address challenges.

Multidisciplinary scientific expertise and cross-disciplinary regulatory science training address inefficiencies and challenges posed by novel products. In pharmaceutical innovation, to facilitate fewer postapproval timelines, the prioritized values for the pharmaceutical company are speed to market, regulatory burden miniaturization of cGMP manufacturing, innovation flexibility, less R&D expenditure and freedom from regulatory uncertainties like inspections and procrastinated approvals. However, realistic and effective laws and regulations that address the patient's medical needs and necessities is the main objective for pharmaceutical regulations and to promote innovations that address the global disease burden. A company's priorities sometimes clash with those of the regulatory mandates and increasingly, revised legislations attempt to provide an appropriate framework to address these demands. These efforts are intended to promote risk miniaturization, and to explore avenues that would provide a path for correlating clinical trial outcomes to real world populations backed with quality scientific assessment in an effective manner. Companies could intensify strategies that build on technologies that deliver therapeutic solutions with diverse clinical indications to address various patent needs.

European regulators have adopted a complementary approach towards addressing global disease burden by setting priorities based on an evidence-based approach. First, decisions are informed by a collective assessment of burden of disease and clinical efficacy.

These include acute stroke, chronic obstructive pulmonary disease, and Alzheimer's disease. Second, priorities have been based on projections and trends and include antimicrobial resistance and pandemic influenza, whose selection order aligns with the severity of the risk factors. Third, priorities are based on social solidarity. The disease areas include the orphan and neglected diseases. Judgment is based on the ethical and moral values, and theories of social justice that justify its prioritization.

2.8.2 Mergers, Acquisitions, and Outsourcing

Mergers, acquisitions, or comarketing deals are strategies used to address pharmaceutical productivity inefficiencies. The pharmaceutical companies are growing the pharmaceutical value chain networks in emerging markets through capital investments, joint ventures, and collaborations with local companies. Joint ventures with generic manufacturers in emerging markets are intended to capture the value of global generic markets. This is expected to double from $240 billion in 2011 to $430 billion in 2016 [53].

Pharmaceutical firms use their specific strategies and competencies to gain competitive advantage and optimize economic returns. The big pharmas are at the frontlines of technological innovation due to the ability to coordinate cross-disciplinary and cross-functional specializations, and withstand technological instability through learning processes, management expertise, and an ability to undertake and manage multiple technological specializations. Their strengths could be complemented with the parties involved, who mutually agree to capitalize on the synergy between them and the following are examples given here.

In August 2012, 10 big pharmas, namely, Abbott Laboratories, Astra-Zeneca, Boehringer Ingelheim, Bristol-Myers Squibb, Eli Lilly, Glaxo-SmithKline, Johnson & Johnson, Pfizer, Roche's Genentech unit, and Sanofi, launched TransCelerate Biopharma in the United States. It is a non-profit joint venture intended to promote the sharing of their complementary strengths toward a more cost-effective model of R&D. The union is expected to set the stage for eliminating the major limitations encountered in clinical development [54,55].

A company with specialty research devotes less time to general prediscovery and discovery research but concentrates rather on the preclinical and clinical work. The company partners with other companies with enhanced abilities in these areas. For example, Humira, a full human monoclonal antibody for the treatment of rheumatoid arthritis, is a product of a collaboration between Abbott and Cambridge Antibody Technology (cambridgeantibody.com). Abbott took advantage of the drug-discovery tools at Cambridge to complement its intrinsic strengths.

Amgen, Genentech, Genzyme, and Biogen merged with other companies to become large integrated companies or "big biotechs." This is in part due to having commercialized high value orphan drugs for relatively rare, life-threatening diseases, and in small part due to their successful partnerships with the stakeholder pharmaceutical companies [56].

A shift in the pharmaceutical business model that is currently in vogue is the outsourcing of some aspects of the drug discovery projects to laboratories in developing countries. This international engagement, especially with the low-income countries, is no longer a concern as the increasing technological revolution is bringing novelties to these foreign sites, with laboratories that are increasing in sophistication. Special consideration is the much lower operating cost when compared to those of the United States and the European Union. The cost effectiveness plays a role in sustaining the business. Other needs include educational training. It has helped to raise new and well-informed scientists to help drive the healthcare industry forward. For example, in April 2013, Sanofi launched a €20 million new logistics hub in Casablanca, Morocco, for distribution of Sanofi drugs to Moroccan and sub-Saharan African markets. Collaboration agreements have the major objective of clinical education related to standard of care for type 1 diabetes patients, which are, first, training clinical professionals of immediate-need specialties and public awareness in favor of mental disorders and epilepsy. Training professionals to help promote the development of Moroccan pharmaceutical industry was part of the plan including building collaboration networks. Collaboration agreements were signed with the Ministry of Trade, Industry and New Technologies and the Ministry of Health of Morocco [57].

New business models that incorporate venture capital firms bear the risk of early stage R&D to try to settle the problematic high monetary investments toward their successes. Even though it places a demand on the pharmaceutical companies to share the profits of successful products, it allows a concentration on the key requirements for a new therapeutic advance.

Companies are increasingly moving towards a more competitive environment by diversifying into biologics, vaccines, over-the-counter medicines, branded generics, and other care products. Professional intelligence will mean assessing the risk–benefit profile of a compound that enables a decision on the compounds to prioritize. The pharmaceutical industry is taking new innovation paths leading to "open innovation" models. Innovation networks are incorporating leading academic researchers and biotechnology and pharmaceutical companies to boost drug R&D.

2.8.3 Pharmaceutical Research and Development

R&D productivity has been a role model for translating cutting-edge science into promising practical value. However, the slump in R&D has been a recurring issue. Strategies applied to enhance R&D are creating a value-driven drug development to strengthen the pipeline by mitigating the risks in drug development while providing the valued and purposeful drug candidates deemed fit for regulatory approval. It might entail R&D reorganization that dissects and discerns various elements for thorough comprehension of the system as required for bringing a change. This will certainly upgrade efficiencies and performance of the organization. A business model based on this will capture value from early stage technology converting it to economic value [58].

Another strategy is data management. Efforts have been directed to ensure adequate handling of the increasing body of information being generated for accessibility; integrating modeling and analytics, like bioinformatics, cheminformatics, engineering, mathematical modeling, and optimization statistics and data sciences. Virtual libraries are expected to be part of larger and more focused libraries, brought about by new techniques in drug discovery. The breaking down of distinct steps of the R&D value chain by industry players and outsourcing of the others are part of the revitalization process. This enables a faster time to market, reduced operating and production costs, and improvement in quality standards. Restructuring is expected to attract new business models with an open door for new entrants and alliances. For example, GlaxoSmithKline, in its bid to refine its approach to R&D, divided its drug development teams into smaller and more focused groups that incorporate a focus on results with a view to creating and sustaining value [59]. The purpose was to benefit from cross-functional collaboration.

2.8.4 New Avenues of Personalized Medicine: Application of Pharmacogenomics Technology in Drug Development

A satisfactory drug's safety profile lowers cost and protects the safety of the patient population. Most importantly, it gives confidence to the responsible practitioner that a new drug's safety profile has been fully defined. Personalized medicines allow a more specific targeting of a drug to the responder populations who exhibit less adverse effects and positive responses to the drug therapy to save money invested in a nonresponsive population. The field of pharmacogenomics provides a new avenue for effective drug design targeted to the patient population and certain promising outcomes have been reported recently. For example, in May 2013, two advanced skin cancer drugs, Tafinlar and Mekinist, that target skin cell tumors with mutations to the BRAF gene were approved by the FDA for GlaxoSmithKline. The BRAF gene mutation accounts for half of all skin cancer cases. In addition to a molecular diagnostic test, a "THxID BRAF mutation test" was developed by French company bioMérieux. The diagnostic test was used in clinical trials to identify patients with the BRAF gene mutation to produce a more directed drug therapy against the disease [60,61].

2.8.5 Drug Repositioning/Repurposing

A plethora of unapproved drug compounds that could not be marketed are being redirected to other therapeutic applications by a process known as repositioning or repurposing. This has been considered a high growth opportunity as these drugs have been derisked and thus would require significantly less R&D investment; it also avails for the pharmaceutical company the privilege to extend the patent protection.

2.8.6 Building the Pharmaceutical Ecosystem

Effective integration of all aspects of the pharmaceutical ecosystem will lead to high performance standards. For example, a cross-functional team of professionals concerned with drug discovery could work out a proof of concept in the clinical phase to design a compound capable of filling the gaps in regards to patient, regulator, and payer needs. This will enhance productivity and lower total healthcare costs and technological "spillovers" that will benefit the general society.

2.9 CONCLUDING REMARKS

Pharmaceutical innovation has tapped into the advancing science and technology revolution, which still continues to provide an enabling environment for drug creation and access. However, it has not reached its full potential. There is a need for optimistic innovators who focus on disease areas of genuine unmet need to harness the fit-for-purpose technologies, create the right therapy for a targeted patient population, and, most importantly, to offer a substantial and commendable contribution to global medical needs.

The analyses of various pharmaceutical activities are drawn from various daily reports, reports from pharmaceutical and biotechnology industry analysts and industry monitors and other professionals in the form of government publications, webpages, journal, newspaper, and magazine articles.

REFERENCES

[1] Zycher B, DiMasi JA, Milne C. The truth about drug innovation: thirty-five summary case histories on private sector contributions to pharmaceutical science. Medical Progress Report 2008; No. 6. Available from: http://www.manhattan-institute.org/html/mpr_06.htm

[2] Cohen FJ. Macro trends in pharmaceutical innovation. Nat Rev Drug Discov 2005;4. Available from: www.nature.com/reviews/drugdisc

[3] Sadat T, Russell R, Rmit MS. Shifting paths of pharmaceutical innovation: implications for the global pharmaceutical industry. Int J Knowledge Innov Entrep 2014;2(1):6–31.

[4] Walters D, Lancaster G. Implementing value strategy through the value chain. Manag Decision 1985;38(3):160–78.

[5] Hamilton WF, Vilà J, Dibner MD. Patterns for strategic choices in emerging firms: positioning for innovation in biotechnology. California Manag Rev 1990;32(3):73–86.

[6] Matthew H, Peter K. The World's Ten Best-Selling Drugs. Forbes; 2006.

[7] The pharmaceutical and biotech industries in the United States [Internet]; 2014. Available from: http://selectusa.commerce.gov/industry-snapshots/pharmaceutical-industry-united-states [accessed 01.11.2014].

[8] DeNavas-Walt C, Proctor B, Smith J. Income, poverty, and health insurance coverage in the United States: 2012. U.S. Census Bureau; 2013.

[9] Friedrman J, Gerlowski DA, Silberman J. What attracts foreign multinational corporations? Evidence from branch plant location in the United States. J Reg Sci 2006;32(4):403–18.

[10] Buente M, Danner S, Weissbäcker S, Rammé C. Pharma Emerging Markets 2.0: How Emerging Markets Are Driving the Transformation of the Pharmaceutical Industry. New York, NY: Booz & Company; 2013.

[11] Innovation.org, Great moments in innovation [Internet]; 2014. Available from: http://www.innovation.org/index.cfm/nonav/Great_Moments_in_Innovation [accessed November, 2014].

[12] National Institute of Allergy and Infectious Disease. Tuberculosis (TB), age of optimism [Internet]; 2014. Available from: http://www3.niaid.nih.gov/topics/tuberculosis/Research/researchFeatures/history/historical_optimism.htm [accessed 01.11.2014].

[13] Innovation.org, Great moments in innovation [Internet]; 2014. Available from: http://www.innovation.org/index.cfm/nonav/Great_Moments_in_Innovation [accessed 01.11.2014].

[14] NIH, National Institute of Allergy and Infectious Disease, Tuberculosis (TB), age of optimism [Internet]; 2014. Available from: http://www3.niaid.nih.gov/topics/tuberculosis/Research/researchFeatures/history/historical_optimism.htm [accessed 03.11.2014].

[15] Kaplan W, Laing R. Priority medicines for Europe and the World. World Health Organization Department of Essential Drugs and Medicines Policy; 2004. Available from: http://whqlibdoc.who.int/hq/2004/WHO_EDM_PAR_2004.7.pdf

[16] Bradley S, Weber J. The pharmaceutical industry: challenges of the new century. Harvard Business School; 2003. Available from: http://www.ramos.utfsm.cl/doc/169/sc/Casopharmaceuticalindustry.pdf

[17] Hewitt J, Campbell DJ, Cacciotti J. Beyond the shadow of a drought. Life and Health Sciences; 2011. Available from: http://www.oliverwyman.com/content/dam/oliver-wyman/global/en/files/archive/2011/OW_EN_HLS_PUBL_2011_Beyond_the_Shadow_of_a_Drought(3).pdf

[18] Scannell JW, Blanckley A, Boldon H, Warrington B. Diagnosing the decline in pharmaceutical R&D efficiency. Nat Rev Drug Discov 2012;11:191–200. ("Why drug development is failing – and how to fix it" published later in 2012).

[19] Munos B. Lessons from 60 years of pharmaceutical innovation. Nat Rev Drug Discov 2009;8:959–68.

[20] Ahmed R. The patent cliff: implications for the pharmaceutical [Internet]; 2014. Available from: http://triplehelixblog.com/2014/07/the-patent-cliff-implications-for-the-pharmaceutical-industry/#sthash.ILnShoIC.ReC80vJx.dpuf [accessed 03.11.2014].

[21] Top 10 best-selling drugs of the 21st century [Internet]; 2014. Available from: http://www.genengnews.com/insight-and-intelligenceand153/top-10-best-selling-drugs-of-the-21st-century/77899716/ [accessed 04.11.2014].

[22] This patent cliff 2014 chart shows how much revenue big pharma will lose [Internet]; 2014. Available from: http://triplehelixblog.com/2014/07/the-patent-cliff-implications-for-the-pharmaceutical-industry/#sthash.ILnShoIC.dpuf [accessed 03.11.2014].

[23] Tse MT, Kirkpatrick P. 2012 in reflection. Nat Rev Drug Discov 2013;12:8–10.

[24] Gupta RR, Gifford EM, Liston T, Waller CL, Hohman M, Bunin BA, Ekins S. Using open source computational tools for predicting human metabolic stability and additional ADME/TOX properties. Drug Metab Dispos 2013;38(11):2083–90.

[25] Hohman M, Gregory K, Chibale K, Smith PJ, Ekins S, Bunin B, Hohman. Novel web-based tools combining chemistry informatics, biology and social networks for drug discovery. Drug Discov Today 2009;14:261–70.

[26] PhRMA members leading the way in search for new medicines and cures [Internet]; 2014. Available from: http://www.phrma.org/about#sthash.B8mtKP0E.cpiALkJl.dpuf [accessed 06.11.2014].

[27] Treatment advances transform HIV/AIDS [Internet]; 2014. Available from: http://innovation.org/timelines/treatment-advances-transform-hiv/aids [accessed 05.11.2014].

[28] Innovative treatments for rheumatoid arthritis improve the lives of patients [Internet]; 2014. Available from: http://innovation.org/gallery/innovative-treatments-for-rheumatoid-arthritis-improve-the-lives-of-patient [accessed 04.11.2014].

[29] Chronic leukemias: survival rates [Internet]; 2014. Available from: http://www.un.org/millenniumgoals/reports.shtl. http://innovation.org/chronic-leukemias-survival-rates-rise [accessed 07.11.2014].

[30] The Millennium Development Goals Report 2014 [Internet]; 2014. Available from: http://www.un.org/millenniumgoals/reports.shtl [accessed 07.11.2014].

[31] Challenge and opportunity on the critical path to new medical products. Innovation Stagnation. U.S. Department of Health and Human Services. Food and Drug Administration; 2004. Available from: http://spores.nci.nih.gov/applicants/guidelines/guidelines_full.html#1b

[32] Eggermont A, Newell H. Translational research in clinical trials: the only way forward. Eur J Cancer 2001;37.

[33] Rowett L. U.K. initiative to boost translational research. J Natl Cancer Instit 2002;94(10).

[34] Kaitin KI. Deconstructing the drug development process: the new face of innovation. Clin Pharmacol Therapeut 2010;87(3):356–61.

[35] Del Lino J. Discussion point: should governments buy drug patents? Eur J Health Econ 2007;8:173–7.

[36] Grunberg E, Schnitzer RJ. Studies on the activity of hydrazine derivatives of isonicotinic acid in the experimental tuberculosis of mice. Q Bull Sea View Hosp 1952;13:3–11.

[37] Pletscher A. The discovery of antidepressants: a winding path. Experientia 1991;47:4–8.

[38] Booth B, Zemmel R. Prospects for productivity. Nat Rev Drug Discov 2004;3:451–6.

[39] Friedman MA, Woodcock J, Lumpkin MM, Shuren JE, Hass AE, Thompson LJ. The safety of newly approved medicines: do recent market removals mean there is a problem? JAMA 1999;281(18):1728–34.

[40] Cockburn I. The changing structure of the pharmaceutical industry. Health Affairs 2004;23(1):10–22.

[41] Drews J. Drug discovery: a historical perspective. Science 2000;287(5460):1960.

[42] Kaitin KI, Eve SR. Explaining the drug drought. PharmExec.com 2010 [Internet]; 2014. Available from: http://www.pharmexec.com/pharmexec/Explaining-the-Drug-Drought/ArticleStandard/Article/detail/687358 [accessed 05.11.2014].

[43] Horrobin DF. Modern biomedical research: an internally self-consistent universe with little contact with medical reality? Nat Rev Drug Discov 2003;2(2):151–4.

[44] Hammer O. Lessons learned from Sanofi-Aventis's Phase III failure. Seeking-Alpha [Internet]; 2014. Available from: http://seekingalpha.com/article/250527-lessons-learned-from-sanofiaventis-s-phase-iii-failure [accessed 09.11.2014].

[45] Top 10 clinical trial failures of 2012 [Internet]; 2014. Available from: http://www.genengnews.com/insight-and-intelligenceand153/top-10-clinical-trial-failures-of-2012/77899765/ [accessed 09.11.2014].

[46] Paul SM, et al. How to improve R&D productivity: the pharmaceutical industry's grand challenge. Nat Rev Drug Discov 2010;9:203–14.

[47] Rice LB. Federal funding for the study of antimicrobial resistance in nosocomial pathogens: no ESKAPE. J Infect Dis 2008;197:1079–81.

[48] Boucher HW, Talbot GH, Bradley JS, et al. Bad bugs, no drugs: no ESKAPE! An update from the Infectious Diseases Society of America. Clin Infect Dis 2009;48:1–12.

[49] Rice LB. Progress and challenges in implementing the research on ESKAPE pathogens. Infect Control Hosp Epidemiol 2010;31(Suppl. 1):S7–S10.

[50] Gilbert DN, Guidos RJ, Boucher HW, Talbot GH, Spellberg B, Edwards JE Jr, Scheld WM, Bradley JS, Bartlett JG. The 10 × '20 initiative: pursuing a global commitment to develop 10 new antibacterial drugs by 2020. Infectious Diseases Society of America. Clin Infect Dis 2010;50:1081–3.

[51] Tallman G, Brock J. Pipeline or pipe dream: new antibiotics for multidrug-resistant gram-negative bacilli. Infectious Disease News; 2013. Available from: http://www. healio.com/infectious-disease/emerging-diseases/news/print/infectious-disease-news/%7B2d636304-7271-44d3-98a7-fd061a787883%7D/pipeline-or-pipe-dream-new-antibiotics-for-multidrug-resistant-gram-negative-bacilli

[52] Leisinger KM. Meeting the global health challenge: the role of the pharmaceutical industry. Making It Magazine; 2012. Available from: http://www.makingitmagazine. net/?p=6046

[53] Paul SM, Mytelka DS, Dunwiddie CT, Persinger CC, Munos BH, Lindborg SR, Schacht AL. How to improve R&D productivity: the pharmaceutical industry's grand challenge. Nat Rev Drug Discov 2010;9:203–14.

[54] McBride R. 7 Major pharmas unite with academics in €196M discovery effort [Internet]; 2013. Available from: http://muse.jhu.edu/journals/ens/summary/v007/7.3rooij.html [accessed 10.11.2014].

[55] Burrill GS. Biotech2013 - Life Sciences – Capturing Value. Beijing, China: Burrill & co; 2013.

[56] Rooij AV. Shaping the industrial century: the remarkable story of the evolution of the modern chemical and pharmaceutical industries. Enterprise Soc 2006;7(3):624–6.

[57] Sanofi reinforces its presence in Morocco [Internet]. Press Release; 2013. Avaliable from: http://www.bloomberg.com/article/2013-04-17/a0xAyJyVL7J4.html [accessed 11.11.2014].

[58] Chesbrough H, Rosenbloom RS. The role of the business model in capturing value from innovation: evidence from Xerox Corporation's technology spin-off companies. Ind Corp Change 2002;11:529–55.

[59] Finn BM, Sutherland CF. The pharmaceutical industry: where it is, how it got here, where it needs to go, how to get there. Int J Med Market 2004;4(4):361–9.

[60] Carroll J. UPDATED: GlaxoSmithKline bags genetic vaccine developer Okairos for $325 million [Internet]. 2013. FierceBiotech. Available from: http://www. fiercebiotech.com/story/glaxosmithkline-bags-genetic-vaccine-developer-okairos-325-million/2013-05-29 [accessed 12.11.2014].

[61] FDA OKs bioMérieux diagnostic for GSK's cancer drugs [Internet]; 2013. FierceMedical Devices. Available from: http://www.fiercemedicaldevices.com/story/fda-oks-biom-rieux-diagnostic-gsks-cancer-drugs/2013-05-29 [accessed 12.11.2014].

CHAPTER 3

Cash Flow Valley of Death: A Pitfall in Drug Discovery

Odilia Osakwe

Contents

3.1 Introduction	58
3.2 Product Valuation as an Investment Decision-Making Tool	59
3.3 Challenges Associated with the Valley of Death	60
3.3.1 Organization Proportions and Impact in Drug Discovery	60
3.3.2 Vulnerability of Biotech and Small Companies	61
3.3.3 Key Research Activities in the Stage of Lowest Funding	62
3.3.4 Unpredictability of Pharmaceutical Innovation Science	63
3.3.5 Academic Discovery and Research Limitations	64
3.3.6 Target Selection	65
3.4 Firms Involved in the Pharmaceutical Value Chain	66
3.4.1 Big Pharmaceutical Industries (Big Pharma)	66
3.4.2 Biotechnology-Based Industries (Biotech)	66
3.4.3 Biopharmaceutical Industries	66
3.4.4 Contract Research Organizations	67
3.5 Strategies for Bridging the Valley of Death and Innovation Failure	67
3.5.1 The Changing Drug Discovery Landscape	67
3.5.2 Product Forecasting	68
3.5.3 Investment in the Discovery Science	69
3.5.4 Advancing Corporate Productivity: Partnerships	69
3.5.5 Communication	71
3.5.6 Importance of the Biotechnology Incubators	72
3.5.7 Addressing Investment Limitations	72
3.6 Funding Models	74
3.6.1 US Financing Models	74
3.6.2 Canadian Financing Models	75
3.7 Nongovernmental Funding Models	76
3.7.1 Large Pharmaceutical Companies	76
3.7.2 Venture Capital	76
3.7.3 Public-Venture Philanthropy	76
3.7.4 Angel Investment	76
3.7.5 Private-Corporate Investment	77
3.7.6 Crowdfunding	77

Social Aspects of Drug Discovery, Development and Commercialization Copyright © 2016 Elsevier Inc.
http://dx.doi.org/10.1016/B978-0-12-802220-7.00003-X   All rights reserved.

3.8 Other Financial Concepts   77
    3.8.1 Not-for-Profit/Nonprofit Organizations   77
    3.8.2 Cash Flow   78
    3.8.3 Cash Flow Return on Investment   78
    3.8.4 Derisking   78
3.9 Private–Public Sector Groups   78
    3.9.1 National Centre for Advancing Translational Sciences   78
    3.9.2 Innovative Medicines Initiative   79
    3.9.3 European Federation for Pharmaceutical Sciences   79
    3.9.4 The Centre for Drug Research and Development   79
References   79

3.1 INTRODUCTION

The pharmaceutical industry is highly capital-intensive; it costs up to $1.5 billion to produce a new drug. This is a common challenge to every drug manufacturer or sponsor, whether the discovery program succeeds or fails. Drug discovery and development projects reach a financial hiatus as the drug development companies are challenged with waning interest from investors or venture capitalists, which severely affects business stability [1]. The initial stages of the product lifecycle, the prediscovery research, are mostly undertaken at academic and other not-for-profit research and development (R&D) institutes, mostly funded by the government (Figure 3.1). Promising discoveries are usually transferred to the biotechs, drug development centers, or pharmaceutical companies for further development. For small companies or biotechs that partake in novel therapeutic areas or uncharacterized targets, high initial costs are incurred toward establishing the development project, which suffers from insufficient funding leading to negative cash flows [2]. Prospective investors gauge the economic status of the bio/pharmaceutical company using pipeline drugs as value indicators, which informs investment decisions. In addition to the technical and market risks, inflation and tightening of government budgets further deter venture financing that had previously sustained the industry.

According to investopia, Valley of Death is the high probability that a start-up firm will die off before a steady stream of revenue is established. Within the pharmaceutical enterprise, this is referred to as the period of separation between basic research and Phase II of the clinical trials that demonstrates PoC, due to funding limitations that hinder pipeline progression to commercialization.

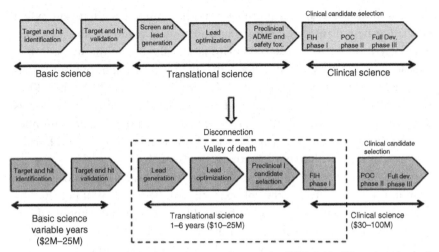

Figure 3.1 *Drug Discovery and Development Progression With Critical Functions Locked in the Valley of Death.* This pipeline productivity problem is now often called the Valley of Death and reflects a disconnect between the translation of new discoveries into clinical candidate compounds suitable for optimization prior to human clinical use.

During this period, funding is hardly enough and leaves the firm in a financially unsafe situation; pipeline progression is very slow and risk of investment is high due to future uncertainty as the lead drug compound has not been established and clinically validated. Typically, additional funding is always sought to derisk the Valley of Death in order to streamline the progression of transitional research to clinics. Due to poor venture financing, the companies increasingly seek alternatives that are more demanding or challenging to obtain.

3.2 PRODUCT VALUATION AS AN INVESTMENT DECISION-MAKING TOOL

Valuations in deal negotiations require prioritization of diseases of interest by assessing the payer environment and standards of care in each disease area. New technologies and business plans of the emerging business are assessed by investors such as the venture capitalists. Several stages of pharmaceutical R&D are used as indicators of the probability of success (PoS) of a product. Early stage companies and investors usually focus on Phase II, proof of concept (PoC). When this stage is successful, it gives the assurance to proceed and expand its private financing from early stage venture capitalists that opt to invest at higher valuations [4]. Venture capitalists opt for the business models that appear promising and have used it as a template when evaluating new plans. The product valuation must demonstrate a new opportunity in order to arouse the curiosity and interest of the investor. If it appears unsatisfactory and unconvincing, the investor might opt out [5]. As reported by the US National Venture Capital Association in October 2011, around 59 out of 150 venture capital firms started cutting down investments in the area of life sciences and this is expected to continue for more number of years. Numerous venture capital firms, for example, Prospect and Excalibur, have already withdrawn investments in biotech.

The risks of early stage projects are technically, regulatorily, and economically associated. Technical concerns are the selection of poorly validated targets or an inability to identify suitable drug-like lead compounds for optimization, suboptimal clinical efficacy, toxicity or poor drug metabolism and pharmacokinetics (PK) results, and clinical safety. Economic effects are hyperinflation, tightening of budgets, and insufficient exit opportunities through public offerings – a way of cashing out investment. Pharmaceutical regulatory control is the reason for the onerous and years-long Food and Drug Administration (FDA) approval process and delay of commercialization that lead to drug shortages. The biotechnology industry has encountered failures in large numbers, which substantially supersede that of the pharmaceutical industry, both technically and commercially. For example, in the United Kingdom, the former venture capital model is comprised of stages of funding to an initial public offering, which the exit strategy phased out. Because these are not publicly traded, the shares could not be sold with ease. The venture capitalists had no access to the wealth of the company so they used the exit strategy to cash out their investment. When this model phased out, investment became less attractive [6,7] especially with a history of costly and risky venture with attrition typically around 75% for Phase II clinical trials.

3.3 CHALLENGES ASSOCIATED WITH THE VALLEY OF DEATH

3.3.1 Organization Proportions and Impact in Drug Discovery

Organization size and capacity have an inverse relationship with their ability to adapt to change. Large multinational biopharmaceutical companies have problems of scale. Their major strength is financial and human resources, but at the other end of the spectrum, the culture of management hierarchies, meetings, commitments, and some competition over resources sometimes deter effectiveness. In the modern era of large-scale "-omic" discoveries based on genomes or protein profiles from whole organisms, pharmaceutical companies that specialize in these endeavors cannot keep up [8]. In contrast, the smaller companies, particularly the biotechs, are much less populated and have a trimmer organizational structure. These downsized companies are usually staffed with creative people that are closer to addressing the problem. They adapt better, are flexible, and can quickly respond to a changing environment. This close-knit interactive framework permits a closer and faster approach to tackling problems. In this regard, the big pharmas are changing the organization structure, breaking into smaller units with particular specialty to create a "masterpiece" that stems from a divided network rather than a whole. One example is the Centers of Excellence Drug Discovery, which was created by GSK, and which has the autonomy to focus on specific therapeutic areas within the company. It has further been subdivided into smaller discovery performance units, much similar to the biotech companies operating the similar business models. This is one way of combating the issue of low productivity.

However, few firms can afford to undertake extensive and exhaustive research; they lack the breadth and depth of knowledge needed to create new drugs. This is the major roadblock of small firms or biotechnology industries. Partnerships have been sought for R&D outsourcing that drive better outputs and productivity.

3.3.2 Vulnerability of Biotech and Small Companies

Early drug development is a daunting task as it requires constant adaptation to undesirable changes in such environments [9]. The most common difficulties are experienced at seed and start-up stages of R&D when the investment risk is high, which deters potential investors that are risk averse – the fear of lack of profitability [10]. Early discovery activities that focus on disease targets are understood through various disciplines such as biochemistry, microbiology, physiology, pathology, as well as observational studies of health interventions, etc. These are only pivotal and with no immediate commercial value and hence not attractive to the big pharma and private investors. Since prediscovery and discovery research are highly explorative, large companies are more likely to focus on late stage technologies. Fragmentation of industries is the consequence of this, leading to the surrender of discovery research by the big pharmas in an attempt to concentrate on clinical trials and marketing that relies on their well-established distribution channels. The larger companies have stronger financial stability against high risk projects, and a wider and more comprehensive range of studies, with better and sounder mechanisms, resources, and experience.

Focusing on the early stages of drug development makes it impossible to project a future outcome as far as 10 years ahead as the seeds of actions are not harvested until years later. And pipeline delay could reach 7 years, further hindering investment potentials by venture capitalists. Early discovery projects are most often taken by the smaller or biotech companies. These are mostly selected from within novel therapeutic areas or indications and involve building the product scope and operating in unexplored and unproven categories. For a start-up company that has not demonstrated its marketing experience, the prospect of higher financial success would be a base consideration for undertaking high risk projects of such kind [11,12].

Even though the small companies are susceptible to higher risks, they hold greater growth opportunities associated with undertaking a novel drug development project. The potential for high financial rewards depends on the therapeutic areas of interest. A predominant chronic disease would be well recognized and highly rated. Some examples especially are the chronic indications like cancer, inflammation, or cardiovascular disease. However, if diagnosis is rare or slightly improved over already existing drugs, this is less predictable. Rating the size of a potential market might not be very clear and depends on a lot of factors as mentioned earlier. Major pharmaceutical companies establish several drugs in the pipeline even though some are more valued than others, in order to spread the risks [13,14]. With established products in sales, these companies are more immune to losses since a portion of sales funds R&D. Estimates from a product in sales are used to determine the weight of the market share it gains, cost, and effectiveness in relation to its competitors.

3.3.3 Key Research Activities in the Stage of Lowest Funding

Translational science mainly plays the role of transforming activity into clinical effectiveness by refining the pharmaceutical properties, determining the preclinical toxicology, and optimizing. The translation of basic biological discoveries into clinically viable applications involves acquiring in-depth understanding of the pathogenesis of a disease prior to finding the target and cognate active compound with optimized properties. Once the target has been identified, developed assays would be used to evaluate pharmacological effectiveness, assay quality, reproducibility, selectivity, specificity, solubility, permeability, and metabolic stability. Bursts of huge data are screened out using high throughput screening technologies to filter out lots of targets at this stage to potentially eliminate unexpected failures due to unpredictable factors, such as toxicological findings in later studies.

The effect of such a rigorous process at an early stage is to achieve greater awareness. It takes several years to accomplish this. Once validated, the transforming drug modulator molecules progress into high-content lead series. A hit molecule that satisfies preclinical candidacy would have the desirable properties that lead to a clinical assessment of the data in the human population in clinical trials. This is crucial information that could be further formulated into safe doses in patients, establishing pharmacokinetic (PK)/pharmacodynamic (PD) modeling and clinical PoC, and full clinical development. These are key activities in modern drug discovery. The decisions or information garnered in this process determine the fate of the drug discovery program and is the premise for the companies' early project-portfolio management strategy, success, and failure. These activities are not strictly government sponsored and seek other investment strategies that rely on the effectiveness and therapeutic promise of these pipeline activities in order to attract funding.

3.3.4 Unpredictability of Pharmaceutical Innovation Science

In the pharmaceutical industry, most of the proposed research projects are based on speculative research ideas and are initially high risk. There is no guarantee of success once a candidate reaches the development pipeline; success is mostly a matter of probability until it progresses toward the late stage research when a proof of biological efficacy has been established (Figure 3.2).

More than 70% of observed innovation failures in Phase II are technical risks and the rest are nontechnical, which are mostly strategic and commercial. The technical risks encountered throughout the discovery pipeline correlate with the ability to achieve optimal chemical druggability or an ability of a drug molecule to modulate a drug target, which satisfies the physical, chemical, and biological properties of a desired drug. A typical technical challenge would be a target approach that complements high throughput screening for structure–activity correlations that might not meet the criteria for clinical efficacy. Some highly frequent technical problems in drug discovery are: the multifactorial chronic diseases that could not be approached with only a single target due to extensive and complicated biological networks; animal models that do not exactly translate to humans; and adverse events or toxicity that could surface with chronic use – a fact that could not be detected during clinical trials. These aspects are considered in parallel

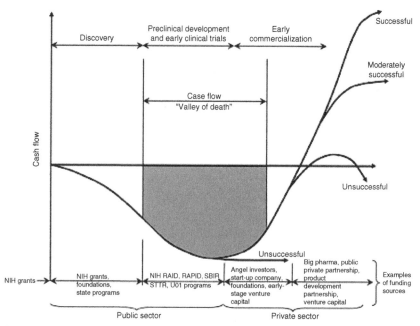

Figure 3.2 *The Path of Cash Flow Through the "Valley of Death," Showing the Most Prominent Funding Organizations and Stage in Drug Development.* RAID, rapid access to interventional development; SBIR, small business innovative research; RAPID, rapid access to preventive intervention development; STTR, small business technology transfer. *Source: Ref. [3].*

with the societal, marketing, and business needs in order to be deemed competitive and attract investment opportunities [15].

3.3.5 Academic Discovery and Research Limitations

In the drug discovery cycle, academic professionals build the hypothesis, gather evidence, and generate the molecular prototypes for further development. Their interest lies in scholarly publications that render the opportunity for professional growth as opposed to locking up the wealth of knowledge in silos pending the seemingly unending duration of the drug discovery program. Publications of stepwise findings that underpin National Institutes of Health (NIH) grant consideration is a high preference since academic accomplishment has been measured based on frequency of scholarly publications and impact [16]. This has compromised growth in translational research and has been considered a deviation from the industry based performance metrics which consider invention disclosures, patents and licenses.

In general, research techniques differ to some extent when compared to that of the industry. For example, academia would use a less stringent format as opposed to the strict reproducibility considerations, as opposed to the use of high throughput screens that is the hallmark of early stage drug discovery in the industry. Academic drug discovery programs lack the technical and scientific capability to further the development of molecules to therapeutic leads due to lack of the required facilities that meet the industrial standard. The expertise and available resources are critically lacking.

3.3.6 Target Selection

The greatest pitfall in drug development is upstream experimental oversight due to misguided target selection affecting all the development processes [17,18]. The initial difficulty encountered in discovery research is multiplicity of biological functions or mechanisms of a potential drug target that could further lead to toxicity in model organisms and humans. Poor target selection results in poor therapeutic outcomes, costs, or fund expenditure and competitiveness. The patient population versus health care provider's willingness to pay for a course of treatment determines the extent of revenue recovered over the commercial lifetime of a drug and depends on its competitiveness or therapeutic success. However, finding the right target and clinical efficacy for a named indication has been a major hurdle, leading to economic failure due to fewer drugs or poor performance of drugs reaching the market and also leading to a bias over drugs that show exclusive financial success [19–21].

3.3.6.1 A Case for Alzheimer's Disease

The number of cases Alzheimer's in USA is over 5 million; thus, market size in an affluent country is important. If every one of those patients was given a drug at $5000 per year, this would produce $25,000 billion, which is a remarkable return. If the health care providers, which are the governments and managed care organizations, are willing to pay for new medicines to support R&D efforts, it is because it costs governments 10 times more in hospital cases and they would rather direct some funding to R&D. Higher prices for drugs tend to be balanced by savings in the health care system, which has worked out strategies to promote less hospitalization and an improved quality of life. Cost–benefit considerations or valuations are performed by the commercial departments of biopharmaceutical companies, governments and academic departments that are committed to the maximization of value for every money spent.

3.4 FIRMS INVOLVED IN THE PHARMACEUTICAL VALUE CHAIN

Firms involved in the pharmaceutical value chain are being categorized based on their competences, according to the level of involvement with drug discovery and development, availability of tools and technologies, and combined forms. The primary purpose for these firms is to create and distribute drugs and other health care products.

3.4.1 Big Pharmaceutical Industries (Big Pharma)

Pharmaceutical industries have been characterized as firms that discover, develop, manufacture, distribute, and market pharmaceutical products. Pharmaceutical drugs are referred as small molecule drugs which are most often derived from chemical synthesis Big pharmas are rather multinational pharmaceutical companies with huge operating costs in the order of tens of millions to billions over a wide geographical area. They are the major contributors to the pharmaceutical global business with high revenue streams that prosper the economy. They engage in large therapeutic areas, with solid marketing and sales abilities, strengthened through huge revenues that are directed to the areas of marketing and sales that help to accelerate distribution of products to the consumer. They are often publically listed in the international stock exchanges and have a shareholder base [22].

3.4.2 Biotechnology-Based Industries (Biotech)

Biotechnology is the process of creating products with biological activity, bacteria, yeast, or other cells, which are manipulated to enable the production of proteins of interest to a commercial quantity. Although Biotech industries are players in the national market for medicines, big biotechs follow a separate regulatory agency and federal code of regulations as their products are aseptically processed and their operations are classified as higher risk. Currently, portfolio extensions incorporate small molecule drugs in choice therapeutic areas. Small biotechs usually initially exist as spin-offs, which can be acquired or outlicensed depending on the capital availability [23]. There is a slim divide between biotechnology and pharmaceutical companies. Some biotechnology firms have been categorized with pharmaceutical companies when they expand their capabilities, for example, Genzyme and Amgen [24]. They are principally distinguished by their core technologies.

3.4.3 Biopharmaceutical Industries

The term biopharmaceutical refers to pharmaceutical companies that develop and produce biotechnology-based products with the capacity

Table 3.1 Example of contract research services [25]

Biology services	Chemistry services	Screening services	Lead optimization services
Protein structural analysis Determining protein–protein interactions Functional genomics	Providing building blocks Compound synthesis and purification Process research Bioinformatics	Assay development Secondary screening Library design	Early absorption distribution metabolism excretion/ toxicity Compound analogs and structure–activity relationships

to complete the product pipeline from development to marketing. The different types of biotechnology companies are therapeutics, diagnostics, agriculture, medical device, and platform technology [26].

3.4.4 Contract Research Organizations

Contract research organizations (CROs) are outsourcing firms, vendors that undertake more precise and focused R&D functions for the pharmaceutical or biotech industry. Their specialization in certain aspects of the development process or specific therapeutic fields underscores expertise in those areas. They are more mistake-proof, well-experienced professionals that offer preclinical, clinical, and regulatory activities for drug development and commercialization. CROs consist of classes of full-service, multinational, publicly traded firms. Midsized CROs are site management contractors, which provide the clinical team, physician investigators, and patient support for clinical trials at the site. CROs can render an administrative function in clinical trials or affiliate with an established project. Their main function is to close the "time-to-marketing" gap through effective application of innovation, engaging in a full spectrum service for the small biotech companies' clinical trial activities (Table 3.1).

3.5 STRATEGIES FOR BRIDGING THE VALLEY OF DEATH AND INNOVATION FAILURE

3.5.1 The Changing Drug Discovery Landscape

With rising drug discovery cost and increasing demand for new and improved forms of health care, the industry has been exploring avenues to achieve optimal value from R&D budgets to boost productivity. Pharm R&D is taking a more holistic approach to drug development with extensive information sharing, reforming of business models, introducing new portfolio management solutions, vertical and horizontal integration and expansion, incremental adaptation of the pharmaceutical quality system, project management, and communication of science.

3.5.2 Product Forecasting

Product forecasting refers to predicting the degree of success of the new drug product in the marketplace. It determines product awareness, distribution, price, ability to fulfill unmet needs, and competitive alternatives. In the early stage of drug discovery, a foreknowledge of attributes of the drug compound is essential in order to understand the marketing prospects of the drug product. This helps to allocate capital prudently, by targeting diseases and drugs with a high prospect of reimbursement.

The narrowing of the chance that discovery will focus attention on areas of interest to development can be addressed through the use of the target product profile (TPP). The application of TPP is critical in valuing the future of a drug in the development process. Key information is the definition of disease and diagnosis, incidence of disease, patient types and characteristics; disease and patient segments and how they will be identified in clinical practice; market size, structure, and dynamics; and trends and barriers. Identifying potential drug candidates would entail consulting the clinicians to gain insights into new products that their originator lacks. Academic physicians' experts, with their wealth of knowledge of both disease and patients, could facilitate drug positioning mainly through the privilege of access to new classes of pharmaceutical agents during very early clinical development. This helps the drug developer to see how a new clinical utility could open new markets. Understanding the unmet medical needs and therapeutic competitiveness offers meaningful advantage over alternative or existing treatments for the same condition. The attributes include target population, dosage form, and safety and efficacy over the existing treatments; toxicity, contraindications, stability, and more. These attributes are to be well reflected in the project design at an early stage. Knowing that new projects in development are often characterized as "high risk," well-executed product forecast and commitment to low-cost development, marketing and risk handling preparedness increases the PoS of the pharmaceutical firm. The validity of technical data in support of the TPP establishes competitiveness and a well-differentiated product for market success.

3.5.3 Investment in the Discovery Science

Focus is increasingly being shifted to the rudimentary aspect of drug discovery, the early discovery research, which is essential to pipeline progression. There is increasing vertical integration to enhance capabilities across the pharmaceutical value chain. Robust biological/biomedical research would require strengthening of the key partnering disciplines (chemistry, chemical biology, systems modeling, etc.) to ensure that the biological targets selected have the best chance of delivering successful PoC studies. These areas are being further reinforced by incorporating technically adept professionals who have in-depth understanding of disease, animal and *in vitro* testing capabilities, and relationships with experience. Also knowledgeable and experienced medicinal chemists are increasingly being engaged with academic centers of drug discovery to support development of sound and quality drug candidates by the academic laboratories and to help abrogate the innovation attrition factors.

3.5.4 Advancing Corporate Productivity: Partnerships

3.5.4.1 *Big Pharma – Early Stage/Biotech Company Partnerships*

Industry partnerships or collaborations have become an important revenue stream for early stage and small biotech companies, which is acquired through licensing, marketing deals, or collaborations on discovery stage or preclinical projects requiring joint research efforts with big pharma [27]. This has the potential to address lapses in R&D through strengthening the internal capabilities to provide access to expertise in R&D, making it more efficient and cost-effective. Even though it is not the only requirement in achieving the ultimate market success, collaborations have contributed to superior performance of most firms. Even though the biotech companies do not possess as many overarching business capabilities as the big pharma, they have ideas, unique abilities about the project that could adequately complement these areas of underachievement, as in the case of big pharma. They offer the advantage of shared risks, pooling of knowledge, resources and expertise, expansion of capabilities and spreading out tools for productivity and cost miniaturization, accelerating project progression, and better and more efficient technology utilization [28]. To satisfy these needs, big pharma has increasingly engaged in developing relationships with early stage/biotech companies to spread the risk and the options that permit technology accessibility and more opportunities. For example, in Pharmaceutical Shared-Risk programs, Eli Lilly rejected the old model of full company integration to a "fully integrated network" model that leverages the expertise of multiple sectors (academia, government research institutes), to reduce costs and increase the probability of success (PoS) and risk sharing to create new avenues for academic and nonprofit funding.

For merged companies, properly allocating functions and granting each partner adequate independence creates more flexibility and room to enhance performance. It grants the participants an opportunity for growth and high performance standards. For example, Roche, as the leading owner of Genentech, allows such flexibility, which has appreciably played out in terms of both innovation and profits. Individual inventors and academic researchers can work synergistically to cultivate unexplored knowledge for the benefit of all. Biotech companies now generate revenues from a milestone and royalty-based model to turn over development of assets as a form of alliance. This is a way of early outsourcing of revenue to build and sustain the company [28]. The royalties are attractive because the technical and nontechnical risks are shared with the collaboration partner. Both parties split the values of the project combining their capabilities, which are instrumental for growth particularly since potential investors are being repelled by the uncertainty of a drug still in development.

The pharmaceutical industries and biotech companies that focus on R&D engage in target validation using the in-house chemical and biological knowledge base. More than 1000 partnerships have been formed between 1993 and 2000 [29,30]. Many spinouts from publicly funded health research at universities are providing high-quality science and innovation within their firms to help attract pharmaceutical multinational enterprises (MNEs), investors, venture capitalists, and other funders.

Merck and the Vaccine and Gene Therapy Institute of Florida are collaboration partners who discover and validate targets for HIV therapy and also biomarkers for efficacy. The California Institute for Biomedical Research is a nonprofit organization collaborating with academics around the globe. It was sponsored by Merck with a $90 million plan over 7 years [31].

3.5.4.2 Industry–Academic Partnerships

Translating upstream research into product requires a well-established collaboration between academics and industries. Through these partnerships, professionals at the academic institutions with unique skills in assay design for target identification tap into the extensive database and libraries of potentially therapeutic molecules provided by the pharmaceutical companies. Also, experienced medicinal chemists from the research laboratories in the academic sector work jointly with pharmaceutical industry experts who are more inclined to development, risk, and marketing strategies.

In the United States, the landmark legislation, the Bayh-Dole Act, promotes partnerships while strengthening the path of advancing basic research to commercialization. Government intervention in drug discovery R&D was a roadmap to enable the promising research discoveries of academic investigators and business people with proven intellectual abilities and innovative ideas in creating new medicines. The government provides the infrastructure and funds to harness the intellectual resources for the public good. The partnering centers have a mutual interest, which is critical to ensuring a robust national research capacity. Academic principal investigators, postdocs, and Pfizer scientists work jointly on research projects within the Centers for Therapeutic Innovation laboratory and also in the academic laboratories. This facilitates the transfer of tacit knowledge and enables the inventor team and the licensee to better synchronize their commercialization efforts. The scope of research spans from PoC, the translational research leading to over 300 million investments through 5 years [32]. Collaboration between clinicians and drug discovery groups is expected to address the cost, timescale, and risk associated with clinical PoC studies to increase the PoS. These enable the building of a more flourishing environment to the investor community. Adequate consultation with the respective persons would promote well-informed commercial decisions, market identification, commercial skills, and access to pilot and demonstration facilities.

3.5.5 Communication

Research capabilities would become redundant without efficient communication across the drug development groups. Poor coordination among the research centers leaves gaps in productivity due to lapses in output [33,34]. Thus, early communication across the sectors, including regulatory authorities, funders, industry, academia, and investors, is an ongoing endeavor, intended to facilitate an understanding of the proposed strategies prior to investments in the drug development projects. Insurance claims data help to improve the efficiency of delivering drugs, tailored to the patient at the right time. Early communications pertaining to standards for drug reimbursement have advanced drug design and clinical studies. Incorporating the necessary clinical parameters and disease-specific knowledge for the purposes of commercialization and reimbursement that are understood and transparent is essential so that research and clinical efforts can be targeted toward the expected end. Beginning with the end in mind is always an important consideration.

External and internal cross-functional communication boosts innovation and would leverage the best minds across the world to enable a better handling of grave issues encountered in research. Large scale information sharing helps to break technological impasse [35]. Open source has been established to enable drug developers to pool highly priced and valued information gathered from top class experts, which is published under a public license at no cost as a way of sharing pivotal ideas that boost pharmaceutical R&D. The shared information is open source, delivered in an incremental, cumulative manner across companies, institutions, areas of expertise, and platforms of research for nonprofit use by all.

3.5.6 Importance of the Biotechnology Incubators

Biotechnology incubators provide financial and managerial support to entrepreneurs and early stage start-up companies. This is achieved with consulting companies and institutional investors, venture capitalists, and business angels. The incubation of technology-based start-up ventures is based on R&D projects. Due to increasing problems associated with high risk product portfolios, potential markets, and team development, biotechnology incubators have been differentiated by the scope, objectives, and business models. The incubators expedite business development through supplying start-up risk capital to help reduce cost, time, and early stage risks in development. For example, the Taube-Koret Center (TKC) functions as a nonprofit biotechnology incubator [36]. Promising therapeutic solutions on Huntington's disease, as well as Alzheimer's disease, Parkinson's disease, and more, were achieved through the effort of the Koret Foundation and Taube Philanthropies. TKC operates in the same way as a biotechnology company and simulates an industry environment, providing the academic institutions the opportunity to move their discoveries [37].

3.5.7 Addressing Investment Limitations

Increase of investment of public funds has provided a pathway to derisking projects that can attract the investors to release more funds. Derisking the proposition to investors has been done by introducing cofinancing measures, tax incentives for investment that support seed and early stage discovery projects, collaboration on R&D projects, and research clusters together with academic institutions. Tax-based incentives to private investors offer seed and start-up funds. Increased public funding for public/private partnerships has been achieved through programmers like

US Enterprise Development programs that promote linkages and partnerships between investors and entrepreneurs. There is also public funding in areas in dire medical need. Translational research grants are available, such as SMART funds from the Technology Strategy Board. Examples of regional funds are European collaborative programs or local/regional funds. The Technology Strategy Board and Technology Transfer Offices are established research initiatives covering the critical points along the pharmaceutical value chain.

3.5.7.1 In the United States

The emerging NIH, National Center for Advancing Translational Sciences (NCATS) is aimed at supporting the creation and enhancement of innovative methods and technologies for development, testing, and implementation of health care products addressing diseases and conditions. The complementary role of the center is important as it strengthens the already existing translational research being carried out at NIH in the public and private sectors. Nonprofit and commercial institutions receive extensive support through the NIH-FDA Regulatory Science Initiative, which is a highly competitive funding source that is focused on research relating to novel technologies and approaches to regulatory review of drugs, biologics, and devices. The US-sponsored NIH Rapid Access Interventional Development (RAID) pilot program is an NIH Roadmap initiative to support preclinical development of small molecule drug candidates that include bulk active pharmaceutical ingredient (API) synthesis and support, formulation development, analytical assays, good manufacturing practice of clinical supplies, safety tests, development and validation of animal PK, and toxicology. This program is currently available to investigators at academic, nonprofit, and Small Business Innovative Research (SBIR)-eligible institutions. There is also the SBIR and Small Business Technology Transfer (STTR) program with similar objectives, all directed toward promoting innovation. As seen in Figure 3.2, as the development process advances, the potential for surviving candidates to become a drug rises in proportion to increasing expenditure for development of target of interest [38–40]. The Clinical and Translational Science Awards program [41] provides infrastructure grants for academic medical institutions that engage in translational research mostly in US centers with expertise in preclinical science, clinical trials, comparative effectiveness research, training, and community engagement.

3.5.7.2 In the United Kingdom

Series of policies for bridging the Valley of Death were proposed by the UK government. Government investments are utilized for the transforming of research as a way of enhancing the climate for commercialization of research. Some of the measures are supplementing the venture capital investments, reforming the tax system, actively supporting the small-to-medium enterprises (SMEs), and technology. The Small Business Research Initiative supports innovative ideas from small companies and others through public procurement [42]. The Stratified Medicines Innovation Initiative supports the strategies that help accelerate and improve development of high-quality clinical candidates. It proactively addresses this problem through collaborations that support the discovery phase, to bridge drug discovery and clinical research and increase the potential of commercialization of research [43–44]. The establishment of the High Value Manufacturing Catapult Centre initiative was to improve innovation risk and lack of productivity in drug discovery while fostering a strong link between university research and commercialization through financial support that provides access to facilities for the SMEs [45]. These initiatives where stimulated by UK failing venture capital investments resulting in low start-up establishments, which was substantially reduced to £677 million in 2009, from £930 million in 2000 [46].

3.6 FUNDING MODELS

Industry, government, and academia are the major sources of R&D funding. The largest source of funding, which is the industry's funds, are directed toward internal industry-related research effort and sponsorships. The next source of funding is federal funding, which is dedicated to external research efforts and the federal-sponsored subsidiaries, which include federally funded R&D centers and managed by industry, university, or nonprofit operators.

3.6.1 US Financing Models

The Brookhaven National Laboratory and the Defense Advanced Research Projects Agency (DARPA) are located in the United States. DARPA funds the development of many technologies for use by the military and have been cited as a successful model [47]. Also, nonprofit organizations such as philanthropists, research institutes, academic institutions, etc., have the least amount of R&D dollars.

3.6.2 Canadian Financing Models

Support for life sciences basic research comes from different funding mechanisms within federal organizations such as Health Canada, Agriculture Canada, the Canadian Food Inspection Agency, the Department of Foreign Affairs and Trade, and Environment Canada. The Canadian Institutes of Health Research promotes federal science and technology strategies in Canada [48]. Ontario Venture Capital is a joint initiative between the Ontario provincial government and the major institutional investors to promote investment in Ontario-based venture capital and growth equity funds; it has operating costs of about $163 million [49]. The Canadian Biotechnology Strategy is a federal strategy for financially supporting Canadian biotechnology enterprise, regulatory systems for biotechnology, and the Genomics R&D program. It invests more than $65 million per year [50]. The Natural Sciences and Engineering Research Council of Canada supports innovators and academicians with varied levels of funding [51]. The Canada-National Research Council of Canada is the Government of Canada's premier R&D organization. It oversees the operation of 19 research institutes, 2 innovation centers, and 4 technology centers across Canada [52].

3.6.2.1 Case for Canada

Several MNEs are spinouts from publicly funded health research at Canadian universities. They seek partnerships and licensing deals with large multinational companies. In addition to the multinational companies, investors, venture capitalists, and other funders to Canada are drawn to the high-quality science culture and innovation. The Business Development Bank of Canada supports Canadian businesses development by providing financing, subordinate financing, venture capital, consulting, and financial security with a focus on SMEs.

The National Research Council's Industrial Research Assistance Program provides a range of technical and business-oriented advisory options and financial support for SMEs engaged in R&D of technological innovations. The Canadian HIV Technology Development Program attracts the SMEs to onward development of HIV vaccines and promotes more intensive efforts or medical solutions to HIV. The Scientific Research and Experimental Development Tax Credit Program is the largest source of federal government support for R&D in Canada. It provides cash refunds and/or tax credits for expenditures on eligible R&D performed in Canada. The Canadian Innovation Commercialization Program uses procurement as a tool for innovation. Its main objective is to enable Canadian companies that are focused on SMEs to support translational science to a practical value.

3.7 NONGOVERNMENTAL FUNDING MODELS

3.7.1 Large Pharmaceutical Companies

The large pharmaceutical companies like Pfizer and GSK make deals with small biotechs that could be in form of mergers, acquisitions, or outlicensing; but priorities change over time. These could be successful or not. Projects could be terminated.

3.7.2 Venture Capital

Venture capital is the capital provided to a company in return for a shareholding and generating a return through sales. It is provided by investors to start-up firms and small businesses with the potential of economic growth, and is of a great utility for start-ups that find it difficult to tap into the capital markets. This would mean high risk for the investor but substantial financial returns are expected. This funding is most often received by a company that has not established a history in their business enterprise, and the venture capitalists have some kind of authority to contribute to making critical decisions pertaining to the company. Examples are financial institutions like banks and groups of wealthy investors.

3.7.3 Public-Venture Philanthropy

Public-venture philanthropy is a form of charitable giving with the intention of investing to accelerate drug discovery research. Recipients are bound to the same guidelines as funding from a for-profit organization. It is expected that return on investment (ROI) flows into other grants. Examples are patient advocacy groups, wealthy individuals, and billionaires.

3.7.4 Angel Investment

3.7.4.1 Private-Angel Investment

Private-angel investment is a small amount of money utilized for R&D to cover the initial operating costs until a regular stream of revenue is established to seek for venture capital funding. It is considered a high risk investment but with the expectation of high returns when the company grows. These early stage financing options are generally regarded as "at-risk" investment, but are often considered as an effort to promote the success of the company. Thus, investments are not very large. Investment usually comes from a variety of sources, individual entrepreneurs, academic licensing departments, and angel investors. These investors obtain returns when companies go public, which can last for several years from start-up.

3.7.4.2 Public-Angel Investment

Public-angel investments come from more lenient investors who provide funding with flexible terms and have an interest in company officials rather ROI. They understand the risks and expect only a minute portion of their early stage investment to yield a return.

3.7.5 Private-Corporate Investment

Private-corporate investment is directed at small or biotech companies by covering the licensing fees, research expenses, or purchase of stocks; it is a way of acquiring some kind of authority or right to the marketed drugs.

3.7.6 Crowdfunding

Crowdfunding is small capital obtained from several individuals to finance a new business venture. It could be generated from social media or friends and family. Crowdfunding is used to expand the pool of investors of a company. This is regulated in the United States because so many new businesses fail leaving the high risk investment at a loss.

3.8 OTHER FINANCIAL CONCEPTS

3.8.1 Not-for-Profit/Nonprofit Organizations

Not-for-profit organization refers to the organization that does not earn profits for its owners and thus does not distribute profits to it owners. The revenues or money received from different sources are applied toward pursuing the objective of the organization. Not-for-profit organizations are expected to be self-sustaining. Philanthropic seed funding is often required but there are no investors or shareholders who might desire a return. Not-for-profit status is a mechanism for research institutes to monetize (or sell for money) their intellectual property assets. These are academia funded by governments, industrial grants, charities, medical research charities, and philanthropic research foundations. Examples of not-for-profit pharmaceutical companies in the United States are the Institute for One World Health – seed funding from the Bill and Melinda Gates Foundation; Cystic Fibrosis Foundation Therapeutics, Inc.; Gladstone Institutes; and the Taube-Koret Center. In Canada, Genome Canada is a federal fund source committed to fostering the operation of genomics and proteomic research [53].

3.8.2 Cash Flow

Revenue or spending leads to a change in the cash account in a given period of time. Cash inflow is money going to the company from financing, operations, investments, or donations. Cash outflow is expenses or investments. Cash flow is often used by analysts to determine the financially stability of a company. When outflows exceed inflows, this results in negative cash flow.

Cash flow is intended to establish a case for launching a chosen drug development program. A value-added indicator (VAI) helps the managers of a company to make an investment decision. Net present value (NPV) calculation is performed and is the current value of all revenues and expenditure over time, also known as present values or discount rate. A positive value brings a go decision while a negative value means a no-go decision as it will only amount to a loss. The risk-adjusted NPV takes into consideration the risk of the particular stage of drug development. Different therapeutic areas have different risk-adjusted values. Also ROI is a form of VAI.

3.8.3 Cash Flow Return on Investment

Cash flow ROI is estimated as the market value of capital employed. Free cash flow is possible when minimal expenses are made during the setting up of the company.

3.8.4 Derisking

Derisking is applied to any operation or activity that potentially mitigates risks.

3.9 PRIVATE–PUBLIC SECTOR GROUPS

3.9.1 National Centre for Advancing Translational Sciences

NCATS is supported by the NIH to promote innovative methods and technologies for diverse therapeutic areas. It was established in 2012 with a running budget of US$575 million. The NCATS Strategic Alliances Office aims to support industry and academia interactions and partnership with other NCATS laboratories and scientists including universities, pharmaceutical companies, and biotechnology companies. Experts predict that NCATS could help rescue the Valley of Death situation [54].

3.9.2 Innovative Medicines Initiative

The Innovative Medicines Initiative (IMI) was established in 2008 by the European Federation of Pharmaceutical Industries and the European Commission. It is the largest public–private partnership, created to improve development strategies in Europe. It is concerned with the development of tools to predict efficacy, safety, and the management systems in the drug development program [55]. It supports a public–private partnership initiative that encourages competitors to apply for government funds. The IMI is an open innovation program with a mandate to improve the drug development process. An implementation plan with a €2 billion budget was provided by governments and industry participants.

3.9.3 European Federation for Pharmaceutical Sciences

The European Federation for Pharmaceutical Sciences was established with a mandate of advancing the interests of scientists in industry, academia, government, and other institutions engaged in drug research, development, regulation, and policymaking in Europe.

3.9.4 The Centre for Drug Research and Development

The Centre for Drug Research and Development is Canada's national, not-for-profit drug development and commercialization center. It was established to derisk discoveries of publicly funded research while providing investment opportunities for the private sector to bridge the Valley of Death in drug discovery [56]. The National Chemical Genomics Centre has a screening capacity equivalent to that of a major pharmaceutical company [57]. The Molecular Libraries program is an NIH Roadmap Initiative that is focused on promoting chemical biology research that applies high throughput screening that identifies viable small molecules with promising drug-like characteristics [58].

REFERENCES

[1] Graul A, Revel L, Rosa E, Cruces E. Overcoming the obstacles in the pharma/biotech industry: 2008 update. Drug News Perspect 2009;22:39–51.
[2] Dickson M, Gagnon JP. Key factors in the rising cost of new drug discovery and development. Nat Rev Drug Discov 2004;3(5):417–29.
[3] Steinmetz KL, Spack EG. The basics of preclinical drug development for neurodegenerative disease indications. BMC Neurol 2009;9(Suppl. 1):S2.
[4] Lehoux P, Daudelin G, Williams-Jones B, Denis J-L, Longo C. How do business model and health technology design influence each other? Insights from a longitudinal case study of three academic spin-offs. Res Policy 2014;43:1025–38.

[5] Pierrakis Y. Venture capital - now and after the dotcom crash. Research report. NESTA 2010.

[6] Ernst and Young. Beyond borders: matters of evidence. Global Biotechnology Industry Report; 2013. Available from: http://www.ey.com/Publication/vwLUAssets/Beyond_borders/$FILE/Beyond_borders.pdf [accessed 08.12.2014].

[7] Butler D. Translational research: crossing the Valley of Death. Nature 2008;453:840–2.

[8] Dosi G. Technological paradigms and technological trajectories: a suggested interpretation of the determinants and directions of technological change. Res Policy 1982;11(3): 147–62.

[9] Down M, Blackburn T. The challenges of the changing drug discovery model. Drug Discov World 2012. Available from: http://www.ddw-online.com/business/p191021-the-challenges-of-the-changing-drug-discovery-model-fall-12.html. [accessed 14.12.2014].

[10] Teece D. The competitive challenge: strategies for industrial innovation and renewal. Science 1987;239(4845):1320–1.

[11] Tegarden LF, Lamb WB, Hatfield DE, Ji FX. Bringing emerging technologies to market: does academic research promote commercial exploration and exploitation. IEEE Trans Eng Manage 2012;59(4):598–608.

[12] Collins FS. Reengineering translational science: the time is right. Sci Transl Med 2011;3:90cm17.

[13] Pober JS, Neuhauser CS, Pober JM. Obstacles facing translational research in academic medical centers. FASEB J 2001;15:2303–13.

[14] Hopkins AL, Groom CR. The druggable genome. Nat Rev Drug Discov 2002;1:727–30.

[15] Roberts SF, Fischhoff MA, Sakowski SA, Feldman EL. Perspective: transforming science into medicine: how clinician–scientists can build bridges across research's "Valley of Death". Acad Med 2012;87(3):266–70.

[16] Guild PF. Commercializing inventions resulting from university research; analyzing the impact of technology characteristics on subsequent business models. Technovation 2011;31:151–60.

[17] Bridging the "Valley of Death": improving the commercialization of research. House of Commons Science and Technology Select Committee inquiry Royal Society of Chemistry Response. House of Commons Science and Technology Committee. Eighth Report of Session 2012-13. Available from: http://www.publications.parliament.uk/pa/cm201213/cmselect/cmsctech/348/348.pdf [accessed 08.12.2014].

[18] Curry S, Brown R. The target product profile as a planning tool in drug discovery research. Pharmatech 2003;67–71. Available from: http://www.fda.gov/downloads/drugs/guidancecomplianceregulatoryinformation/guidances/ucm080593.pdf [accessed 08.12.2014].

[19] Tebbey PW. Target product profile: a renaissance for its definition and use. J Med Market 2009;9(4):301–7.

[20] Spilker B. Guide to Drug Development. A Comprehensive Review and Assessment. New York: Wolters Kluwer, Lippincott Williams & Wilkins; 2009. p. 976.

[21] Available from: http://www.pmlive.com/top_pharma_list/global_revenues

[22] Robins-Roth C. From Alchemy to IPO: The Business of Biotechnology. Cambridge, MA: Perseus Publishing; 2000.

[23] The Economist. Climbing the helical Staircase 29 March 2003; 8317:3-7.

[24] Spilker B. Guide to Drug Development. A Comprehensive Review and Assessment. New York: Wolters Kluwer, Lippincott Williams & Wilkins; 2009. p. 121 [chapter 12].

[25] Outsourcing in Drug Discovery: The Contract Research Organization (CRO) Market, 6th ed. April 30, 2014. 200 Pages – Pub ID: KLI5237347.

[26] Taunton-Rigby A. Does biotech need pharma? Drug Discov Today 2001;6:1131–3.

[27] Gottinger H, Umali CL. Strategic alliance in global biotech pharma industries. Open Business J 2008;1:10–24.

[28] Rai AK. Fostering cumulative innovation in the biopharmaceutical industry. Berkeley Tech L J 2001;813:815–8.

[29] Higgins MJ. The allocation of control rights in pharmaceutical alliances. Soc Sci Res Netw 2006. Working Paper No. 918980.

[30] Latest News: Merck partners with academic scientists and biotechnology entrepreneurs to create the California Institute for Biomedical Research (Calibr). Available from: http://www.merck.com/licensing/our-partnership/Calibr-Licenses-partnership.html [accessed 08.12.2014].

[31] Advancing medical breakthroughs. Available from: http://www.pfizer.com/partnering/partnership_highlights/

[32] Mullard A. Partnering between pharma peers on the rise. Nat Rev Drug Discov 2011;10:561–2.

[33] Vernon JA, Golec JH, Dimasi JA. Drug development costs when financial risk is measured using the Fama-French three-factor model. Health Econ 2010;19(8): 1002–5.

[34] Hollingsworth JR. In: Stapleton D, editor. Creating a Tradition of Biomedical Research. New York: Rockefeller University Press; 2004. p. 17–63.

[35] Taube-Koret Center Annual Report. Available from: http://www.gladstoneinstitutes. org/u/sfinkbeiner/taube-koret/Resources.html [accessed 09.12.2014].

[36] Finkhbiner S. Bridging the Valley of Death of therapeutics for neurodegeneration. Nat Med 2010;16(11):1227–31.

[37] Yua H, Adedoyin A. ADME-Tox in drug discovery: integration of experimental and computational technologies. Drug Discov Today 2003;8(18):852–61.

[38] Penzotti JE, Landrum GA, Putta S. Building predictive ADMET models for early decisions in drug discovery. Curr Opin Drug Discov Devel 2004;7:49–60.

[39] Kennedy T. Managing the drug discovery/development interface. Drug Discov Tech 1997;2:436–41.

[40] Steele SJ. Working with the CTSA Consortium: what we bring to the table. Sci Transl Med 2010;2:63mr5.

[41] Pugsley MK. Challenging current paradigms in early drug development – innovative approaches to safety pharmacology. Available from: http://www.aptuit.com/Media/Default/Verona/Symposium/Paradigms-2012/Presentations/Michael_Pugsley_lecture_May16.pdf [accessed 09.12.2014].

[42] Tendering for public sector contracts. Available from: http://www.businesslink.gov.uk/bdotg/action/layer?topicId=1074033478 [accessed 09.12.2014].

[43] ChemistryInnovation annual report 2011. Available from: https://connect.innovateuk. org/web/case-studies [accessed 09.12.2014].

[44] BIOCHEM project. Available from: http://www.biochem-project.eu/ [accessed 09.12.2014].

[45] United Kingdom Parliament – Parliament UK. Available from: http://www.publications. parliament.uk/pa/cm201012/cmselect/cmsctech/writev/valley/valley42.htm [accessed 09.12.2014].

[46] Henderson J. The role of corporate venture capital funds in financing biotechnology and healthcare: differing approaches and performance consequences. Available from: https://www.imd.org/research/publications/upload/Henderson_WP_2007_02_Level_1.pdf [accessed 09.12.2014].

[47] Defense Advanced Projects Agency; 2012. Available from: http://www.darpa.mil [accessed 09.12.2014].

[48] Canadian Institutes of Health Research. Available from: http://www.cihr-irsc.gc.ca/e/193. html [accessed 09.12.2014].

[49] Ontario Venture Capital Fund. Available from: http://www.ovcf.com/ [accessed 09.12.2014].

[50] Natural Sciences and Engineering Research Council of Canada. Available from: www.nserc-crsng.gc.ca [accessed 09.12.2014].

[51] National Research Council Canada. Available from: www.nrc-cnrc.gc.ca [accessed 09.12.2014].

[52] Available from: http://www.ncats.nih.gov/research/rare-diseases/bridgs/bridgs.html

[53] Genome Canada. Available from: www.genomecanada.ca [accessed 09.12.2014].

[54] National Centre for Advancing Translational Sciences (NCATS). Available from: www.ncats.nih.gov [accessed 09.12.2014].

[55] Innovative Medicines Initiative (IMI). Available from: www.imi.europea.eu [accessed 09.12.2014].

[56] The Centre for Drug R&D (CDRD). Available from: www.cdrd.ca [accessed 09.12.2014].

[57] Inglese J, Auld DS, Jadhav A, Johnson RL, Simeonov A, Yasgar A, Zheng W, Austin CP. Quantitative high-throughput screening: a titration-based approach that efficiently identifies biological activities in large chemical libraries. PNAS 2006;103(31):11473–8.

[58] Molecular Libraries Program. Available from: http://mli.nih.gov/mli/ [accessed 09.12.2014].

SECTION II

Drug Discovery Cycle I: Discovery and Preclinical Drug Development

4. Prediscovery Research: Challenges and Opportunities   85
5. The Significance of Discovery Screening and Structure Optimization Studies   109
6. Preclinical *In Vitro* Studies: Development and Applicability   129
7. Animal Utilization in Drug Development: Clinical, Legal, and Ethical Dimensions   149
8. Pharmaceutical Formulation and Manufacturing Development:
   Strategies and Issues   169

CHAPTER 4

Prediscovery Research: Challenges and Opportunities

Odilia Osakwe

Contents

4.1 Introduction	85
4.2 Models of Human Disease Biology	88
4.2.1 Target-Based Drug Discovery	88
4.2.2 Phenotypic Drug Discovery	89
4.3 Diseases Considered in Biopharmaceutical Research and Development	91
4.4 Modern Trends in Drug Discovery	91
4.4.1 Extracellular RNA Communication as an Emerging Paradigm in Drug Discovery	91
4.4.2 The Applicability of Systems Biology in Drug Discovery	92
4.4.3 The Omics Technology	93
4.4.4 Network: A Systems Biology Approach to Drug Discovery	95
4.4.5 Mapping the Disease Association Networks	96
4.4.6 Polypharmacological Profiling: A Novel Approach to Drug Discovery	98
4.4.7 Multiple Transporters Drug Targeting	101
4.5 Current Challenges in Early Drug Discovery	101
4.5.1 Setbacks in Identification and Selection of New Targets	101
4.5.2 Network/System Biology Application-Limitations	103
4.5.3 The Impact of the Pharmaceutical Ecosystem	104
4.5.4 Effect of Size and Capability	104
References	105

4.1 INTRODUCTION

Drug therapies are generated through manipulation of the activity of human proteins, known in the industry as targets that have been implicated in disease pathways. Pharmaceutical firms have encountered several roadblocks in the drug discovery of novel drug molecules, especially those that work against new targets.

Prediscovery research investigations are carried out to understand disease and its causes at the level of cell genes and proteins in order to identify novel targets of therapeutic value. Many diseases are modulated at

Social Aspects of Drug Discovery, Development and Commercialization Copyright © 2016 Elsevier Inc.
http://dx.doi.org/10.1016/B978-0-12-802220-7.00004-1   All rights reserved.

the gene level. A well-understood genetic root of a disease enables the determination of risk factors to recommend a therapy. For example, genes could be activated or deactivated by drugs or totally replaced through gene therapy. The advent of molecular science brought remarkable break-throughs in disease diagnosis and therapy. The understanding of the disease mechanism provides the first "green light" to seeking intervention and possible treatment options. The Human Genome Project, which discovered the 3 billion bases of human DNA, enabled an advanced understanding of human biology and is the foothold for the "omics" technology that has revolutionized the science of drug discovery. The project moved the fledgling field of genomic science, characterized by its slow pace and cost, toward an enhanced and highly efficient approach currently applied in biomedical research [1,2]. The posthuman Genome Project era enabled identification of compounds that could interact with molecular targets at low concentrations [3]. Gene manipulation in various forms – knock-ins, knockouts, transgenic systems, and gene expression profiles – can be used to accelerate the discovery process where target function and drug mechanisms of action at the molecular level are discernible (Figure 4.1). For example, sickle-cell anemia is an inherited mutation in a gene for hemoglobin, the red blood pigment, leading to its dysfunction and distortion of the red blood cells, giving them a sickle shape. They clump together and block the blood vessels. Gene therapy that replaces this gene could lead to a total cure.

A human cell contains about 100,000 different proteins while the genome contains only 30,000–40,000 genes in all the cells [4]. Metabolic proteins or enzymes are a part of the cell composition, actively involved

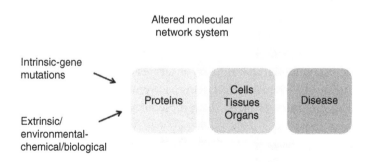

Figure 4.1 *Perturbations in Human Disease.*

with building and breaking down substances that energize physiological processes. Signaling proteins are important inter- and intracellular communicators. The activities of these proteins are vital to cellular, tissue, and organ function. Thus, they are the principal functioning biological molecules in living systems. They are the primary drug targets, having been involved in many human diseases.

The concept of disease is due to disturbances of function (Figure 4.1), which can be treated if there is an understanding of disease mechanisms that helps to define the disease phenotype and which can be measured. Many diseases are very complex and multifactorial. Understanding disease factors and targets involves discerning the molecular pathways, signaling, metabolic and regulatory networks of the cell's tissues, organs, and the entire organism.

Certain molecular substances exhibit a regular pattern of frequent association with certain diseases. These provide hints for the selection of drug targets and are often involved in the metabolic or signaling pathway specific to a disease condition or pathology, or to the infectivity or survival of a microbial pathogen. A drug compound is essentially configured according to the molecular structure of its target, which has the ability to modulate its activity and combat the disease of interest. This is an important application in drug discovery and has been the framework for identifying new disease drug targets, and biomarkers for complex diseases.

In the twentieth century, biology focused on a reductionist approach to determining systemic functions and discerning disease pathways, an approach that was based on the activities of individual components of a living system. However, the advent of high throughput technologies, such as genomics and proteomics, has permitted the study cells as systems, leading to a conceptual re-evaluation of the fact that cells are a collection of individual cellular components that have previously been based on the function of individual molecules and chemical properties of molecules that make up the cells. The conventional conception is that the function of the biological systems is mostly network based, in other words, stems from the whole and not parts. This has been dubbed "emergent" properties because they emerge from the whole and are not properties of the individual parts. A recent change of focus toward "systems biology/network medicine or network pharmacology" is a widely accepted phenomenon in drug discovery.

The major strategies employed in basic discovery research and their relevance will be discussed in subsequent sections.

4.2 MODELS OF HUMAN DISEASE BIOLOGY

4.2.1 Target-Based Drug Discovery

A target is any molecule such as a gene or protein that is associated with a disease pathway and that could be modulated in order to improve the disease condition. Target identification refers to determining the cause of disease inhibition or activation of a protein or pathway in order to identify potential drug targets.

Target identification is fundamental to understanding of cellular pathways underlying disease pathogenesis and/or pathophysiology (Figure 4.2). Any gene product could be a target. For example, RNA expression data can potentially be used to construct a theoretical linkage between many proteins and a disease. The Human Genome Project discovered 20,000–25,000 genes in human genomes out of which about 3000 genes have been considered druggable, and are prioritized depending on the ability to change disease pathology using drug compounds. However, posttranslational modifications, alternative splicing, and protein complex association account for an excessive number of different proteins available in the human "targetome."

Identifying new targets for common diseases from a pool of new targets has not materialized. In addressing these questions, an increasing number of drug targets are being added to the database. These targets could be enzymes, receptors, hormones, nuclear receptors, nucleic acids, and ion channels, and these could be narrowed to the best "druggable" target, which is

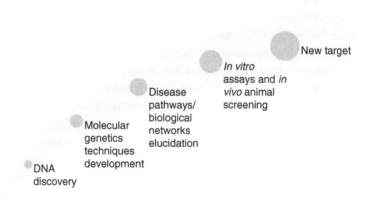

Figure 4.2 *The Process of Target-Based Drug Discovery.*

referred to as those that possess recommended attributes associated with successful drug candidates. Most often, individual molecules that hit a useful set of multiple targets are chosen [5–7]. Since the completion of the Human Genome Project, target-based drug discovery has dominated modern pharmaceutical research due to its complementary advantage over phenotypic drug discovery.

Determining the network for complex diseases is challenging. For example, no single gene has been identified as the only cancer gene. A typical cancer patient would have several mutations in up to 300 genes, which is a daunting complexity for the medical researcher [8]. Also there is multiplication of false positives, a common experience in studies of this nature [9].

Target Drug Discovery (TD2) was established for the screening of external molecules in target-based assays to find compounds with therapeutic potential and collaboration possibilities [10]. It was pointed out that a target-centric approach for first-in-class drugs without optimization of the mechanism of action might lead to failure and a drop in productivity [11].

Some of the problems with target identification is that it has not completely optimized the number of druggable targets with well-defined active sites that could be manipulated or inhibited with small molecule drugs. Targets might be acting as transcription factors, structural components of key complexes inside the cell, or with unknown function. This is leading to a shift in focus toward a more direct drug discovery approach involving screening of compound libraries through phenotypic assays.

The following are target areas for drug development:
- Central nervous system – Alzheimer's disease, Parkinson's disease, affective disorders
- Cardiovascular and metabolic diseases
- Atherosclerosis/thrombosis, type 2 diabetes, obesity
- Oncology – tumor growth molecules, cell signaling receptors
- HIV/AIDS – targets in viral lifecycle
- Infectious diseases – hepatitis B and C
- Autoimmune and inflammatory diseases – multiple sclerosis, arthritis, psoriasis, inflammatory bowel disease
- Asthma, chronic obstructive pulmonary disease (COPD)

4.2.2 Phenotypic Drug Discovery

Disease phenotype is based on signs and symptoms of disease mechanism or pathogenesis. Some diseases are easier to detect than others because the causative organisms can be easily known. A typical example is infections.

For a drug company to pursue research in this area, epidemiological data of the morbidity and mortality are taken into consideration, linking the phenotype to a genotype. This normally begins by discovering the organs or tissue involved and a measureable function to discern change of activity, followed by finding the malfunctioned protein and other biomolecules that drive these chemical and electrical signals through body cells; their activities provide the first line of information used in the design of small molecules that interact with the drug target. Some examples are receptors, ligands, small molecule hormones, neurotransmitters, peptide hormones, growth factors, cytokines, trophic factors, vitamin D, chemokines, steroid hormones, retinoids, neuromodulatory peptides, thyroxin, and cortisol.

The phenotypic screen is usually more physiologically relevant since cells that are intact in their natural environment are used. Primary hits identified in this process could target different types of proteins such as receptors, transcription factors, enzymes, and the signaling pathways. The finding of the associated molecules could help the tracing of the cell mechanism, and the upregulated or deregulated proteins along the biological network or pathway. This phenomenon has been instrumental in the discovery of many drugs but without the knowledge of their mechanism of action [12]. Certain therapeutic areas are more prone to phenotypic screening like infectious and the central nervous system diseases whereas target based areas are more aligned with oncology. Thus, no method could be universally applicable as every format has its niche. However, most new molecular entities were discovered through target-based screening. Through case study analysis, among several key considerations for selecting a therapeutic area or need is the unmet medical need, based on clinical manifestations like symptoms reported or observed, what populations are affected, progression of the condition, and the severity of the disease based on literature or clinical reports. Decision is informed by obtaining information about alternative therapies, compliance and tolerance, evidence, and the strength of the information accrued.

The phenotypic-centered approach does not include disease mechanism studies since the screening assays could generate a good readout if properly designed [13] and the outcomes of which could lead to prototype design when establishing the structure–activity relationships. These are more suitable for the discovery of drugs for rare diseases and neglected diseases, being a rather faster approach to save time and cost as the pharmacological properties of the drugs are known. The obtained information can be used for a new drug development program following the validation of a new target. In this regard, the current trend is redirecting efforts toward phenotypic drug discovery [14]. The Big Pharma is seeking to invite academic and biotech professionals for collaborations. The Lilly-sponsored Phenotypic Drug Discovery (PD2) initiative was established for the screening of external molecules in phenotypic modules to find compounds with therapeutic potential and collaboration possibilities [15].

4.3 DISEASES CONSIDERED IN BIOPHARMACEUTICAL RESEARCH AND DEVELOPMENT

Decision on a therapeutic area is based on both humanitarian and commercial interest considerations. Selection of a disease area is mostly based on relevance to:

- Unaddressed disease conditions or those with limited alternatives such as stroke, chronic obstructive pulmonary disease, Alzheimer's disease, osteoarthritis, hearing loss, dementias, low back pain, and rare (orphan) diseases.
- Diseases that are widespread globally, for example, cancer, cardiovascular disease, HIV/AIDS, diabetes, depression, pneumonia, and neonatal conditions.
- Diseases for which existing drug therapy is ineffective are suboptimal. These are infections due to antibacterial resistance and pandemic influenza.
- Neglected tropical diseases, for example, malaria and tuberculosis.
- Infectious diseases, which mainly affect people in low- and middle-income countries, for example, HIV/AIDS, tuberculosis, and malaria.

Current pharmaceutical efforts have not sufficiently addressed these conditions. In addition, these are diseases where basic research is needed to establish biomarkers.

4.4 MODERN TRENDS IN DRUG DISCOVERY

4.4.1 Extracellular RNA Communication as an Emerging Paradigm in Drug Discovery

Extracellular RNA (exRNA) communication has extended drug discovery capabilities for a more effective identification of reliable drug disease targets to effect a cure. Extracellular RNA communication is carried out through cell-to-cell signaling. RNA plays a primary role of translating genes to proteins and the control of protein expression inside cells. A recent discovery found that RNA is secreted outside cells, thus, exRNA, could migrate out of the cell to other parts of the body, acting as a signaling molecule to communicate with other cells and also carrying information from cell to cell throughout the bodily systems. This has enabled the understanding and discerning a wide spectrum of diseases. But the success rate would depend on the competence in discerning the exRNA biology. A collaborative, cross-cutting National Institutes of Health (NIH)-funded Extracellular RNA Communication program was coined in 2012 to help accelerate application and full utilization in drug discovery. Scientists are investigating the exRNA processes throughout the entire spectrum of translational research from discovery to the clinics. They are actively searching for diverse ways for exRNA cell targeting and possible alterations in diseased conditions for their use as biomarkers, or indicators of a disease to help strengthen early disease discovery [16].

4.4.2 The Applicability of Systems Biology in Drug Discovery

Drug discovery traditionally is based on animal models, cells, and tissue screens while molecular biology-based technologies define molecular targets and enable the scaling down and narrowing of the range of screening tests. The so-called "reductionist target-based approach" is mainly focused on distinct aspects of the whole organism, which are the groups of tissues, cells, molecules, and molecular interactions. Such endeavors did not take into consideration the interdependency and cross-interaction of macromolecules, which form complex networks with properties that extend beyond individual functions.

Drug discovery researchers are increasingly departing from the path of traditional techniques to parallel models, combining and integrating all data for a more comprehensive evaluation for drug discovery applications. The growing recognition of integrated biological systems lends itself to the application of a systems biology analytical technique as a suitable method to describe the complexity of human diseases, to streamline the drug development process [17,18]. The emergence of systems biology can be traced historically as far back as molecular biology, which has slowly evolved to its full development and application over the past decade, coinciding with the concomitant introduction of modern high throughput and computation technologies, the utility of internet systems in the processing of data, and the appearance of other applications in rational drug discovery.

Systems biology can be defined as "the study of an organism, viewed as an integrated and interacting network of genes, proteins and biochemical reactions, which give rise to life." System biology focuses on physiology and diseases across the complex interaction networks at all levels of the cellular organization to the whole organism [19,20]. As translational research is premised on the complexity of human biology, system biology permits the comprehension of the complex biological systems (e.g., DNA and RNA in different forms, proteins and posttranslational modifications, interaction networks, organelles, cells, tissues, organs, human populations, and environments), to enable the development of predictive models of human disease. The cell could be termed a "micro living system" with the many strata of biology and components that carry out intra-, extra-, and intercellular functions in a complex network of interactions.

A functional interdependency between the molecular components in a human cell reflects in the perturbations of the complex intracellular and intercellular network involved in diseases (Figure 4.1). This molecular complexity requires the unraveling of disease pathways, and relationships among different disease phenotypes. Their molecular signatures suggest interactions that may play a role in disease etiology. Multicomponent analysis that integrates data from multiple biological levels is the key to the comprehension of the behavior of complex systems.

The application of systems biology has led to a tremendous improvement in drug discovery research as it has enabled the generation of highly diverse and extensive high throughput data of the system components through the thorough investigation of the complex molecular pathways for better prediction ability [19,21,22]. In recent years, systems biology has incorporated integration of data from multiple omics technologies to reduce data complexity and to further enhance the predictive network models such as chemical structure, protein sequence, structure and expression; genome and gene; biological network; pharmacokenetics (PK); and pharmacodynamics (PD). An example of the application of systems biology in clinical medicine is the RNA expression profiles of diffuse B cell lymphoma. The lymphoma's genetic profile led to an unprecedented discovery for a disorder once considered a single entity, but which was identified in the three different genetic profiles: germinal-center B cell-like, activated B cell-like, and type 3 diffuse large B cell lymphoma [23]. The study of drug mechanisms and drug combinations has been made possible through system biology to identify the enhancement of the creating drug's effectiveness by using combination drugs that augment their effects [24].

4.4.3 The Omics Technology

Omics refers to study areas in biology with the ending "-omics," such as genomics, proteomics, or metabolomics. Omics technology focuses on characterization and quantification of series of biomolecules associated with the structure, function, and dynamics of an organism. The application of omics technology provides extensive information about changes across the hierarchical levels of organizations of the whole organism, which is probed in cell-based assays, animal and clinical studies. It is useful in mapping the genotype origin in diseases at the level of genes, proteins, and cells. Examples of omics tools used in drug discovery are genomics, epigenomics, transcriptomics, proteomics, metabolomics, pharmacogenomics, phosphoproteomics, and herbalomics (definitions given later). Genomics (genes) could be interpreted as "what to expect," transcriptome (RNAs) as "what occurs," the proteome (proteins) as "what is responsible for the occurrence," and metabolome (sugars, nucleotides, amino acids, lipids – the metabolites) as "the outcome." The metabolites enable determination of function or the disease phenotype. These are discerned through systems biology and organized through informatics [25].

The omics platform has been helpful in establishing associations between multitarget networks and drug action, which is widely applicable in drug design. It has helped to reveal the biological function of the gene product, as high throughput technologies have contributed to the rising number of data generated. It has opened new avenues, increasing the efficiency of biomarker discovery, important signaling molecules associated with various physiological processes and early detection of diseases that would shape and refine diagnosis and treatment of disease.

All the data types, including genomics information, are the foundation for constructing models of cell signaling, pathway and disease networks that unravel novel drug targets and clinical efficacy. Data reduction typically involves sorting, which are grouped based on statistical definitions with methods such as clustering, factor analysis, or others. These permit the connection of results to external information and to integrate multiple sources of data. Natural language processing is a high throughput technology that enables generation of massive structured and codified data, applicable for clinical applications that promote efficiency in drug development and outcomes. It has been used for refining the information generated from human systems.

4.4.3.1 Definitions
- Genomics – sequencing, organizing, and analysis of function and structure, and mapping the genomes (the complete set of DNA within a single cell of an organism).

- Epigenomics – reversible modifications of the DNA or histones that lead to nongenomic changes of mRNA expression. Typical epigenetic changes are histone modifications, which are essential in cell differentiation and development.
- Transcriptomics – discovery of whole genome gene expression profile of a disease and mRNA transcripts produced in a cell or tissue system.
- Pharmacogenomics – identification of the genetic variation in a group of individuals to inform design of drugs customized to their genotype.
- Proteomics – detecting global targets and candidate proteins' network target response to a drug. These could be proteins, receptors, enzymes, structural cell components – measurement of proteins in a given system.
- Phosphoproteomics – protein phosphorylation as a posttranslational modification essential in cell signal transduction. Protein phosphorylation plays a key role in regulation of signaling pathways.
- Metabolomics – studying the effect of drugs from metabolites, which are small biomolecules in the cells or cellular biomolecules, for example, lipids nucleotides, peptides, and hormones.
- Herbalomics – identifying potential benefit and toxicity of herbal components with therapeutic value. Herbalome chips are platforms in which arrays of compounds are screened for their binding to key peptides as well as doing the multicomponent, multitarget coordination research.

4.4.4 Network: A Systems Biology Approach to Drug Discovery

Network-based drug discovery drives the application of systems biology and computational technologies as powerful tools for multitarget drug discovery and development of network medicine. Currently, the concept of network-based drug discovery is attracting a great deal of attention in biomedical and pharmaceutical research due to its potential in advancing drug discovery [26–31].

Beyond traditional approaches that rely on individual molecules or pathways, network systems biology offers an opportunity for integration of biological complexity and multilevel connectivity linking genes to drugs. Understanding the potential targets for new drugs is based on experimental pharmacology, when there is a working hypothesis of a molecular mechanism underlying the pathophysiology. Causal network modeling investigates series of biological cause and effect statements to identify network components prior to initial observations [32]. It incorporates multiple omics and other experimental systems to streamline the predictive power of drugs.

Network analysis enables simultaneous incorporation of both the expected effects (the target or pathway of interest) and off-target effects. This type of integrated system further clarifies the path to personalize the application of medicine, enabling drug quality and innovation success, and expanding the application of existing ones to find new uses. The network-based approach takes into consideration the whole human system of diseases and contributing factors, linking molecular biology and clinical manifestations. This principally involves discerning molecular networks such as protein interaction networks, metabolic networks, regulatory networks, and RNA networks. These are the platform for probing molecular substances and disease associations in order to find new patterns that lead to medical therapy. Networks serve as templates for integrating all the multiple levels of complexity for drug–protein interaction to help to identify single-, multitarget, and network drug target candidates (Figure 4.3).

Computer simulations build mathematical and graphical models that account for the behavior of the system perturbations, offering a holistic approach that generates organ system-level responses for selection of targets for drug design. This incorporates all network constituents; integrated protein and metabolite measurements, and automation of cell-based assays that unify a broad range of disease-relevant human biology as a foundation for further target validation and prototype design.

4.4.5 Mapping the Disease Association Networks

Disease mapping techniques have been used since the turn of the nineteenth century to track diseases and origins. There has been a growing interest in disease mapping in the last decade, particularly with the additional developments in statistics and computerized information system

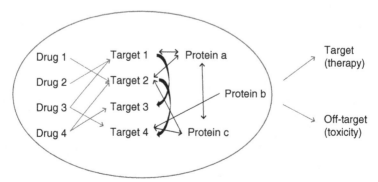

Figure 4.3 *Model of Complex Drug Interactions.*

technology, which has further streamlined disease mapping. Mapping the molecular association networks relies on genetic changes as a foundation in tracking all the change of state or functions of the associated proteins, pathways, and diseases. Research is currently expanding from probing of the biological network itself to a newer approach based on text/reports on previously conducted studies. Groups of molecular substances identified by statistical analysis of these networks have been reported as verifiable groups of molecular substances and appropriate frameworks for analyzing and visualizing large-scale, complex relationships among molecular networks and diseases [33]. The utility of data from previous reports has provided a wide database for identifying major players in clinical diseases and molecular associations. Most importantly, elucidation of networks of diseases based on molecular more integrated than focusing on a single disease itself. This has also been recommended as a potential for providing a conceptual basis for the association of experimental with theoretical knowledge [34].

4.4.5.1 Genome-Wide Association Studies

Introduction of genome-wide association studies (GWAS) enabled the evaluation of DNA or genome markers of individuals in order to find genetic variations associated with a particular disease. Earlier research methodologies relied on sequencing individual genomes with exceptional phenotypes and studies of epigenomic regulation of gene expression. There is an increasing inclination toward the utility of systems biology-based techniques that assess proteomes, metabolomes, and cellular pathways. Evidently, this has favored the pathway to establishing clinical efficacy [35]. High volume and highly diverse data on gene product interactions, mostly generated with high throughput technology, are integrated to produce functional association networks. Clinical samples for individuals with disease phenotype are scrutinized for possible genes that could be linked to disease: protein–protein physical interactions could be correlated with functional associations of genes that expressed the proteins. This is a necessity in drug discovery as it helps to clarify certain ambiguities associated with similar clinical phenotypes that exhibit genetic differences and differences in response. An earlier study reported the similarities in phenotypic side effects that were used to deduce the possibility of the sharing of a target by two drugs. This study required the application of 746 marketed drugs with a network of 1018 side effects, which identified 11 out of 13 implied drug–target interactions that had an associated inhibitory effect [36].

GWAS provides information about genetic risk factors, genetic variants that show disease susceptibility, drug targets-associated pathways, and those that are "druggable" targets, the gene variants of already approved drugs and also those that are strongly linked to variable clinical manifestations when exposed to certain marketed drugs [37,38]. For example, GWAS has enabled the identification of 1100 genetic risk factors for common diseases [37,39].

4.4.5.1.1 Relevance of GWAS in Pharmacogenomics

Pharmacogenomics is the study of the effect of genetic variations on individual responses to drug therapy. Early discovery research requires finding intra- and interindividual expression of proteins. Such information is used to define drug development activities throughout the development lifecycle, which could be achieved through the application of pharmacogenomics. Understanding an individual's genetic component is crucial to personalized medicine as it gives the assurance of greater efficacy and safety. Application of pharmacogenomics in early stage disease models will enable selection of drug molecules that are effective in a metabolic heterogeneous environment. This takes into account genetic heterogeneity, metabolic variation, and epigenetic modulation that could be tackled in the early stages of the drug discovery process. Thus, drug molecules could be optimized for binding selective genetic variants, rather than a one-size-fits-all genetically heterogeneous patient population.

Research could selectively aim at targets with an effect on multiple diseases, such that whole-genome sequencing could help to unravel individuals with gene mutations that lead to protein malfunction, which are explored for the development of therapy. When a drug that interacts with numerous targets, losing one target might not exert a significant effect on the drug action. This variation might be more effective to the single target model of drugs and would not be applied in the development of drugs that only engage single targets. In multitargeting, this strategy would be helpful as it could be tailored to a target population that shows a high response and less adverse effects. Details about pharmacogenomics will be dealt within Chapter 10.

4.4.6 Polypharmacological Profiling: A Novel Approach to Drug Discovery

Polypharmacology is a term that is used to describe compounds that interact with multiple targets. A recurring issue in drug discovery is drug compounds acting on multiple targets; this has been termed as being "blind" to other connected processes. The high throughput screening, computations structure-based approaches have evolved around the single-target approach. Drug compounds acting on other targets have been attributed to adverse effects. There is an increasing paradigm shift from one-drug-target to one-drug-multiple-targets drug design. Instead of focusing on a single target, the newer strategies are evaluating varied levels of polypharmacology to identify the enhancing or undesired effects, and to determine its activity with antitargets [40]. Polypharmacological analysis of multiple targets (i.e., preferred macromolecules with which the drug is intended to interact) is important in drug development as it allows a more precise prediction of all the on- and off-target effects in order to determine the potential adverse effects of an intervention (Figure 4.3). Engagement of multiple targets by a drug molecule could be either beneficial (for repurposed drugs) or harmful (toxic). Certain drugs do possess multitargeting activities.

Aspirin is an analgesic drug popularly known for its pain relieving or fever reduction activity. However, it also acts as an anti-inflammatory medication to treat rheumatoid arthritis [41], pericarditis [42], and Kawasaki disease [43]. Additionally, it has been used in the prevention of transient ischemic attacks [44], strokes, heart attacks [45], pregnancy loss [46], and even cancer [47]. The rapid increase in molecular data generated in the postgenomic era has inspired a greater need for polypharmacological research to be fully incorporated in drug discovery. The omics technologies are also being incorporated [48,49]. Polypharmacology represents a gateway to the rational design of the next generation of less toxic therapeutic agents to improve their effectiveness [50]. In addition, polypharmacological approaches are beneficial in the discovery of unknown off-targets for the existing drugs (also known as drug repurposing) [51]. Polypharmacological studies also require systematic integration of the multidisciplinary data from computational modeling, synthetic chemistry, *in vitro/in vivo* pharmacological testing, and clinical studies. Computational identification of combinations of drug targets has been a helpful way of selecting the most viable drug target [52].

Polypharmacological approaches help to increase the efficiency of drug action when developed with individual molecules that hit a useful set of multiple targets [6,7,53]. A single drug can act on multiple targets of a single disease pathway, or multiple targets associated with multiple disease pathways. For complex diseases, multiple drugs could act on different targets of a network to regulate various physiological/pathological processes [54].

The systems biology approach – investigating the drug–target interactions in the context of a molecular network – helps to deduce the polypharmacological relations among drugs and proteins [55–58]. Thus, systems biology approaches that are integrated with polypharmacology are being frequently used to identify new off-targets [59–61]. The polypharmacological phenomenon represents an important advancement in drug discovery as it enables the development of multitarget therapeutics agents to maintain an optimal balance of drug activity while uncovering the new off-targets and side effects for drugs: an emerging paradigm with a potential of transforming our next-generation pool of marketed drugs [62].

Polypharmacology has enabled the prediction of the activity of 656 marketed drugs on 73 unintended side effect targets, with confirmations on about half these predictions [63].

A polypharmacology approach allowed the identification of proteins linked by drug–target binary associations from a list of the US Food and Drug Administration-approved drugs. Moreover, polypharmacology has been credited for its speed and extensive capabilities in the identification of drug targets, which also opens up avenues to repurpose the existing drugs.

The use of "cocktails," in other words multiple or single-drug molecules that engage different targets, has been employed in disease therapy such as HIV. For example, antiretroviral triple cocktail therapies for AIDS control can simultaneously suppress HIV fusion, while interfering with viral protein translation and transcription by using an HIV fusion inhibitor, a protease inhibitor, and a reverse transcriptase inhibitor, thus conferring resistance and preventing its maturity. This is a mechanism for minimizing a patient's viral load down to almost basal levels and restoring white and red blood cells toward normal levels [64]. Until today, numerous polypharmacology-related problems do exist especially in modeling and rational design of multitargeting agents, which is highly cumbersome to accomplish.

4.4.6.1 The Road Ahead for Polypharmacology

A major advantage offered by the early application of polypharmacology is that it facilitates early decision making. Early decisions proactively address downstream complications, which stand to save financial losses and time. The ICH regulatory guidelines, ICH S7A guidelines require "secondary PD studies" to investigate the effects of a substance not related to its desired therapeutic target. Polypharmacology belongs under this category and this study is undertaken to inform the selection and design of safe drug compounds and for its application in the interpretation of *in vivo* safety pharmacology and toxicology studies. Understanding of the pharmacological safety properties of a drug could help the pharmaceutical company to outcompete the existing therapies for a disease, while offering advantage over its competitors and, most importantly, the promise of overall safety to the patients.

In an effort to strengthen the polypharmacology in drug discovery, academic–industry collaborations are been undertaken, which could elevate progressive research into potential adverse effects or drug toxicity in drug discovery. The NIH-based National Clinical Assessment and Treatment Service has launched programs to identify new uses for existing agents developed by the pharmas [65]. Ultimately, there is a growing expectation that sophisticated and comprehensive polypharmacological approaches will emerge to fine tune the rational design of more potent and less toxic multitargeting agents to address the current experimental limitations and complexity.

4.4.7 Multiple Transporters Drug Targeting

Transporters are required to deliver drugs to the site of action and are particularly important due to this special role. Their ability to transport natural, endogenous metabolites predicates design of drugs with the attributes of structural similarity with metabolites in such a way that permits recognition and shuttling by these physiological transporters. Hence, the study of transporters and intracellular behavior is an important aspect of drug development. For a drug that can access multiple transporters, a knockout of only one is not likely to show a phenotypic effect, or require applying the polypharmacology phenomenom to discriminate, which transporters are involved.

4.5 CURRENT CHALLENGES IN EARLY DRUG DISCOVERY

4.5.1 Setbacks in Identification and Selection of New Targets

Identification and selection of novel drug targets has not been very promising as only a few identified targets have therapeutic value. Previously, a change in gene regulation was sufficient for target identification but with the increasing acceptance of the "expanded networks" concept following the introduction of the system biology paradigm, target identification must be based on consolidation of gene expression data along with other (global) information.

In discovery research, the differential expression of a protein in a diseased condition showing a change from normal cells or tissues is an initial signal that might prompt further investigation as a crucial target in the disease pathogenesis. Sometimes, the mRNA levels are not in the same proportion with the protein concentrations. There could be many complicated and varied posttranslational mechanisms that transcribe mRNA into protein that are not controlled; error and noise in these experiments are ambiguities that might affect the integrity of generated data [66,67]. The observed activity levels of expressed proteins do not correspond to quantity and could differ significantly. Some proteins are nonfunctional after being expressed, which could require further processing or agents for further modifications. This could introduce variations as the concentration of the agents and activity levels are not controlled. Spatial and temporal expression of proteins is another source of variability that could lead to differing protein expression and functionality due to cell type and time dependence. Early tumor cells will differ from tumor cells in advanced stage, which are clearly distinguishable through the lining of endothelium of the tumor blood vessels. These could confound identification of proteins as drug targets.

In selecting new targets, polypharmacological approaches have greatly improved drug discovery but challenges still exist that require improved methodologies. Finding the druggability of the identified targets using the omics technology has added another level of complexity in the rational design of compounds that would meet the expectation of having all the required binding regions of proteins in the intracellular space [68]. Establishing the relevance of network models to human disease biology can also be challenging. A model that proves very effective in one system might not be reproducible in another system. The utilization of tissue and plasma samples from a disease population can play a role in validating the target hypothesis but effectiveness depends on the particular disease studied [69,70]. Most of the time, it could be helpful in particular, for chronic diseases that have not been well characterized. The target-centric approach is well suited for the high throughput screens needed to define the structure–activity relationships of the lead molecules, but in some cases this could only demonstrate a suboptimal efficacy and safety profile. Thus, blind trust in high throughput technologies may lead to unknown limitations.

Systems biology, which enables the determination of biological complexity at the level of the entire system, is a very promising strategy in drug discovery. However, due to the extent of connectivity between the genome, proteome, the entire cell systems, the molecular architecture, and entire functionality of the cell system, all this information adds more depth toward the understanding of the processes involved. This requires investigating the genes, other cells, and environmental influences at the biological level, such as polygenic diseases. The multifactorial nature of disease involving this web of molecular interactions must be well investigated to exclude flaws for efficient unraveling of the molecular pathways to describe diseases at a higher level or dimension. Thus, without knowledgeable scientists with a higher degree of specialization in the appropriate field, deficiency in skills might affect output standards. Certain technology platforms might demand more specialized skill sets.

Advances in discovery research technology have pioneered recent breakthroughs in the enhancement of the drug discovery process, marked by observed success in many areas, including biologics, but this has not settled the recurring drug attrition rates as there are still a limited number of valid targets [71]. Most of these approved drugs have similar mechanisms (e.g., ceftobiprole, with 15 similar agents) as the active moieties on structures bind to the same receptors. Often, the same or closely related mechanisms are repeated and could be verified by using the date of first registration of a US adopted name, available from the United States Pharmacopeia dictionary [72].

4.5.2 Network/System Biology Application-Limitations

Advances and modernizations in biological techniques and incorporation of system biology provide a growing knowledge of biological regulatory mechanisms and data volume, which is rapidly increasing. But this has not sufficiently served the purpose as a complete understanding of the systems-level biology has not been achieved. The omics techniques, even though they are high throughput and efficient, may not adequately detect all changes in the system under investigation as they are not all–encompassing. Systematic or methodology defects might influence the integrity of data and hence, inappropriate experimental design may generate erroneous data. Well-conducted studies mainly rely on the proficiency of the laboratory analysts – poorly constructed networks might include incomplete inclusion of data from proteins and interactions and also choice measurement parameters that could lead to methodological artifacts. Certain elements of biological systems might not be thoroughly represented. There has also been a focus on selected families for the application of systems biology approach.

An impediment to biological investigations in drug discovery is that the human genome is not known in its entirety, that is to say, not all of the genome had been cloned. A consequence of this is that biological models are not all-encompassing and predictions are not all-inclusive. This means that disrupting an agent or protein in a pathological pathway could lead to a variety of possibilities; it could negate, promote, or alter other pathways that are not known. Even though the models are a representation of the organ systems, knowledge gaps still exist. What is the probability that these changes could lead to an expected result?

4.5.3 The Impact of the Pharmaceutical Ecosystem

Drug discovery projects are highly influenced by the strength of the ecosystem, which is comprised of stakeholders who make decisions that strongly impact target selection, for example, health-related social groups, law and health policy makers, investors, patients/doctors, drug regulators, and potential payers (see Introduction). These types of influences have been disclosed through social audits. The internal groups are, from top to bottom, the chief executive officer and the board members who approve the proposals including the disease areas and research budget. A consensus has to be reached among the top personnel of the company including the marketing and financial leaders or directors before embarking on such a project. A well-informed decision requires a team of experts, well knowledgeable in the area, and must not be biased or subjected to particular motives.

For example, following the approval of a drug discovery research and development (R&D) project, a research portfolio will be established, which includes the selected indication or therapeutic area and projects. This mostly is debated among the responsible personnel, the senior scientists or managers, and the research directors. Approval of a project is based on the ability to show significant improvement over existing ones or that it holds high prospect for success (although not entirely predictable as some of the low rated projects have amounted to huge returns on investment).

4.5.4 Effect of Size and Capability

Bio/pharmaceutical organizations of different capacities engage in discovery and development of therapeutic agents. Company size and financial power influences the number of targets pursued. For example, a start-up or biotech might be working on four targets while a multinational pharmaceutical company might be working on 40 targets, which, intuitively, will require a higher research investment and which in turn, increases the probability of success. This is why the biotech or small pharmaceutical companies grapple with lack of funding or reach operational hiatus, prompting an exhaustive search for alternative means of company survival. Thus, time and capital are of a paramount value and these important elements have a major impact on the prospect for functional breakthrough.

REFERENCES

[1] Collins FS, Morgan M, Patrinos A. The human genome project: lessons from large-scale biology. Science 2003;300:286–90.

[2] Battelle Technology Partnership Practice, Economic Impact of the Human Genome Project [Internet]; 2011. Available from: http://www.battelle.org/publications/humangenomeproject.pdf [accessed 06.01.2015].

[3] Drews J. Drug discovery: a historical perspective. Science 2000;287:1960–4.

[4] Yeh R, Lim LP, Burge CB. Computational inference of homologous gene structures in the human genome. Genome Res 2001;11(5):803–16.

[5] Paolini GV, Shapland RH, Van Hoorn WP, Mason JS, Hopkins AL. Global mapping of pharmacological space. Nat Biotechnol 2006;24:805–15.

[6] Hopkins AL. Network pharmacology: the next paradigm in drug discovery. Nat Chem Biol 2008;4:682–90.

[7] Metz JT, Hajduk PJ. Rational approaches to targeted polypharmacology: creating and navigating protein-ligand interaction networks. Curr Opin Chem Biol 2010;14:498–504.

[8] Barabási AL. The network takeover. Nat Phys 2012;8:14–6.

[9] Schadt EE. Molecular networks as sensors and drivers of common human diseases. Nature 2009;461:218–23.

[10] Available from: https://openinnovation.lilly.com/

[11] Swinney DC, Anthony J. How were medicines discovered? Nat Rev Drug Discov 2011;10:507–19.

[12] Kell DB. Genotype: phenotype mapping: genes as computer programs. Trends Genet 2002;18:555–9.

[13] Zheng W, Natasha Thorne N, McKew JC. Phenotypic screens as a renewed approach for drug discovery. Drug Discov Today 2013;18(21–22):1067–73.

[14] Lee JA, Berg EL. Neoclassic drug discovery: the case for lead generation using phenotypic and functional approaches. J Biomol Screen 2013;18(10):1143–55.

[15] Available from: http://www.pd2.lilly.com

[16] Available from: http://www.ncats.nih.gov/research/rare-diseases/trnd/trnd.html

[17] Barabási AL, Gulbahce N, Loscalzo J. Network medicine: a network-based approach to human disease. Nat Rev Genet 2011;12:56–68.

[18] Silverman EK, Loscalzo J. Network medicine approaches to the genetics of complex diseases. Discov Med 2012;14:143–52.

[19] Hood L, Perlmutter RM. The impact of systems approaches on biological problems in drug discovery. Nat Biotechnol 2004;22:1215–7.

[20] Butcher EC, Berg EL, Kunkel EJ. Systems biology in drug discovery. Nat Biotechnol 2004;22:1253–9.

[21] Weston AD, Hood L. Systems biology, proteomics, and the future of health care: toward predictive, preventative, and personalized medicine. J Proteome Res 2004;3:179–96.

[22] Kohl P, Noble D. Systems biology and the virtual physiological human. Mol Syst Biol 2009;5:292.

[23] Rosenwald A, Wright G, Chan WC, Connors JM, Campo E, Rosenwald A, Wright G, Chan WC, Connors JM, Campo E, Fisher RI, Gascoyne RD, Muller-Hermelink HK, Smeland EB, Giltnane JM, Hurt EM, Zhao H, Averett L, Yang L, Wilson WH, Jaffe ES, Simon R, Klausner RD, Powell J, Duffey PL, Longo DL, Greiner TC, Weisenburger DD, Sanger WG, Dave BJ, Lynch JC, Vose J, Armitage JO, Montserrat E, López-Guillermo A, Grogan TM, Miller TP, LeBlanc M, Ott G, Kvaloy S, Delabie J, Holte H, Krajci P, Stokke T, Staudt LM. The use of molecular profiling to predict survival after chemotherapy for diffuse large-B-cell lymphoma. N Engl J Med 2002;346:1937–47.

[24] Phillip CJ, Giardina CK, Bilir B, Cutler DJ, Lai Y, Kucuk O, Moreno CS. Genistein cooperates with the histone deacetylase inhibitor vorinostat to induce cell death in prostate cancer cells. BMC Cancer 2012;12:145.

[25] Available from: http://metabolomics.se/Images/Research/Sy

[26] Barabási AL, Gulbahce N, Loscalzo J. Network medicine: a network-based approach to human disease. Nat Rev Genet 2011;12:56–68.

[27] Ideker T, Krogan NJ. Differential network biology. Mol Syst Biol 2012;8(565):1–9.

[28] Isserlin R, Emili A. Nine steps to proteomic wisdom: a practical guide to using protein-protein interaction networks and molecular pathways as a framework for interpreting disease proteomic profiles. Proteomics Clin Appl 2007;1(9):1156–68.

[29] Li J, Zhu XY, Chen JY. Building disease-specific drug-protein connectivity maps from molecular interaction networks and PubMed abstracts. PLoS Comput Biol 2009;5(7):1–15.

[30] Margineanu DG. Systems biology impact on antiepileptic drug discovery. Epilepsy Res 2012;98(2–3):104–15.

[31] Zhao ZM, Kier LB, Buck GA. Systems biology: molecular networks and disease. Chem Biodivers 2012;9(5):841–7.

[32] Schlage WK, Westra JW, Gebel S, Catlett NL, Mathis C, Frushour BP, Hengstermann A, Hooser AV, Poussin C, Wong B, Lietz M, Park J, Drubin D, Veljkovic E, Peitsch MC, Hoeng J, Deehan R. A compatible cellular stress network model for non-diseased pulmonary and cardiovascular tissue. BMC Syst Biol 2011;5:168.

[33] Hu X, Zhao D, Strotmann A. Mapping molecular association networks of nervous system diseases via large-scale analysis of published research. PLoS One 2013;8(6):e67121.

[34] Suthram S, Dudley JT, Chiang AP, Chen R, Hastie TJ, Butte AJ. Network-based elucidation of human disease similarities reveals common functional modules enriched for pluripotent drug targets. PLoS Comput Biol 2010;6(2):e1000662.

[35] Visscher PM, Brown MA, McCarthy MI, Yang J. Five years of GWAS discovery. Am J Hum Genet 2012;90:7–24.

[36] Campillos M, Kuhn M, Gavin AC, Jensen LJ, Bork P. Drug target identification using side-effect similarity. Science 2008;321(5886):263–6.

[37] National Human Genome Research Institute – a catalog of published genome-wide association studies. Available from: http://www.genome.gov/gwastudies

[38] The Pharmacogenomics Knowledge Base. Literature analysis by R. Ranganathan and C. Woods. Available from: http://www.pharmgkb.org

[39] Manolio TA. Genome wide association studies and assessment of the risk of disease. N Engl J Med 2010;363(2):166–76.

[40] Merino A, Bronowska AK, Jackson DB, Cahill DJ. Drug profiling: knowing where it hits. Drug Discov Today 2010;15(17-18):749–56.

[41] Berman J, Haffajee CI, Alpert JS. Therapy of symptomatic pericarditis after myocardial infarction: retrospective and prospective studies of aspirin, indomethacin, prednisone, and spontaneous resolution. Am Heart J 1981;101(6):750–3.

[42] Durongpisitkul K, Gururaj VJ, Park JM, Martin CF. The prevention of coronary artery aneurysm in Kawasaki disease: a meta-analysis on the efficacy of aspirin and immunoglobulin treatment. Pediatrics 1995;96(6):1057–61.

[43] Grundmann K, Jaschonek K, Kleine B, Dichgans J, Topka H. Aspirin non-responder status in patients with recurrent cerebral ischemic attacks. J Neurol 2003;250(1):63–6.

[44] Amory JK, Amory DW. Dosing frequency of aspirin and prevention of heart attacks and strokes. Am J Med 2007;120(4):e5.

[45] Daya S. Recurrent spontaneous early pregnancy loss and low dose aspirin. Minerva Ginecol 2003;55(5):441–9.

[46] Baron JA. Aspirin and cancer: trials and observational studies. J Natl Cancer Inst 2012;. djs338.

[47] Schmid A, Blank LM. Hypothesis-driven omics integration. Nat Chem Biol 2010;6(7):485–7.

[48] Joyce AR, Palsson BO. The model organism as a system: integrating "omics" data sets. Nat Rev Mol Cell Biol 2006;7(3):198–210.

[49] Boran ADW, Iyengar R. Systems approaches to polypharmacology and drug discovery. Curr Opin Drug Discov Devel 2010;13(3):297–309.

[50] Oprea TI, Nielsen SK, Ursu O, Yang JJ, Taboureau O, Mathias SL, Kouskoumvekaki L, Sklar LA, Bologa CG. Associating drugs, targets and clinical outcomes into an integrated network affords a new platform for computer-aided drug repurposing. Mol Inform 2011;30(2-3):100–11.

[51] Achenbach J, Tiikkainen P, Franke L, Proschak E. Computational tools for polypharmacology and repurposing. Future Med Chem 2011;3(8):961–8.

[52] Paolini GV, Shapland RH, van Hoorn WP, Mason JS, Hopkins AL. Global mapping of pharmacological space. Nat Biotechnol 2006;24:805–15.

[53] Reddy SA, Shuxing Z. Polypharmacology: drug discovery for the future. Expert Rev Clin Pharmacol 2013;6(1):10.

[54] Auffray C, Chen Z, Hood L. Systems medicine: the future of medical genomics and healthcare. Genome Med 2009;1(2):90. Capobianco E. Ten challenges for systems medicine. Front Genet 2012;3:193.

[55] Hood L, Flores M. A personal view on systems medicine and the emergence of proactive P4 medicine: predictive, preventive, personalized and participatory. New Biotechnol 2012;29:613–24.

[56] Mardinoglu A, Nielsen J. Systems medicine and metabolic modelling. J Intern Med 2012;271:142–54.

[57] Wolkenhauer O, Auffray C, Jaster R, Steinhoff G, Dammann O. The road from systems biology to systems medicine. Pediatr Res 2013;73:502–7.

[58] Zhao S, Iyengar R. Systems pharmacology: network analysis to identify multiscale mechanisms of drug action. Ann Rev Pharmacol Toxicol 2012;52(52):505–21.

[59] Boran AD, Iyengar R. Systems approaches to polypharmacology and drug discovery. Curr Opin Drug Discov Devel 2010;13(3):297–309.

[60] Dar A, Das T, Shokat K, Cagan R. Chemical genetic discovery of targets and anti-targets for cancer polypharmacology. Nature 2012;486(7401):80–4.

[61] Boran AD, Iyengar R. Systems pharmacology. Mount Sinai J Med 2010;77(4):333–44.

[62] Xie L, Xie L, Kinnings SL, Bourne PE. Novel computational approaches to polypharmacology as a means to define responses to individual drugs. Ann Rev Pharmacol Toxicol 2012;52(52):361.

[63] Lounkine E, Keiser MJ, Whitebread S, Mikhailov D, Hamon J, Jenkins JL, Lavan P, Weber E, Doak K, Côté S, Shoichet BK, Urban L. Large-scale prediction and testing of drug activity on side-effect targets. Nature 2012;486(7403):361–7.

[64] Allison M. NCATS launches drug repurposing program. Nat Biotechnol 2012;30(7):571–2.

[65] Tian Q, Stepaniants SB, Mao M, Weng L, Feetham MC, Doyle MJ, Yi EC, Dai H, Thorsson V, Eng J, Goodlett D, Berger JP, Gunter B, Linseley PS, Stoughton RB, Aebersold R, Collins SJ, Hanlon WA, Hood LE. Integrated genomic and proteomic analyses of gene expression in mammalian cells. Mol Cell Proteomics 2004;3:960–9.

[66] Szallasi Z. Genetic network analysis in light of massively parallel biological data acquisition. Pac Symp Biocomput 1999;5–16.

[67] Swinney DC, Anthony J. How were new medicines discovered? Nat Rev Drug Discov 2011;10:507–19.

[68] Paul SM, Mytelka DS, Dunwiddie CT, Persinger CC, Munos BH, Lindborg SR, Schacht AL. How to improve R&D productivity: the pharmaceutical industry's grand challenge. Nat Rev Drug Discov 2010;9:203–14.

[69] Andersen MR, et al. Trends in the exploitation of novel drug targets. Nat Rev Drug Discov 2011;10:579–90.

[70] Knowles J, Gromo G. Target selection in drug discovery. Nat Rev 2003;2(1):63–9.

[71] Pammolli F, Magazzini L, Riccaboni M. The productivity crisis in pharmaceutical R&D. Nat Drug Discov 2011;10:428–38.

[72] The USP Dictionary of USAN and International Drug Names. US Pharmacopeial Convention; 2010.

CHAPTER 5

The Significance of Discovery Screening and Structure Optimization Studies

Odilia Osakwe

Contents

5.1 Introduction	109
5.2 Screening Tools in Drug Discovery	110
5.2.1 High Throughput Screening in Drug Discovery	110
5.2.2 Setbacks in HTS Application	112
5.2.3 Bioassays	112
5.3 In Silico Models in Drug Discovery and Design	114
5.3.1 Virtual Screening	115
5.3.2 Computer-Aided Drug Design	116
5.3.3 Structure–Activity Relationship in Drug Discovery	118
5.3.4 Pharmacophore Models of Drug Targeting	120
5.3.5 Cheminformatics and Bioinformatics Technology	122
5.4 From Hit to Lead: Summary of Compound Optimization in Drug Discovery	123
References	126

5.1 INTRODUCTION

The last 20 years have seen a major change in drug development processes due to incremental introduction of new technologies, which contributes to competencies in design, screening, and identification of new chemical entities leading to evolution of a rapid, integrated, and highly targeted process. With the increasing incorporation of the systems biology paradigm in drug discovery, complexity of cellular function has intensified the drug discovery processes. Nevertheless, incremental introduction of technological tools has widened the available options, facilitating the study of the simultaneous function of multiple gene products and enabling a better understanding of the cellular function. Increasing technological introductions, for example, the "omics" tool, have widened the scope of drug discovery research, increasing the ability to explore the biological networks, with enhanced capabilities in finding disease drug targets. The increasing ability to link

Social Aspects of Drug Discovery, Development and Commercialization Copyright © 2016 Elsevier Inc.
http://dx.doi.org/10.1016/B978-0-12-802220-7.00005-3 All rights reserved.

diseases to proteins (in physiological or pathophysiological environments) has led to an exponential rise in drug targets as they continue to escalate in the order of 1000 targets for a single disease associated protein [1], requiring more extensive efforts in handling the growing compound population and vast chemical space [2].

The emergence of computations and related technologies has sparked an enthusiasm to embrace rational approaches, thus *in silico* technology has become an integral part of industrial and academic research. Computer-assisted design has prompted a better handling of the highly diverse molecules investigated, further facilitating the precise identification of optimal drug candidates with better prospects for success. High throughput screening has helped in the screening of extensive data sample populations to reduce time and cost and which allow better control over experimental complexity [3]. The "informatics" technology has improved data organization, leading to elaborate data analysis and display, greatly providing an enabling environment for pharmaceutical innovation and new medical solutions.

The current explosion in technological contributions has enabled the disease process to be better understood and evaluated for drug targets, and increase the number of diseases targeted by the drug developers. Despite the promises offered by advancing technology, adaptation of existing methods to address the scale of the genomics era has been a challenge, leading to much difficulty in creating new drugs [4]. The previous chapter dealt with the initial early discovery research, which is mostly concerned with the techniques for exploring the pathogenic pathways to finding drug targets. This chapter will discuss the tools involved in compound optimization toward the selection of a lead drug compound that is taken to the preclinical stage of the drug discovery program. The strategies, relevance, prospects, and setbacks will be discussed.

5.2 SCREENING TOOLS IN DRUG DISCOVERY

5.2.1 High Throughput Screening in Drug Discovery

High throughput screening (HTS) is one of the leading technological breakthroughs in drug discovery. The pharmaceutical industry strictly depends on HTS for generating hits from the explosive library of the compound database. The stepwise screening strategy tends to eliminate both compounds that fail the standard criteria and the probability of errors generated [5]. Robotic and automation technology permits handling of an enormously large number of compounds. Robotic liquid handlers are tailored technologies for micropipetting at blistering speeds, well suited to over a million screening assays conducted within 1–3 months. Since initial screens always need validation and optimizations for any drug discovery approach, the relevance or usefulness of HTS is not directly determined. In general, due to project complexity, a number of procedures and techniques confirm function and delivery of the right drug compound that is not directly attributable to HTS. An important part of cell-based HTS is high content screening, which has drawn interest because of its multiplexing ability and the efficiency in enabling detection of functional cell characteristics [6]. High throughput experimental technologies have stimulated increasing incorporation of the systems' point of view in cellular and molecular biology, promoting the study cells as systems.

HTS has been instrumental to the empirical approach to drug discovery, which is based on trial and error but not on any prior known biological properties or mechanism of action. It has been dedicated to early drug discovery processes, but is now increasingly being integrated to downstream processes of lead optimization, encouraging scientists and engineers to streamline workflows with reduced timelines [7]. The changing drug discovery program that incorporates parallel programs (which is shifting from the earlier sequential process of the past) allows much of the information generated to be utilized concurrently, and thus increases the number of compounds generated through robotic systems. The multidimensional workflow and use of low-volume assays underlie its cost effectiveness. Increased miniaturization, through micro- or nanochip-based approaches and on-bead screening, has helped to expand its capabilities. Solid-support-on-bead screening has reduced reactions to nanoscale levels, making it easier to process large datasets within a short period of time. Thus, high throughput screening is no longer a concern [8].

Larger databases provide a greater variety of options and more insight into possible leads during the critical stages of the discovery process. The timely access of information allows a more managed and distribution system. The statistical computations and algorithms are proven standards that permit better organization of HTS data for high performance [9,10].

Development of the Molecular Libraries Initiative, the Molecular Libraries and the Screening Center Network, and eventually the Production Center Network was part of the National Institutes of Health Roadmap program strategy to advance chemical biology. This led to the setting up of translational- and chemical-screening programs at academic screening centers in many US universities. All contributed to generating diverse chemical libraries and the development of novel chemistries based on HTS. These tools are indispensable in advancing understanding of complex biology for target and disease pathway identification and are well-validated potential medical therapies [11,12].

5.2.2 Setbacks in HTS Application

A known fact is the effectiveness of HTS in the discovery of new chemotypes in translational research, which has enabled the progression of compound optimization studies. But still, productivity decline has not been completely addressed. Sound performance of HTS also depends on the target classes, which is very limiting as the broad screening approaches remain ineffective for certain subclasses like Class B G-protein-coupled receptors. As a major contributor to finding drug leads, HTS has often been criticized for its "dead end" lead compounds [13,14]. Certain compounds in the HTS libraries are too complex, making it difficult to access the cellular protein targets for these compounds [15]. This is because not all the hits harbor the required structural features following the primary screening [16]. The problem of compound solubility in physical stability could limit HTS effectiveness.

In HTS, the number of hits multiplies with the number of compounds screened but since the budget for HTS is always limited to cover the cost for screening a huge number whole collection this could reach millions of compounds. The postgenomic era inspired technological novelty that led to a burst in the number of therapeutic targets, which are mostly large-molecule modulators. Heightening increase in cost of innovative therapies and tightening of budgets are continuing to shape policy decisions throughout the world. This has pressurized bio/pharmaceutical research and development (R&D) to actively generate new molecular entities as fully developed commercialized drugs [17].

5.2.3 Bioassays

Biological assays are biological experimental methods for screening potential bioactive molecules for the identification of structural leads and the prediction of potentially useful pharmacological activity or therapeutic potential that informs compound development. These assays are often carried to assign biological properties to the compounds. The biologically active moieties are validated and then screened in series in more specific or secondary assays.

Primary bioassays are the first line of screening that identifies possible bioactivity. These assays are usually high capacity, low cost, and rapid. Potential drug targets in the form of recombinant proteins are expressed in these cells and then measured with linked secondary messenger systems in order to measure functional response. It is very useful in determining whether a drug is an agonist or antagonist at the target.

Cell-based assays are specifically used to detect a functional response [18]. It is generally applicable to selected target categories such as membrane receptors, ion channels, and nuclear receptors, and is mostly based on mammalian cell lines overexpressing the target of interest. These receptors have been shown as specific sites of action of the biochemical messenger systems. Primary cell systems are increasingly being employed for compound screening [19]. Cell-based assays offer the advantage associated with its applicability in evaluating human targets when the human cell systems are in use. If a drug exhibits a functional response, then biochemical assay is initiated. The functional assay can enable determination of efficacy, toxicity, and allosteric effectors (distant actors) in the primary screen. Challenges for cellular assays include the need to keep low dimethyl sulfoxide concentration and cell culture volume. Identifying off-target activities would need additional exhaustive steps to rectify the problem.

Biochemical assays are focused on measuring the compound–target affinity. They also are applicable to both receptor and enzyme targets [20]. They do not provide any information on the pharmacological mechanism of the drug action, like determination of an inhibitory or stimulatory (agonists or antagonists) action but utility is based on the assumption that human binding activity will be equivalent at the native human target. The relevance becomes obvious when tested in functional *in vitro* or *in vivo* assays.

The use of cell-based and biochemical assays has been debated elsewhere [21]. Pharmacologists utilize bioassays to identify biological properties of drug compounds under early development. As the discovery program progresses, from early exploratory research to clinical evaluation, the experiments become more extensive since the molecules become increasingly complex, and are scrutinized more intensely as the drug discovery cycle approaches the clinical stage. This is a time when a wide range of biopharmaceutical properties of the compound are optimized by the chemist requiring intact physiological systems and testing of absorption, distribution, metabolism, elimination, and toxicity (ADMET) properties over the massive data generated with combinatorial chemistry.

5.3 *IN SILICO* MODELS IN DRUG DISCOVERY AND DESIGN

Biology has experienced an increased use of highly sophisticated systems mathematics and computer simulations leading to growing application of *in silico* techniques. *In silico* refers to the use of computers to perform biological studies. Its usefulness in human biology has improved drug discovery inquiry at the biological level – *in silico* tools simulate responses at the scale of disease manifestation in both cell and tissue or organ [22,23].

Computer models take into consideration the complex processes that utilize what is known about the properties of each component in the system and their interconnectivity [24]. Thus, computer models are applicable in rational drug design, which solely depends on the existing biological and pharmacological properties of compounds. Series of compounds with such qualities are screened for the selection of the most viable candidates. *In silico* organisms are computer representations of their *in vivo* models. These methods are both algorithm and network based. An algorithm tool can be used to determine the number of drug combinations in a data screening. For example, the algorithm can minimize the number of trial experiments in the order of tens of thousands of possible combinations. It could be utilized for the identification of a well worked out drug combination and the core disease causative pathways. Computational experiments can now analyze the integrated networks associated with the host mechanisms, mostly the pathological pathways, to assign therapeutic strategies using parallel models. Certain considerations such as efficiencies, toxicities, and other side effects of drugs enable the managing of diseases from a system perspective [25].

Some examples are screening models called Medicinal Algorithmic Combinational Screen, and quantitative composition-activity relationship of herbal formulae. The network-based biological computational tools are applied through mathematical modeling of biological pathways to determine the higher level cellular effects of the multitarget drugs. The integrated Network Target-Based Identification of Multicomponent Synergy model, which can transfer correlations between drugs to the interactions among their molecular targets [26,27], emphasizes its applicability as a data-modeling technique.

The utility of the *in silico* technology has further improved the detection of the toxicological effects of drug compounds [28]. The *in silico* approach has also extended the possibilities of drug repurposing through integrated networks [29,30]. This approach evaluates the genetic variations that contribute to variable responses to drugs for individualized medicine application and for the prediction of disease susceptibility [31].

5.3.1 Virtual Screening

The increasing difficulty experienced in the biological screening of billions of compounds is the reason for the application of computer-aided drug screening approaches in drug discovery, named virtual screening (VS). VS is a set of computer methods that screen large chemical databases in virtual HTS (from a virtual library) to select compounds for synthesis, allowing structure-based screening of up to 100,000 molecules per day using parallel processing clusters. This approach has been applied in the early stages of discovery to prioritize chemicals for evaluation of biological properties to enable a mechanistic understanding of these predictions and to know the potential activity levels. VS was initially intended to save costs and as substitute for HTS, but the clarity of the role of each can be increasingly seen as rather complementary. Recent developments have taken advantage of both, particularly in finding compound leads [32]. The role of VS in hit (bioactive molecules) identification strategy cannot be underestimated as its utility is becoming more obvious, just as HTS and VS have both been actively applied as an integrated technique for hit and lead identification [33].

In VS, a library containing a large number of molecular compounds of about 10^5–10^7 molecules is downsized by a computational algorithm to about 10^0–10^3 that are tested experimentally. Ranking compounds according to pharmaceutical relevance has been made possible due to its ability to predict the putative binding affinities between small molecules and biological receptors with potential therapeutic qualities [34]. A parallel approach allows multiple protocols to be carried out synchronously to generate integrated data. VS has served unique roles to enable identification of compounds when there is lack of biological assays for HTS, leading to the use of homology modeling to produce a receptor-based pharmacophore model allowing selection of molecules for validation.

Focused or knowledge-based screening is applied with a selection of smaller subsets of molecules from a chemical library. The selected candidates would be those that show some activity at the target protein and that would be based on what is known about the protein or earlier reports or literature, and has led to the utility of pharmacophores and molecular modeling to conduct virtual screens of compound databases [35]. VS is dependent upon how well the known structural information about both, the target and the small molecules being docked, could provide leading information needed for effective screening. The target is probed for the presence of an appropriate binding pocket [36] with the known target–ligand cocrystal structures or using *in silico* methods to identify novel binding sites [37]. For fragment screening, high concentration screens generate small molecular weight compound libraries with high quality and viable protein structures that progress through the discovery path. The academic community and small pharmaceutical companies have benefited from VS as it is less expensive than HTS, and still as efficient or even better.

There are a number of challenges associated with VS technology. For example, medicinal chemists are not fully involved with the initial optimization process that involves VS. This could lead to errors that might only be discovered further downstream the drug discovery process. Publication of drug compounds of such (as successful) masks early discovery of underlying problems that might be discovered later and hence affecting its effectiveness [38]. Recent changes include the increasing incorporation of medicinal chemists into academic programs in order to promote cross-functional or multidisciplinary interaction and active engagement that provide complementary skills.

Limited understanding of the complexity of living organisms deters the ability to establish or build ideal compound libraries, which also depends on the nature, stage, and goal of the project being pursued. Increasing knowledge gathered from the past lessons has brought up further inquiries requiring possible solution pathways that could allow creation of viable library collections [39]. The high cost and amount of time needed to attain the goals of screening compounds, might not directly yield commensurate outcomes. Success also depends on the quality of the compounds screened [39–41]. In addition, management of the facility and the level of expertise of the personnel handling the computer-related projects and appropriateness in data handling are concerns [42].

5.3.2 Computer-Aided Drug Design

Computer-aided drug design (CADD) has been credited to the modern patterns in compound characterization in drug discovery following its inception in 1981 [43]. It represents an advancement when compared to HTS as it requires minimal compound design or prior knowledge, but can yield multiple hit compounds among which promising candidates have been elected. The typical role of CADD in drug discovery is to screen out large compound libraries into smaller clusters of predicted active compounds (Figure 5.1), enabling optimization of lead compounds by improving the biological properties (like affinity and ADMET) and building chemotypes from a nucleating site by combining fragments with optimized function.

Clustering has been applied as a means to select representatives from screening libraries [44]. Screening hits include molecules that specifically

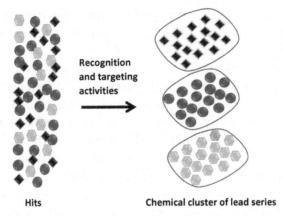

Recognition
and targeting
activities

Hits   Chemical cluster of lead series

Figure 5.1 *Screening of Drug-Like Compounds into Activity Criteria.*

bind to the target in addition to a greater number of nonspecific compounds requiring a triaging process to filter these out (Figure 5.1). Thus, such a large library that contains a number of possible hits is further downsized and clustered into series.

Computational chemistry algorithms have been developed to group hits based on structural similarity, which is necessary to ensure that compounds are adequately sorted over a broad spectrum of chemical classes. Thus, selection of hits would be based on chemical cluster, potency, and factors such as ligand efficiency (which gives an idea of how well a compound binds for its size).

The increasing application of diverse computerized methods in drug discovery has enabled a better handling of data associated with a large number of compounds screened against the target molecules or proteins for leads. Computational tools help to define and elaborate the strength of interaction between ligands and targets, and have been instrumental in the identification of lead molecules from databases. Nevertheless, the lack of specificity leads to low hit rate for HTS, which could limit its applicability and efficiency in screening large compound libraries. CADD is a more targeted approach to the generation of "hits" when compared with traditional HTS. It enables the elucidation of the molecular basis of therapeutic activity and possible derivatives, and those variables that could be applied or improved for generating an optimal drug compound, thus leading to prioritization of the actives without requiring extensive development and validation prior to use, as in the case of assay HTS. The CADD approach has played a vital role in the search and optimization of potential lead compounds with a considerable gain in time and cost. It has been applied during various stages in drug discovery: target identification, validation, molecular design, and interactions of drug candidates with targets of interest [45].

CADD can be structure or ligand based. Structure-based CADD seeks the knowledge of the target protein structure in the determination of interaction levels of all compounds being examined. Ligand-based CADD relies on the chemical similarity criteria, and the predictive, quantitative structure–activity relationship (QSAR) models that it creates from the molecules to determine the known active and inactives [46]. QSAR modeling enables understanding of the influence of structural factors on biological activity, using the models and the understanding to construct compounds with improved and optimal biological profiles. Other methods for quantitative description of structural change are comparative molecular field analysis and GRID.

Structure-based CADD is a preferred choice for soluble proteins that could be crystallized, while ligand-based CADD is better suited for compounds with high binding affinity to the target, devoid of off-target effects, and that could be designed with minimal free energy, favorable drug metabolism, and pharmacokinetic/ADMET properties [47]. In general, CADD is better suited for occasions where sparse structural information is available. This is usually the case for membrane protein targets.

5.3.3 Structure–Activity Relationship in Drug Discovery

Structure–activity relationships (SAR) explore the relationship between a molecule's biological activity and the three-dimensional structure of the molecule; computational chemistry is employed only if the target structure is known. Structural-aided drug design uses crystal structures in the design of molecules. It is often used as an adjunct to other screening strategies within big pharma. A compound is docked into the crystal in order to use it to predict where modifications could be added to provide increased potency or selectivity.

Since the early 1980s drug discovery has principally relied on a target protein's structure to aid drug design. One outstanding strategy is design of compounds through design-make-test-analyze involving expert designers from varied pharmaceutical disciplines that interact to simplify the process of a candidate compound that is taken to the synthetic routes. This involves medicinal, computational, synthetic, and physical chemists and also pharmacokinetics (PK) experts on each project [48–50]. Molecular modeling software packages are often useful to identify binding site interactions, but when there is no previous knowledge of the target structure, traditional noncomputational methods of studying SARs are employed.

Drug molecules typically contain several functional groups, which can interact with certain groups in the biological target. The biological targets respond to compound properties and not structure but have to be determined by downstream process for clinical applications. Structure-based computer-aided drug design (SBCADD) is a promising approach in analyzing 3D structures of biologic molecules. The operating principle of SBCADD is based on the notion that a molecule could interact with a specific protein and exert a desired biologic effect, which essentially relies on its ability to favorably interact with a particular binding site on that protein and that any molecule with this ability could exert similar biologic effects. This has allowed elucidation of novel compounds based on their interaction potential with the protein's binding site. Structural information about the target is a prerequisite for any SBCADD project.

Computational tools offer the opportunity to exploit a database containing new, potential compounds, predicted using QSAR models. A combinatorial approach to constructing chemical libraries results in a chemical space different from that of known drugs and natural products. Because of this, QSAR has been useful in guiding the combinatorial library synthesis for libraries that could be screened for targeted drug classes allowing a wide coverage of chemical space with more likely targeted hits [51].

Pharmaceutical researchers use 3D structural techniques such as protein docking and pharmacophore similarity to specify similar biological activities. An enhanced feature of this permits actual visualization of results – compounds can be viewed docked into the protein structure. This enables adequate selection of highly promising compounds that exhibit favorable protein docking and hence potency. Different structures can act at the same biological target to elicit the same biological action, but the chemical structures, which are mostly atoms separated by bonds, are not what is recognized by a biological target. Two molecules devoid of any structural relationship to one other could mimic each other in occupying the same site on a common target but could exhibit very diverse activities at the target. The electrostatic fields are dynamic and change with the orientation or shape of the drug compound and this resultant electrostatic field that aligns with that of the protein target is the reason for target-drug selectivity [52]. The results of SAR studies can provide information on the intermolecular interactions that are established at the binding site.

5.3.3.1 Limitations of SAR Application

Increasing sophistication in drug discovery tools and technologies has still not completely resolved the most crucial need; the preclinical ADME (absorption, distribution, metabolism, and excretion), safety, and toxicity problems that consequently either fail to meet Food and Drug Administration (FDA) approval, or lead to unanticipated health issues while in the market. ADME prediction with the available models has been an arduous task but when not predictive enough, could, at least, guide the drug developer into safer chemical space [53].

For example, it has become a challenge for the chemist to build a chemotype due to the uncertain probability of success since the structural features do not give precise information about compound activity or all the required attributes of a candidate drug [52]. This obviously requires a huge investment, which might be lost if no alternative viable chemotypes are found. Individual (Q)SAR *in silico* toxicological methods do not consider dose and exposure, unless the exposure–response relationship is part of the study. Therefore, it predicts toxicity independently. For example, the aromatic nitro group that triggers a structural alert for carcinogenicity may pass undetected if this fragment is contained in a chemical that is minimally exposed in the system; its prediction remains questionable. Prediction of a toxicology endpoint is more often performed on a parent chemical structure and such experiment that preclude the metabolite, especially in cases where the metabolite is the principal source of toxicity and could be misleading. Such an experiment that does not consider metabolites of parent compounds has implications for the drug discovery process [54,55].

5.3.4 Pharmacophore Models of Drug Targeting

The pharmacophore is a description of the main molecular features necessary for biological activity and their relative positions in space.

Knowing the key binding site interactions and the pharmacophore, the structural features of lead compounds can be modified to give desired properties. A pharmacophore model of the target binding site is based on the sum of the steric and electronic features that underpin optimal interaction of a ligand with its target. Common features normally used to define the pharmacophore maps are acidic and basic groups, partial charges of hydrogen bond acceptors and donors, aliphatic hydrophobic moieties, and aromatic hydrophobic moieties [56]. A pharmacophore feature map is carefully constructed to categorize all functional groups with similar physiochemical properties (i.e., similar ionizability, hydrogen bonding behavior) as one.

Particular feature definitions could be specific atom types at specific locations. These allow the identification of novel scaffolds but also lead to an increase in false positives. These molecular attributes have led to VS, *de novo* design, and lead optimization [57].

Pharmacophore algorithm software packages used for ligand-based pharmacophore generation include Molecular Operating Environment (MOE), Catalyst [58], genetic algorithm similarity program [59], and Phase [60].

5.3.4.1 How Does the Protein Recognize its Binding Partner?

A protein recognizes its cognate binding drug compound by its grooves or indentures or complementary moieties, just like a lock and key, as the antigen–antibody interactions. Also, electron density or electrostatic interactions by nearby charges resulting in electrostatic fields that change along with the conformational change of drug molecule. Hydrophobic effect allows the molecule to aggregate to exclude the polar water molecules; the "Log P" is an index for quantifying these effects. Two molecules with different classes could engage the same biological site when they have the same type of field pattern described. Comparing these fields could match up or find similar biological activities and this is widely applicable in drug discovery and development. Any active compound displays a field pattern and this can be used to virtually screen the database rather than field patterns, which are not based on structures. The library would be commercially available molecules that could be further developed into leads.

5.3.4.2 Limitations of the Pharmacophore Approaches

Knowing that these methods use a statistical approach, molecular descriptors and experimental data are used to model complex biological processes [61]. The rules for drug-likeness [5,6] relying on simple physicochemical properties are also well known and implemented [62]. There are limitations because it relies on the quality of experimental data, which might not always be available [63].

Strategies that consider protein flexibility are the 3D structures of ADMET proteins, molecular docking, and others, which indicate that these proteins are difficult to investigate – partly due to the huge and flexible ligand-binding cavities within them that can interact with a wide range of ligands. *In silico* toxicology prediction has been a rigorous endeavor due to the several toxicological effects resulting from changes in multiple physiological processes [64].

Both internal and external solutions have been proposed, which include regulatory guidance. Another proposed solution is integrated workflow that incorporates combined use of data extraction, quantitative structure–activity relationships, and read–across methods.

Advances in this field are leading to a transition to a new paradigm of the discovery process, as exemplified by the Toxicity Testing in the 21st Century initiative [64].

5.3.5 Cheminformatics and Bioinformatics Technology

Computer technology and biology, particularly genomics, revolutionized drug discovery. This combination has been termed bioinformatics while specialized computational programs that deals with chemical data and the associated tools for prioritizing drug compounds is known as cheminformatics. The introduction of bioinformatics and cheminformatics approaches has been very useful in crucial points of the drug discovery processes for better handling of data associated with complex molecular mechanisms, requiring extensive integration of structure and bioactivity data generated at various points. Their exclusive benefits stem from their ability to scrutinize large data volumes for data uniformity, security, and management, thus islands of data developed and maintained within each department could be exchanged.

These techniques have challenged drug developers to learn more about computers and aspects that interface with the chemistry or biology of drug discovery. Successful integration of such knowledge has resulted in the availability of databases that are the largest in the world. Celera, Inc.'s database of human genome information is reportedly the largest private database in the United States.

Through bioinformatics, there is better control of sequence data derived from the Human Genome Project irrespective of the size and level of complexity, for better results [65]. Its application in data mining has enabled the finding of disease targets, which relies on a wide source of data that is associated with the biological approaches. One example is the genotype with the phenotype, a genetic polymorphism, and the risk of disease progression where amyloid precursor proteins lead to an increase in the formation of the A beta peptide associated with Alzheimer's disease and deposition in the brain [66].

These technologies offer a great deal of confidence in the handling of complex data associated with the intricate molecular mechanisms that require extensive integration of structure and bioactivity data generated at various points in the product lifecycle. However, there are still concerns associated with the management of enormous data generated through analysis of multiple large databases simultaneously, placing a special demand for software, hardware, and behavior developments. Before the inception of bioinformatics and cheminformatics, handling of large individual databases remained a daunting task, which currently is being addressed through the informatics technologies, although the challenges of efficient correlation of such diversified information still exist [67].

The United States National Center for Biotechnology Information has been responsible for keeping databases for genome projects. GenBank, an international collaboration of three databases between the United States, the European Molecular Biology Institute, and the DNA Data Bank of Japan, constantly engages in interchange of database information. This has resulted in problems requiring continual update of records in the old database regarding the use of terms and tags that are not consistent with the new format. Private companies are building web interfaces for their database offerings. Celera and Incyte offer web subscriptions to their proprietary databases and customized analysis tools. It appears that the bioinformatics child will continue to speak the web language.

Bank It is a web submission program that includes the top 100 most-accessed information. Sequin is GenBank's submission program, running on several platforms, with complicated entries and the ability to locate errors such as missing organism information, incorrect coding region lengths, mismatched amino acids, or internal stop codons in coding regions, and more.

Information exchange in drug discovery would have been more constrained if it were not for the increasing application of informatics [68].

5.4 FROM HIT TO LEAD: SUMMARY OF COMPOUND OPTIMIZATION IN DRUG DISCOVERY

Compounds that exhibit a positive response in the biological assays are called "hits." These compounds have the potential of becoming the "leads," if the positive response is continuously maintained. A "hit" molecule can vary in its definition by different researchers. Generally, a hit could be defined as a compound with a desired activity following compound screening.

A "lead" is defined as a hit confirmed by more than one assay *in vitro*, and if possible *in vivo*, in a manner that shows biologically relevant activity that correlates to the target. To be a lead, the compound must show evidence that a SAR can be built around it [2].

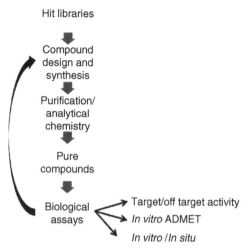

Figure 5.2 *Iterative Process of Compound Design, Synthesis, and Testing.*

Once a drug hit shows a possibility with its target, series of further chemical modifications take place to ensure *in vivo* compliance and adequate functionality. Multiple chemical series are generated based on the structural framework of the hit molecules, leading to an enormous number of compounds with wide chemical and structural diversity. The classical medicinal chemistry approach is used to build a SAR by modifying substituents on a structural scaffold using mostly biochemical knowledge to obtain the desired affinity for the target. Most chemical libraries focus on the chemical series that contain many variations on the same molecular scaffold or molecular backbone. Medicinal chemists utilize many strategies like combinatorial chemistry to introduce structural changes in order to improve a compound's pharmacodynamics properties.

Combinatorial chemistry involves preparation of diverse compounds and structures by synthesis methods. It could be simply defined as a technology involved in the creation of large diversity libraries, speeding up the production of a wide combination of reactive chemical entities. It has aided the construction the chemicals in a way that improve the biological properties that are determined through bioassays (Figure 5.2). Together with HTS it is expected to provide more biological data in the same proportion with the efficiency of the technique used.

As the chemical series are being evaluated, the pharmacological profile further narrows the series and helps to prioritize the hit compounds. Parallel models in drug compound optimization seek to synchronize biological

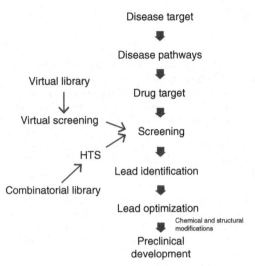

Figure 5.3 *The Pathway Leading to Compound Optimization in Drug Discovery.*

with chemical studies that increasingly transform the drug compounds to become more drug-like for future clinical application. Successive screenings of the drug molecules lead to a more extended HTS of arrayed targets and ligands (Figure 5.3).

The newly found pharmacologically active moieties might not possess the drug-like properties. Thus, as the bioassays are being conducted, the medicinal chemists use relevant robust data as a foundation for decision making on the chemical modification (Figure 5.3), which gives rise to drug-like qualities. Molecular modification often involves adapting the molecular structure into one that has improved drug qualities, which would exhibit properties like potency, minimized side effects, bioactivity, and improved PK. Such data would be used to identify the undesirable activities and to determine SARs at the molecular targets to aid drug design while excluding the undesirable attributes from the chemical series. The modified versions of the lead compound could be synthesized in order to reduce side effects, enhance affinity for one receptor over another, and/or improve activity.

The iterative screening and optimization schemes have taken varied formats, where the building knowledge enables the development process, resulting in a lead compound optimized for potency, selectivity, and PK qualities. When the selectivity profile has been established, and pharmacology attributes and druggability have been duly confirmed for a particular drug, the drug development cycle progresses to the preclinical phase.

REFERENCES

[1] Horrobin DF. Realism in drug discovery – could Cassandra be right? Nat Biotechnol 2001;19:1099.

[2] Drew KL, Baiman H, Khwaounjoo P, Yu B, Reynisson J. Size estimation of chemical space: how big is it? J Pharm Pharmacol 2012;64:490–5.

[3] Fox S, Farr-Jones S, Sopchak L, Boggs A, Wang Nicely H, Khoury R, Biroshigh M. High throughput screening: update on practices and success. J Biomol Screen 2006;11:864–9.

[4] Lahana R. How many leads from HTS? Drug Discov Today 1999;4:447–8.

[5] Coma I, Clark L, Diez E, Harper G, Herranz J, Hofmann G, Lennon M, Richmond N, Valmaseda M, Macarron R. Process validation and screen reproducibility in high-throughput screening. J Biomol Screen 2009;14:66–76.

[6] Nichols A. High content screening as a screening tool in drug discovery. Methods Mol Biol 2007;356:379–87.

[7] Bleicher KH, Böhm HJ, Müller K, Alanine AI. Hit and lead generation: beyond high-throughput screening. Nature Rev Drug Discov 2003;2:369–78.

[8] Houston JG, Banks MN, Binnie A, Brenner S, O'Connell JO, Petrillo EW. Case study: impact of technology investment on lead discovery at Bristol-Myers Squibb, 1998–2006. Drug Discov Today 2008;13:44–51.

[9] Zhang JH, Chung TD, Oldenburg KR. A simple statistical parameter for use in evaluation and validation of high throughput screening assays. J Biomol Screen 1999;4:67–73.

[10] Makarenkov V, Zentilli P, Kevorkov D, Gagarin A, Malo N, Nadon R. An efficient method for the detection and elimination of systematic error in high-throughput screening. Bioinformatics 2007;23:1648–57.

[11] Kaiser J. Industrial-style screening meets academic biology. Science 2008;321:764–6.

[12] Silber BM. Driving drug discovery: the fundamental role of academic labs. Sci Transl Med 2010;2:30cm16.

[13] Posner BA. High-throughput screening-driven lead discovery: meeting the challenges of finding new therapeutics. Curr Opin Drug Discov Devel 2005;8(4):487–94.

[14] Zhang Z, Guan N, Li T, Mais DE, Wang M. Quality control of cell-based high-throughput drug screening. Acta Pharmaceut Sin B 2012;2(5):429–38.

[15] Hann MM, Leach AR, Harper G. Molecular complexity and its impact on the probability of finding leads for drug discovery. J Chem Inform Comput Sci 2001;41:856–64.

[16] Irwin JJ. How good is your screening library? Curr Opin Chem Biol 2006;10:352–6.

[17] Lahana R. Who wants to be irrational? Drug Discov Today 2003;8:655–6.

[18] Michelini E, Cevenini L, Mezzanotte L, Coppa A, Roda A. Cell based assays: fuelling drug discovery. Anal Biochem 2010;397:1–10.

[19] Dunne A, Jowett M, Rees S. Use of primary cells in high throughput screens. Meth Mol Biol 2009;565:239–57.

[20] Hughes JP, Rees S, Kalindjian SB, Philpott KL. Principles of early drug discovery. J Pharmacol Mar 2011;162(6):1239–49.

[21] Moore K, Rees S. Cell-based versus isolated target screening: how lucky do you feel? J Biomol Scr 2001;6:69–74.

[22] Hunter PJ, Borg TK. Integration from proteins to organs: the Physiome Project. Nat Rev Mol Cell Biol 2003;4:237–43.

[23] Noble D. Modelling the heart – from genes to cells to the whole organ. Science 2002;295:1678–82.

[24] Bassingthwaighte JB, Vinnakota KC. The computational integrated myocyte: a view into the virtual heart. Ann NY Acad Sci 2004;1015:391–404.

[25] Wang F, Wong PK. Intelligent systems and technology for integrative and predictive medicine: an ACP approach. ACM Trans Intell Syst Technol 2013;4(2):1–6, article 32.

[26] Li S, Zhang B, Zhang N. Network target for screening synergistic drug combinations with application to traditional Chinese medicine. BMC Syst Biol 2011;5(Suppl. 1):S10.

[27] Vedani A, Smiesko M. *In silico* toxicology in drug discovery – concepts based on three-dimensional models. Altern Lab Anim 2009;37:477–96.

[28] Kuhn M, Campillos M, Letunic I, Jensen LJ, Bork P. A side effect resource to capture phenotypic effects of drugs. Mol Syst Biol 2010;6:343.

[29] Ekins S, Williams AJ, Krasowski MD, Freundlich JS. *In silico* repositioning of approved drugs for rare and neglected diseases. Drug Discov Today 2011;16:298–310.

[30] Mendrick DL. Transcriptional profiling to identify biomarkers of disease and drug response. Pharmacogenomics 2011;12:235–49.

[31] Mah JT, Low ES, Lee E. *In silico* SNP analysis and bioinformatics tools: a review of the state of the art to aid drug discovery. Drug Discov Today 2011;16:800–9.

[32] Tanrikulu Y, Kruger B, Proschak E. The holistic integration of virtual screening in drug discovery. Drug Discov Today 2013;18(7/8):358–64.

[33] Stumpfe D, Ripphausen P, Bajorath J. Virtual compound screening in drug discovery. Fut Med Chem 2012;4:593–602.

[34] Kitchen DB, Decornez H, Furr JR, Bajorath J. Docking and scoring in virtual screening for drug discovery: methods and applications.. Nat Rev Drug Discov 2004;3: 935–48.

[35] McInnes C. Virtual screening strategies in drug discovery. Curr Opin Chem Biol 2007;11(5):494–502.

[36] Hajduk PJ, Huth JR, Tse C. Predicting protein druggability. Drug Discov Today 2005;10:1675–82.

[37] Laurie ATR, Jackson RM. Methods for the prediction of protein-ligand binding sites for structure-based drug design and virtual ligand screening. Curr Protein Pept Sci 2006;7:395.

[38] Prinz F, Schlange T, Asadullah K. Believe it or not: how much can we rely on published data on potential drug targets? Nat Rev Drug Discov 2011;10:712.

[39] Faller B, Ottaviani G, Ertl P, Berellini G, Collis A. Evolution of the physicochemical properties of marketed drugs: can history foretell the future? Drug Discov Today 2011;16:976–84.

[40] Park BK, Boobis A, Clarke S, Goldring CE, Jones D, Kenna JG, Lambert C, Laverty HG, Naisbitt DJ, Nelson S, Deborah A, Nicoll-Griffith R, Scott O, Philip R, Smith DA, Tweedie DJ, Vermeulen N, Williams DP, Wilson ID, Thomas AB. Managing the challenge of chemically reactive metabolites in drug development. Nat Rev Drug Discov 2011;10:292–306.

[41] Bauer RA, Wurst JM, Tan DS. Expanding the range of "druggable" targets with natural product-based libraries: an academic perspective. Curr Opin Chem Biol 2010;14: 308–14.

[42] Leeson PD, St-Gallay SA. The influence of the "organizational factor" on compound quality in drug discovery. Nat Rev Drug Discov 2011;10:749–65.

[43] Van Drie JH. Computer-aided drug design: the next 20 years. J Comput Aided Mol Des 2007;21:591–601.

[44] Bocker A, Derksen S, Schmidt E, Teckentrup A, Schneider G. A hierarchical clustering approach for large compound libraries. J Chem Inform Model 2005;45:807–15.

[45] Kapetanovic IM. Computer-aided drug discovery and development (CADDD): *in silico*-chemico-biological approach. ChemBiol Interact 2008;171(2):165–76.

[46] Kalyaanamoorthy S, Chen YP. Structure-based drug design to augment hit discovery. Drug Discov Today 2011;16:831.

[47] Jorgensen WL. Drug discovery: pulled from a protein's embrace. Nature 2010;466:6–8.

[48] Plowright AT, Johnstone C, Kihlberg J, Pettersson J, Robb G, Thompson RA. Hypothesis driven drug design: improving quality and effectiveness of the design-make-test-analyse cycle. Drug Discov Today 2012;17:56–62.

[49] Andersson S, Armstrong A, Björe A, Bowker S, Chapman S, Davies R, Donald C, Egner B, Elebring T, Holmqvist S, Inghardt T, Johannesson P, Johansson M, Johnstone C,

Kemmitt P, Kihlberg J, Korsgren P, Lemurell M, Moore J, Jonas AP, Pointon H, Pontén F, Schofield P, Selmi N, Whittamore P. Making medicinal chemistry more effective – application of lean sigma to improve processes, speed and quality. Drug Discov Today 2009;14:598–604.

[50] Johnstone C, Pairaudeau G, Pettersson JA. Creativity, innovation and lean sigma: a controversial combination? Drug Discov Today 2011;16:50–7.

[51] Erickson JA, Mader MM, Watson IA, Webster YW, Higgs RE, Bell MA, Vieth M. Structure-guided expansion of kinase fragment libraries driven by support vector machine models. Biochim Biophys Acta 2010;1804:642–52.

[52] Vinter A, Gardner S, Rose S. Overcoming the limitations of chemical structure. Mol Model 2009;59.

[53] Gleeson MP, Hersey AS, Hannongbua S. In-silico ADME models: a general assessment of their utility in drug discovery applications. Curr Top Med Chem 2011;10:11358–81.

[54] Li Q, Jørgensen FS, Oprea T, Brunak S, Taboureau O. hERG classification model based on a combination of support vector machine method and GRIND descriptors. Mol Pharm 2008;5(1):117–27.

[55] Gavaghan CL, Arnby CH, Blomberg N, Strandlund G, Boyer S. Development, interpretation and temporal evaluation of a global QSAR of hERG electrophysiology screening data. J Comput Aided Mol Des 2007;21:189–206.

[56] Acharya C, Coop A, Polli JE, Mackerell AD Jr. Recent advances in ligand based drug design: relevance and utility of the conformationally sampled pharmacophore approach. Curr Comput Aided Drug Des 2011;7:10–22.

[57] Yang SY. Pharmacophore modelling and applications in drug discovery: challenges and recent advances. Drug Discov Today 2010;15:444.

[58] Kurogi Y, Güner OF. Pharmacophore modelling and three-dimensional database searching for drug design using catalyst. Curr Med Chem 2001;8:1035–55.

[59] Jones G, Willett P, Glen RC. A genetic algorithm for flexible molecular overlay and pharmacophore elucidation. J Comput Aided Mol Des 1995;9:532.

[60] Dixon SL, Smondyrev AM, Knoll EH, Rao SN, Shaw DE, Friesner RA. PHASE: a new engine for pharmacophore perception, 3D QSAR model development, and 3D database screening: 1. Methodology and preliminary results. J Comput Aided Mol Des 2006;20:647.

[61] Michielan L, Moro S. Pharmaceutical perspectives of nonlinear QSAR strategies. J Chem Inf Model 2010;50:961–78.

[62] Lagorce D, Maupetit J, Baell J, Sperandio O, Tufféry P, Miteva MA, Galons H, Villoutreix BO. The FAF-Drugs2 server: a multistep engine to prepare electronic chemical compound collections. Bioinformatics 2011;27:2018–20.

[63] Bhogal N, Grindon C, Combes R, Balls M. Toxicity testing: creating a revolution based on new technologies. Trends Biotechnol 2005;23:299–307.

[64] Modi S, Hughes M, Garrow A, White A. The value of in silico chemistry in the safety assessment of chemicals in the consumer goods and pharmaceutical industries. Drug Discov Today 2012;17(3-4):135–42.

[65] Yang Y, Adelstein SJ, Kassis AI. Target discovery from data mining approaches. Drug Discov Today 2009;14:147–54.

[66] Bertram L, Tanzi RE. Thirty years of Alzheimer's disease genetics: the implications of systematic meta-analyses. Nat Rev Neurosci 2008;9:768–78.

[67] Fayyad U. Diving into databases. Database Program Design 1998;11(3):24–31.

[68] Baell JB. Observations on screening-based research and some concerning trends in the literature. Future Med Chem 2010;2:1529–46.

CHAPTER 6

Preclinical *In Vitro* Studies: Development and Applicability

Odilia Osakwe

Contents

6.1	Introduction	129
6.2	Predictability of Preclinical Disease Models	130
6.3	Trends in Preclinical Drug Development	132
6.4	Relevance of ADME/PK Studies	133
	6.4.1 Important Considerations in Evaluating Human Drug Toxicity	135
6.5	Experimental Tools Used in Preclinical Development	135
	6.5.1 In Vitro Systems for Metabolism and Toxicology Studies	135
	6.5.2 Intestinal Absorption Studies Models: Caco-2 Cells	137
	6.5.3 Advances in Cell Culture Systems	138
6.6	Drug eliminating Agents and Mechanisms	139
	6.6.1 Metabolizing Enzymes: CYPs (P450)	140
	6.6.2 Drug–Drug Interactions	141
	6.6.3 Transporters	143
6.7	Application of Zebrafish as a Model Whole Organism: A Landmark in Preclinical Development	144
References		145

6.1 INTRODUCTION

Preclinical development consists of a myriad of development activities that all together prepare the candidate drug for clinical application. For biological preclinical development, lead compounds are subjected to *in vitro* (cell cultures and tissues) and *in vivo* animal experimental systems. Modern *in vitro* and *in vivo* extrapolation techniques aid in establishing a criteria that allows progression from late preclinical development to early clinical drug development. The active compounds are tested in whole organisms to understand the effect in real time and to determine the toxicity profile. The use of laboratory animals is informed by its relevance – a high degree of similarity in genetic constituents with certain species that makes them

Social Aspects of Drug Discovery, Development and Commercialization
http://dx.doi.org/10.1016/B978-0-12-802220-7.00006-5

the most "relevant" to humans whenever possible. Animal models provide certain toxicity information fundamental for initiating clinical studies.

In the preclinical phase, the biologically yet incompetent development candidates are screened for pharmacokinetic (PK) and pharmacodynamics (PD) properties to support the process of validating clinical efficacy and these are based on the absorption, distribution, metabolism, and excretion (ADME) properties.

The use of *in vitro* and *in vivo* systems help to proactively address cost issues and human tragedy that could have been associated with a novel drug candidate with limited biological characteristics and which cannot be extrapolated to humans. It is intended to minimize the attrition rates and to improve clinical candidate selection based on safety criteria, toxicology, and exposure behavior of the new chemical entity. A recent report indicated that human-based experimental systems are useful in predicting human drug toxicity and those *in vitro* systems with primary cells, especially from human organs, play a crucial role in the evaluation of human-specific drugs [1]. Safety pharmacology is of crucial importance in this stage of drug development. The primary goal is to evaluate possible risks and early toxicity markers, which is a precondition for the design of clinical study protocols. The most important role of preclinical pharmacology studies is to identify the starting dose for Phase I clinical trials. In these studies, the safety profiles of lead compounds are evaluated through a battery of assessment assays adapted to determining side effects of new agents.

There are gaps in finding the postapproval unexpected adverse events when the drug must have been exposed to wider populations and timelines. This emphasizes the unpredictability that relies on patient response and preclinical toxicology findings. This chapter will describe the preliminary toxicological and pharmacological investigations to understand the behavior of drugs *in vivo* using a model organism and other biological platforms.

6.2 PREDICTABILITY OF PRECLINICAL DISEASE MODELS

Most of the predicaments of the early drug discovery projects were mostly attributed to complexity of the biological systems that limit the ability to understand disease networks, which is a major challenge in pharmaceutical research and development (R&D). Unexpected toxicity issues emerged due to multiple targeting of drug molecules, giving rise to both known and

unknown pharmacological activities. The high interconnectivity characteristic of the metabolic pathways is the reason for the resultant high level of
interconnectivity within the dynamic processes and thus it is not surprising
that blocking a pathway would lead to unanticipated effects due to extensive and divergent functions. If a single point mutation in a functional gene
leads to numerous consequences, then, in a diseased state, a multilevel-based
investigation would be required. The reason is that a whole unit (and not a
single molecule like a protein) in the higher molecular organization, such as
the cell, is involved. Thus, preclinical safety assessment conducted in healthy
participants might seemingly be normal but with unknown hidden effects,
which most often could be observed later as rare or idiosyncratic responses
in the wider subpopulation. This has been a major reason why predictive
accuracy of many toxicology models and safety assays remains uncertain,
requiring more refined strategies to be able to generate data with more accuracy and reliability.

An intracellular-level preclinical evaluation is usually performed within
the context of its native environment comprising all the processes that relate
to function and response. Therefore, its predictive correlation to the *in vivo*
function is essential. The essential elements that define its function are indispensable in building a viable model with which to probe drugs for proper
prediction of function. One major problem is that many cell lines that are used
in these studies are selected due to economic advantage or ease of handling,
and sometimes would be a preferential choice over those that are difficult to
handle but possess more endearing qualities in terms of clinical relevance. Neglecting the essential attribute means neglecting the very basis for its structure
and function, which is important for generating valid results [2]. For example,
primary cells are more difficult to maintain, as they require a more complex
tissue culture medium than the commonly used cell lines like cancer/Hela
cell lines. The primary cells might add more variability as they have very
short passage numbers requiring a change of lineage. Results from replacement cell lines do not essentially replicate themselves [3]. Cellular models do
show varied predictability and some have failed *in vitro/in vivo* correlation, a
major limitation in transforming such knowledge into a disease model in the
drug discovery process. A chromosomal aberration has been correlated with
increased passage numbers further distorting the experimental outcomes [4].
Certain advances in the cell culture systems are being introduced in an effort
to mitigate these issues as discussed in this chapter.

Attrition rates have been blamed on a large number of experiments
that are mandatory requirements and which must pass the stringent

conditions stipulated by regulations prior to Investigational New Drug and New Drug Application filing [5–7]. The widespread failure in Phase I first-in-human studies has been in part attributed to unacceptable PK [8], which led to the emergence of the DMPK activities to upgrade the ADME works toward better laboratory outputs and more promising drug candidates.

6.3 TRENDS IN PRECLINICAL DRUG DEVELOPMENT

Advances in preclinical investigations have added a new level of sophistication, which is a critical contribution to the progress. Allometric scaling has strengthened the assurance that PK data from animal studies could be translated or extrapolated to humans. The differences in PK processes is assumed to reflect the species-wide differences like weight and lifespan, thereby permitting a quantitative projection of human PK parameters. Earlier on, logic reasoning was an instrument used to make unreliable inferences deducted from animal PK data. The increasing availability and characterization of human-derived reagents utilized in *in vitro* drug metabolism studies laid the foundation for the application of ADME in drug discovery today [9].

Prediction algorithms have improved significantly from simple equations to complex physiologically based PK modeling. The prediction of simple parameters, such as volume of distribution (VD), can solely be done using computational methods. Drug transporters are aspects of the ADME science that are being applied for the prediction of target tissue-free concentrations but such an endeavor is awaiting full application. There is a remarkable improvement in the way preclinical studies are conducted to eliminate extraneous uninformative systems, one of which is the utility of biomarkers in predicting undesired effects and as well as potency of dug candidates [10]. Biomarkers have been acknowledged for their highly predictive power that enables the progression of biological evaluations. However, there are shady areas in basic scientific research methods in drug discovery and development, whose full development is still under way and, as such, there are still gaps in overall assessment feasibility with the techniques currently in use. Biomarkers with sparse predictive ability fail to adequately stratify patients to subpopulations, particularly those with slight differences in indications. This further weakens the ability to accurately measure disease susceptibility and progression, leading to difficulty in discerning novel pathways for drug targets and overall weakening of predictive power when using biomarkers.

6.4 RELEVANCE OF ADME/PK STUDIES

Crucial to the determination of the safety and effectiveness of drugs is the exposure–response information that reflects the risk/benefit profile of the drug. PK helps to identify the behavior of drugs upon systemic exposure. Human PK is an essential precondition for qualifying a drug candidate for approval and marketing. As a major requirement for the optimization of exposure and toxicity profile, human PK information is usually included in the marketing label, expressed as dosage and adverse effects. There are various exposure behaviors of drugs, some are well tolerated with low dose-related toxicity and some are more toxic with a higher dose-related toxicity. Exposure–response relationships ultimately guide drug development and regulatory decision making.

ADMET relates to the absorption, distribution, metabolism, excretion, and toxicity characteristics of the drug candidate. These parameters permit an understanding of the ability of the compound to reach the site of action and also the concentration at the site of action, to understand which concentrations are achievable. ADMET-related experiments enable an understanding of the potency, which is the ability to elicit a response at the targeted site of action or pharmacological effect; exposure levels, clinical relevance in target population, the therapeutic window for the indication of interest, and the ability to demonstrate adequate interpatient reproducibility. Aspects of drug disposition in humans include clearance, VD, and impact of genetic polymorphisms on drug disposition. Absorption considerations are half-life, oral bioavailability, effective dose, and passage into target organs. Concentration-versus-time curves are associated with interindividual variability. Drug–drug interactions have implications for toxicity. Oral bioavailability is a fundamental consideration in assigning a dosing regimen. It is the extent of drug absorption or elimination of an orally ingested drug before it reaches the systemic circulation and consequently the site of drug action. Elimination follows a first-pass metabolism pathway where it interacts with the drug metabolizing enzymes. Oral bioavailability data is the key for assigning a dosing regimen. Solubility and permeability are major role players in drug absorption following oral administration.

Knowledge of *in vitro* receptor binding properties of a drug candidate determined during the exploratory and lead optimization studies, and provides the basis for understanding the tolerability and PK of a drug in humans. These directly or indirectly predict human half-life, the time it takes for half of the drug to be cleared from the system, which is normally used to retrospectively assess the suitability of human PK prediction methods. Response refers to the PD response to the drug, which is the biological activity or pharmacologic effect of the drug. In more detail, it is all of the effects of the drug on any physiologic and pathologic process, including effectiveness and those related to adverse reactions. These are presumed mechanistic effects. One example is ACE inhibition which is regarded as an endpoint (outcome), or surrogate effects like effects on blood pressure, lipids, or cardiac output, or biomarkers like receptor occupancy and full range of clinical effects related to either efficacy or safety.

PD studies enable identification of the interaction of drugs with specific transporters involved in the chemical biotransformation in the liver known as metabolism. Interspecies variations in clearance tend to vary, affecting the animal data-based predictions of half-life. However, transporters have been used as a major clearance mechanism as half-life predicted from clearance (and VD) separately has been suggested as more accurate. For oral drugs, the drugs in blood are channeled through the liver en route to the site of therapeutic action. In the liver, the metabolic enzymes interact with the drugs; these enzymes are a diverse species that exist in discreet forms or species, which show special preference or affinity to any drug they bind to. PD effects are generally characterized by an exposure–response relationship of drugs, and genetic differences that lead to changes the exposure–response profile. Exposure refers to PK profile following administration, which expresses the behavior of the drug following ingestion, and is mostly concerned with the rate at which it reaches the site of action and the rate and extent it follows the elimination route. Quantitatively, it refers to the dose and concentrations in plasma or other biological fluid estimated using the parameters such as C_{max}, C_{min}, C_{ss}, and AUC. Response and exposure are the foundation for understanding the PD effects, and determine of the exposure–response relationship between animals and humans. Exposure–response and PK data enable identification of a mechanism of drug action that guides the design of clinical endpoint trials that generate data necessary to assign a dosing regimen, potency, and the time course of drug action. This is important in the selection of dose, dosing interval, monitoring procedures, and important decisions concerning which dosage form (e.g., controlled-release dosage form) to develop. Establishing the exposure information in connection with a disease would be a more guided approach to finding potency and potential toxicity outcomes. Drug interaction refers to a drug activity that is altered by the PK of another drug or its metabolites. Drug interactions also can reflect the additive nature of the PD effect of either drug when taken concomitantly with the other drug.

ADMET screens, for example, the REACH project, were launched so as to reduce the available number of animals used in biomedical experimentation. Traditional modeling methods (like quantitative structure–activity relationships or quantitative structure–property relationships) have been used to determine the ADMET property using variable approaches and experimental data to model the complex biological processes [11–13].

6.4.1 Important Considerations in Evaluating Human Drug Toxicity

- Model organism dependence on toxicity profile
- Contribution of drug metabolism on organ distribution
- Toxicity of the chemical entity, side chains, functional groups
- Adverse effects induced by drug–target and/or drug–drug interactions induced
- Adverse effect induced by interaction with multiple targets – polypharmacology
- The suitability of the model organism used

6.4.1.1 Case

It was discovered that troglitazone alters the gene expression of toxicologically relevant genes instead of the relatively nontoxic structure analogs, rosiglitazone and pioglitazone. The effects of both toxic and nontoxic forms on gene expression enabled the discerning of the mechanisms of toxicity, in an experimentally verifiable way and which is applicable in the prediction of human effects. This knowledge can be applied in the development of biomarkers of toxicity and screening assays for specific toxic liability [14, 15].

6.5 EXPERIMENTAL TOOLS USED IN PRECLINICAL DEVELOPMENT

6.5.1 *In Vitro* Systems for Metabolism and Toxicology Studies

The human systemic hierarchical organization of cells gives rise to tissues, organs, and systems. Thus, their use in isolated environments is believed to reflect the functions of the body (Table 6.1). Cells are fundamental functional units or machinery in the living organisms that perform vital functions to sustain life. Cell cultures are finding increasing applicability in replicating the functions of the organs, *in vitro* systems are comprised of assemblies of various organ-specific cells that exhibit functions close to those in the human body. Cell-based studies could be customized to various

Table 6.1 Toxicity associated with organ-specific cell

Type of toxicity	Organ-specific cells
Liver toxicity	Hepatocytes
Nephrotoxicity	Renal proximal tubule
Cardiotoxicity	Cardiomyocytes
Rhabdomyolysis	Skeletal myocytes
Vascular toxicity	Vascular endothelial cells
Cytotoxicity	Organ specific

kinetic parameters of substrates or inhibitors. *In vitro* cell cultures are employed in evaluation of drug efficacy through monitoring of the biological activity of the drug compound on the cell of interest [16].

Cells grown as monolayers (two-dimensional models) are routinely used model systems for identifying the most viable compounds that progress to preclinical animal studies before advancing to human clinical trials. Growing cells as three-dimensional (3D) models tend to depict more closely the natural environment as they are cocultured with other neighboring cells and cellular components in the physiological microenvironment, in order to make them more clinically relevant.

In vitro experimental cell cultures have greatly enhanced the ability to generate parameters to predict transporter-mediated drug distribution and elimination and the associated drug interactions (Table 6.2). *In vitro* cell cultures increase in complexity from single-gene overexpressing immortalized cell lines to isolated hepatocytes and 3D cultured hepatocyte systems. Cells expressing individual uptake transporters have been widely used to determine potential inhibitory function of a transporter or substrate [17–19]. For compounds that have low passive permeability and/or are

Table 6.2 *In vitro* screening assays for identifying the corresponding function of an orally ingested drug

Assay	Function
Caco-2 permeabililty, PAMPA	Intestinal absorption
P450 inhibition; induction	Drug–drug interaction
Hepatocyte liver microsome metabolism	Hepatic metabolism
Hepatocyte biliary excretion	Bile excretion
Hepatocyte cytotoxicity	Organ toxicity

Source: Adapted from Ref. [20]

efflux transporter substrates, apparent intrinsic clearance in hepatocytes is usually lower than that in enzyme systems, due to lower free hepatocyte. Other types of *in vitro* data that address drug disposition properties (e.g., membrane penetrability, P450 inhibition, others) are also gathered early using high throughput methods.

In vitro screening assays provide the first line of information about the potential effect of the drug compound on the biological system. They eliminate the complexities associated with the use of the whole systems by providing options that would have required extensive experimental work and yet with the promise of reliable conclusions. The cell cultures are pivotal and only used for pilot and backup data for animal studies. The specialized cells of various organs that retain their specific characteristics are important experimental systems for early toxicity screening [21].

Cytotoxicity is concerned with biochemical or physical malfunctions of the important functional organelles or units of the cells, which include mitochondrial functions, lysosomal functions, and cellular metabolites. Mechanisms of known functions are important. Cytotoxicity endpoints are mitochondrial functions and lysosomal functions, cellular metabolite content, and membrane integrity. Another advantage of cellular screens is that they employ the high-throughput screening (HTS) technology, which is deployed when molecular targets could not be tested in an isolated form or due to the extent of patent protection. This allows only a whole-cell system to be tested. Such cellular screens permit the evaluation of multiple targets in a pathway and identification of allosteric effectors, which are early indicators of toxicity.

6.5.2 Intestinal Absorption Studies Models: Caco-2 Cells

Caco-2 cells have been of great utility in intestinal absorption studies due to their exclusive ability to model human absorption characteristics and Caco-2 is the most commonly used intestinal permeability model. Caco-2 cells and intestinal enterocytes cells have enabled the validation of the application of Caco-2 cells in drug absorption studies. Caco-2 cells have special features: they develop into small intestinal cells with tight junctions and microvilli, expressing the drug metabolizing enzymes involved in uptake of the agents crucial in drug metabolism [22,23].

The limitations of Cacao-2 cells are that they are unable to be used in screening of formulations that are sensitive to pharmaceutical excipients since dilution is a poor representation of the original formulation potency and functionality; they have a low tolerability to organic solvents, limiting their use in this kind of permeability study. they are assayed in microwells, which do not represent the whole system; and they do not accurately predict the side or adverse effects, which is a common experience with drugs in the context of the human body or target organ system. The whole intact system encompassing the natural physiological environment comprising discrete functions that integrate into a network of functions could not be recapitulated in the *in vitro* systems, which is critical to identifying toxicity. But since the intestinal absorption in rodents and humans are well correlated, their utility is essential [24]

6.5.3 Advances in Cell Culture Systems

Cellular disease models permit a detailed study of disease processes and therefore this function need to be validated for a better *in vivo* correlation with Organs on a Chip. The complexity of human biology and the networks often requires viewing each isolated case within the context of another and thus highlights the necessity for a multiparametric approach to certain biological investigations. Organs-on-chips are intelligent fabrications that represent the various aspects of the physiological environment. This is applicable for disease modeling and drug discovery tailored to various needs, particularly for the study of drug toxicity and metabolism [25,26]. Compartmentalization-based applications termed "semiconductor processing" have been introduced [27]. For example, the Integrated discrete Multiple Organ Culture system has been introduced to coculture organ-specific cells with interconnection of blood circulation. It is used to evaluate the effect of drugs and metabolites [28]. There have been proposals for creating personalized organs-on-chips, which is already under way [29] not only for individualized screening platforms but to accelerate drug screening in a way that addresses speed and efficiency.

Some recent progress in four areas has been described that covers integrated microdevices for cell culture; 3D cell patterning and culture; multilayered microfluidic structures; and perfusion-based microdevices, as explained in Ref. [30] and as follows.

6.5.3.1 Microwell Array Technology: Cell Function/Toxicity Assays

The utility of microfabrication techniques technology has been applied to cell culture systems with compartmentalization-integrated microwell arrays and cell culture analogs [31]. These were introduced to address the limitation of lack of interconnectivity and interactions of organs in the cell culture format. They are known as "small wells within large wells," wells within a well such that cells form organs that are cultured within the small wells, surrounded by the drug-containing large wells described in [32]. This device permitted the maintenance of the human liver cells' phenotypic functions for several weeks. It allowed the evaluation of gene expression profiles, Phase I/II metabolism proteins, secretion of liver-specific products, and susceptibility to hepatotoxins. Application of this technique shows prospects in overcoming aspects of the preclinical failures in drug discovery.

6.5.3.2 Integrated Microcell Culture Systems

In a similar arrangement, the microcell culture analog (μCCA) approach was developed to create a cell culture environment that is close to that of humans, to improve the credibility of the drug PK and PD profiles [33]. The device consists of separated chambers connected with microchannels to link the different chambers of cultured cells of the liver, tumor, and marrow, to simulate the blood flow. The microenvironment provided by the μCCA was intended to simulate more of the *in vivo* environment in than a conventional monolayer culture.

6.5.3.3 Three-Dimensional Cell Patterning and Culturing

Cell culture systems created to very closely represent the human physiological characteristics are interaction prone, as they produce a fertile environment for cell–cell and cell–matrix interactions [34,35]. This platform is adaptable to variable cell patterning methods.

6.5.3.4 Membrane-Based Multilayer Microfluidic Devices

This technology reproduces the *in vivo* microenvironment of kidney tubular cells. It was created in an attempt to resolve the issue of the lack of a tissue-like microarchitecture in traditional two-dimensional systems. Using this device, cell polarization and cytoskeletal rearrangement studies have been made more predictive [36].

6.6 DRUG ELIMINATING AGENTS AND MECHANISMS

The passage of an orally administered drug onto the site of action is initiated through absorption by the small intestine into the portal circulation driving it to the liver where drug metabolism occurs. The small intestine is the rate-limiting barrier as it metabolizes drugs by several pathways involving both Phase I and Phase II reactions, elicited by the cytochrome P450 (CYP) family of enzymes and the UDP-glucuronosyltransferases (UGTs)r enzymes which limit systemic exposure. The small intestine is regarded as an absorptive organ and may act as a rate-limiting barrier. CYP3A4 is the most abundant P450 present in human hepatocytes as well as the intestinal enterocytes [37–39].

6.6.1 Metabolizing Enzymes: CYPs (P450)

A prominent drug activity in the body is drug metabolism, which is what the body does to the drug. Metabolism refers to the biotransformation of a parent drug by drug-metabolizing enzymes. In addition to bile and renal excretion, drug metabolism contributes to determining the fate of the drug in the body. CYPs are the most popular enzyme studied in drug development. They are the Phase I metabolizing enzymes chiefly involved with oxidation of foreign compounds including the xenobiotics and select medicinal compounds, committing them to the elimination pathway. They could transform nontoxic compounds to toxic reactive intermediates. Drug metabolism is generally regarded in the context of Phase I oxidation. The oxidation activity mostly involves the nonpolar molecules, which are oxidized by the addition of oxygen atoms, usually in the form of a hydroxyl moiety (–OH group). Phase II conjugation involves adding a very water-soluble molecule such as glucose (glucuronidation) or sulfate (sulfation) to the organic group, especially at the –OH site. Early determination of the downstream metabolic effect is a key to successful clinical studies. CYPs play a role in drug–drug interactions through drug activation or inhibition [40,41].

Around 75% of approved drugs are metabolized by CYPs, particularly the five major isoforms [42]. Single nucleotide polymorphism has been attributed to several species, including CYP2D6 and CYP2C9. As discussed earlier, size and flexibility have been attributed to multiple and simultaneous ligand binding. CYP3A4 metabolizes the most active of all the CYPs with a reported metabolizing activity of up to 50% of all drugs [43]. *In silico* methods of modeling ADMET models the protein flexibility, which is a fundamental step in its bioactivity – conformational changes have been reportedly induced by ligand binding. The hepatocytes or liver microsomes are liver cells that are used in clinical trials to model the activity of the metabolizing enzymes [44,45].

6.6.1.1 Assays Used in Evaluating Drug Metabolism

Metabolic assay is used to identify metabolic stability in chemical structures in connection with hepatic metabolism. It evaluates the rate of clearance of a drug using the liver hepatocytes or microsomes. The disappearance of the parent chemical with time is an example of a change. Metabolic profiling involves incubation of drug compounds with *in vitro* hepatic metabolic systems or cells of which the major metabolites are identified with mass spectrometry. The metabolites identified enable structure optimization to prevent a choice metabolite from forming. It is also applicable in the selection of animal species with similar physiology that produce identical metabolites to humans for assigning the "relevant animal species."

6.6.2 Drug–Drug Interactions

The effects of a drug depends on the concentration levels at various sites of drug action (relates to the PD), or the blood or tissue concentration of the drug. Elimination of a drug or its active metabolites therefore affects the concentration at the sites of drug action. This occurs either by metabolism to an inactive metabolite that is excreted, or by direct excretion of the drug or active metabolites. Identifying metabolic drug–drug interactions that elicit these changes enables the determination of the extent to which toxic or active metabolites are formed [46].

One example is the inhibition of the metabolism of a nondrowsy antihistamine, terfenadine, by the antifungal drug etoconazole. Concomitant administration of both terfenadine and ketoconazole lead to fatal cardiac arrhythmia because of the elevated level of terfenadine. Terfenadine has been recalled owing to its drug–drug interaction potential. Ketoconazole is a well-known potent inhibitor of CYP3A4, the P450 isoform responsible for metabolism of terfenadine.

6.6.2.1 Types of Drug–Drug Interactions

There are two types of drug–drug interactions: metabolism driven and absorption and excretion driven. Metabolism-driven drug–drug interaction has been widely characterized as it has the most impact and is the reason why it is the subject of most biological investigations in drug discovery. Metabolism-driven drug–drug interactions can differ among individuals based on genetic variation of a polymorphic enzyme. For example, a strong CYP2D6 inhibitor results in the increase of the plasma levels of a CYP2D6 substrate in subjects who are extensive metabolizers of CYP2D6, but which is reduced in subjects who are poor metabolizers of CYP2D6. This is because there are no available active enzymes to be inhibited. Inhibition of drug interactions for a specific drug may occur based on a combination of drug–drug interactions, which follow multiple interaction mechanisms:

- Simultaneous inhibition and induction of one enzyme transporter by a drug
- Inhibition of drug elimination by inhibitor of the same enzyme that metabolizes the drug
- Inhibition of enzyme/transporter in subjects with varying degrees of impairment of drug eliminating organs (e.g., liver or kidney)

Drug-metabolizing enzyme induction strategies have been used in *in vitro* human liver-based experimental systems to evaluate drug–drug interactions. A drug that can induce any of these enzymes, for example, CYP1A2, CYP2A6, CYP2B6, CYP2C9, and CYP3A4, could cause inductive drug–drug interactions [47]. Drug–drug interaction assays are in general focused on P450 isoforms, with CYPs 1A2, 2A6, 2C8, 2C9, 2C19, 2D6, 2E1, and 3A4 as the major isoforms studied. The same experimental systems are applicable for evaluating drug–drug interactions involving Phase II [46] and transporters [48,49].

Absorption and excretion-driven drug metabolism involves biliary and renal drug transporters and small plasma protein binding (the risk is low; may be important for highly bound drugs with narrow therapeutic windows).

6.6.2.2 Plasma Binding Proteins as Drug Eliminating Compounds

Model plasma binding proteins are human serum albumin (HSA) and alpha 1-acid glycoprotein, known to bind a high number of drugs. Interaction of these types of proteins with drugs leads to elimination of a fraction of the drug in a protein-bound state while the free and unbound portion exerts the therapeutic action. They have important biological roles, mostly in the transport of important biomolecules that are fairly insoluble. Some examples are hormones, vitamins, and fatty acids. These proteins have several binding sites for drugs located in their IIA and IIA domains [50].

The drug's ligands that bind to negatively charged sites are warfarin, azapropazone, and dansylamide [51]. The aromatic carboxylic acids like ibuprofen, diazepam, and arylpropionic acids bind to the smaller site II (the diazepam site), while propofol and oxyphenbutazone, among others, bind within the five other sites identified in the three domains. The drugs that can bind to at least two sites are azapropazone, indomethacin, and fatty acids. The *in silico* 3D HSA paradigm was utilized to terminate binding of methionine aminopeptidase-2 inhibitors plasmaproteins [52,53]. Lipophilicity and the charge of a molecule at physiologic pH affect the ability of a drug molecule to bind to the plasma proteins, but increases with lipophilicity or cationic charge and decreases with increasing anionic charge at physiologic pH [54].

6.6.3 Transporters

Transporters are present with varying abundance in all tissues in the body and play important roles in drug targeting, drug absorption, drug distribution, and elimination. The safety profile of a drug is altered when its concentration or that of its metabolites is affected in various tissues. Transporters are expressed in the renal tubule cells. They play a role in the active renal secretion and reabsorption of endogenous compounds and xenobiotics. A large superfamily of proteins transport molecules across the membrane barriers within the human body and about 48 members have been identified [55]. P-glycoprotein (Pgp) is the most important efflux transporter and very active across the intestinal epithelium and the blood–brain barrier. Verapamil and cyclosporin are examples of drugs transported through the Pgp–efflux pathway. The multidrug resistance protein MRP1 and the MRP2 transporter, as well as multidrug and toxin extrusion proteins, are major transporters on the apical membrane. The synchronous activities of these transporters promote active renal secretion of compounds. Meanwhile, peptide transporter 2 and system L amino acid transporters, etc., are more associated with active reabsorption.

There are marked species differences in transport function and transporter expression of these transporters. Along the proximal tubule is remarkable heterogeneity and this has posed difficulty in prediction of renal elimination of actively secreted compounds from *in vitro* data [56]. A recent study indicated that monkeys are superior to rats and dogs, a notion that is supported by the fact that monkeys are evolutionarily closest to humans, and which is the reason why both uptake and efflux transporters in monkeys have been shown to be more predictive of humans than the other species mentioned [57,58]. They are actively involved in the multidrug resistance effect, an activity that reduces drug potency.

Multidrug resistance protein 1 is a Pgp, the first ABC transporter and the most characterized transport protein. Its role in expelling molecules out of the cell results in reducing the fraction of drug available for the therapeutic function. This is further exacerbated by its broad substrate specificity as it can recognize a wide range of drug compounds regardless of charge distribution or molecular structure. The transporter substrate binds to its high-affinity binding site on the membrane domains resulting in multiple simultaneous binding to ligands in up to seven binding sites [59].

6.6.3.1 UDP-Glucuronosyltransferases

The UDP-glucuronosyltransferases (UGTs) are Phase II enzymes that induce drug metabolism through covalent addition of a glucuronic moiety to a drug or endogenous compound. The three major ones are UGT1A1, UGT1A4, and UGT2B7, which account for 15, 20, and 35% of the UGT-metabolized drugs, respectively [60].

6.7 APPLICATION OF ZEBRAFISH AS A MODEL WHOLE ORGANISM: A LANDMARK IN PRECLINICAL DEVELOPMENT

Zebrafish (*Danio rerio*) as an experimental model has gained wide popularity in recent times and has been widely applied in various stages in drug discovery processes. Due to its cost effectiveness and its close physiological and anatomical semblance with human systems, it has been applied as a viable alternative to well-known mammalian models such as rodents, dogs, and pigs. This close semblance is the reason why it has been applied in the study of molecular mechanisms of diverse human diseases, including cancers, particularly due to ease of handling and manipulation and high reproducibility. The use of zebrafish model systems has created the opportunity to use HTS in the assessment of drug effects based on the physiological and pathological functions with relevance to safety pharmacology/toxicity studies since only milligram or minute quantities are required for screening studies. *In vivo* phenotype-based screening methods for humans could be adapted to zebrafish [61–63]. Its distinguishing features include the development of discreet organs and tissues like bones, muscles, brain, liver, pancreas, kidneys, intestines, nervous systems, and sensory organs, which show stark similarity to those of humans [64–66].

A small *ex utero* zebrafish embryo can permit multiwell or microwell dishes in the HTS of water-soluble chemical compounds. Toxicology studies have utilized 18 different compounds to determine lethal concentrations (IC 50) of drugs, which was comparable between *in vivo* systems [67–70]. In biomedical research, it has been used to study various therapeutic areas like immunology, vascular systems, central nervous systems, musculoskeletal systems, and subjects pertaining to all the vital tissues and organs of the body, since it possesses phenotypic features resembling that of humans. Zebrafish models have improved the determination of toxic or protective effects of various drugs and nanomaterials on internal organs during the developmental stages [71–73]. The regulatory authorities require data from whole organism animal models for IND application. Whole organisms retain the characteristics comparative to the human systems in an *in vivo* model.

REFERENCES

[1] MacGregor JT, Collins JM, Sugiyama Y, Tyson CA, Dean J, Smith L, Andersen M, Curren RD, Houston JB, Kadlubar FF, Kedderis GL, Krishnan K, Li AP, Parchment RE, Thummel K, Tomaszewski JE, Ulrich R, Vickers AE, Wrighton SA. *In vitro* human tissue models in risk assessment: report of a consensus-building workshop. Toxicol Sci 2001;59(1):17–36.

[2] Tilakaratne N, Christopoulos G, Zumpe ET, Foord SM, Sexton PM. Amylin receptor phenotypes derived from human calcitonin receptor/RAMP coexpression exhibit pharmacological differences dependent on receptor isoform and host cell environment. J Pharmacol Exp Ther 2000;294(1):61–72.

[3] Kenakin T. Efficacy at G-protein-coupled receptor. Nat Rev Drug Discov 2002;1(2):103–10.

[4] Dzhambazov B, Teneva I, Koleva L, Asparuhova D, Popov N. Morphological, genetic and functional variability of a T-cell hybridoma line. Folia Biol (Praha) 2003;49(2): 87–94.

[5] Rasgele PG, Muranli FD, Kekeçog˘lu M. Assessment of the genotoxicity of propineb in mice bone marrow cells using micronucleus assay. Tsitol Genet 2014;48(4):39–43.

[6] Legler UF. Experiences with GLP/GCP from the pharmaceutical industry's viewpoint. Methods Find Exp Clin Pharmacol 1993;15(4):233–6.

[7] Spielmann H, Liebsch M. Lessons learned from validation of *in vitro* toxicity test: from failure to acceptance into regulatory practice. Toxicol In Vitro 2001;15(4-5):585–90.

[8] Kola I, Landis J. Can the pharmaceutical industry reduce attrition rates? Nat Rev Drug Discov 2004;3:711–6.

[9] Di L, Feng B, Goosen TC, Lai Y, Steyn SJ, Varma MV, Obach RS. A perspective on the prediction of drug pharmacokinetics and disposition in drug research and development. Drug Metab Dispos 2013;41:1975–93.

[10] Fowler BA. Molecular biomarkers: challenges and prospects for the future. Toxicol Appl Pharmacol 2005;7206(2):97.

[11] Michielan L, Moro S. Pharmaceutical perspectives of nonlinear QSAR strategies. J Chem Inf Model 2010;50:961–78.

[12] Gleeson MP, Hersey A, Hannongbua S. *In silico* ADME models: a general assessment of their utility in drug discovery applications. Curr Top Med Chem 2011;11:358–81.

[13] Van de Waterbeemd H, Gifford E. ADMET *in silico* modelling: towards prediction paradise? Nat Rev Drug Discov 2003;2:192–204.

[14] Kier LD, Neft R, Tang L, Suizu R, Cook T, Onsurez K, Tiegler K, Sakai Y, Ortiz M, Nolan T, Sankar U, Li AP. Applications of microarrays with toxicologically-relevant genes (tox genes) for the evaluation of chemical toxicants in Sprague Dawley rats *in vivo* and human hepatocytes *in vitro*. Mutat Res 2004;549:101–13.

[15] Huh D, Kim HJ, Fraser JP, Shea DE, Khan M, Bahinski A, Hamilton GA, Ingber DE. Microfabrication of human organs-on-chips. Nat Protoc 2013;8(11):2135–57.

[16] Adams CP, Brantner VV. Estimating the cost of new drug development: is it really $802 million? Health Affairs 2006;25:420–8.

[17] Bhatia SN, Ingber DE. Microfluidic organs-on-chips. Nat Biotechnol 2014;32:760–72.

[18] Sharma P, Butters CJ, Smith V, Elsby R, Surry D. Prediction of the *in vivo* OATP1B-1mediated drug-drug interaction potential of an investigational drug against a range of statins. Eur J Pharm Sci 2012;47:244–55.

[19] Soars MG, Barton P, Ismair M, Jupp R, Riley RJ. The development, characterization, and application of an OATP1B1 inhibition assay in drug discovery. Drug Metab Dispos 2012;40:1641–8.

[20] Li AP. Preclinical *in vitro* screening assays for drug-like properties. Drug Discov Today Technol 2005;2(2):179–185.

[21] Varma MV, Chang G, Lai Y, Feng B, El-Kattan AF, Litchfield J, Goosen TC. Physico-chemical property space of hepatobiliary transport and computational models for predicting rat biliary excretion. Drug Metab Dispos 2012;40:1527–37.

[22] Esch MB, King TL, Shuler ML. The role of body-on-a-chip devices in drug and toxicity studies. Annu Rev Biomed Eng 2011;13:55–72.

[23] Gattei V, Aldinucci D, Petti MC, Da Ponte A, Zagonel V, Pinto A. *In vitro* and *in vivo* effects of 5-aza-2'-deoxycytidine (Decitabine) on clonogenic cells from acute myeloid leukemia patients. Leukemia 1993;7(Suppl. 1):42–8.

[24] Dimitrova DS, Berezney R. The spatio-temporal organization of DNA replication sites is identical in primary, immortalized and transformed mammalian cells. J Cell Sci 2002;115:4037–51.

[25] Huh D, Hamilton GA, Ingber DE. From 3D cell culture to organs-on-chips. Trends Cell Biol 2011;21:745–54.

[26] Chen SY, Hung PJ, Lee PJ. Microfluidic array for three-dimensional perfusion culture of human mammary epithelial cells. Biomed Microdevices 2011;13(4):753–8.

[27] Annaert PP, Brouwer KL. Assessment of drug interactions in hepatobiliary transport using rhodamine 123 in sandwich-cultured rat hepatocytes. Drug Metab Dispos 2005;33:294–388.

[28] Ibrahim AE, Feldman J, Karim A, Kharasch ED. Simultaneous assessment of drug interactions with low- and high-extraction opioids: application to parecoxib effects on the pharmacokinetics and pharmacodynamics of fentanyl and alfentanil. Anesthesiology 2003;98(4):853–61.

[29] Anene-Nzelu CG, Peh KY, Fraiszudeen A, Kuan YH, Ng SH, Toh YC, Leo H, Yu H. Scalable alignment of three-dimensional cellular constructs in a microfluidic chip. Lab Chip 2013;13:4124–33.

[30] Three "Organs-on-Chips" ready to serve as disease models, drug testbeds. Available from: http://wyss.harvard.edu/viewpage/484/

[31] Sam H, Chamberlain MD, Mahesh S, Seftonabc MV, Wheeler AR. Hepatic organoids for microfluidic drug screening. Lab Chip 2014;14:3290–9.

[32] Chan CY, Huang PH, Guo F, Ding X, Kapur V, Mai JD, Yuen PK, Huang TJ. Accelerating drug discovery via organs-on-chips. Lab Chip 2013;13(24):4697.

[33] Khetani SR, Bhatia SN. Microscale culture of human liver cells for drug development. Nat Biotechnol 2008;26:120–6.

[34] Wang J, Bettinger CJ, Langer RS, Borenstein JT. Biodegradable microfluidic scaffolds for tissue engineering from amino alcohol-based poly (ester amide) elastomers. Organogenesis 2010;6(4):212–6.

[35] Choi NW, Cabodi M, Held B, Gleghorn JP, Bonassar LJ, Stroock AD. Microfluidic scaffolds for tissue engineering. Nat Mater 2007;6:908–15.

[36] Jang KJ, Mehr AP, Hamilton GA, McPartlin LA, Chung S, Suh KY, Ingber DE. Human kidney proximal tubule-on-a-chip for drug transport and nephrotoxicity assessment. Integr Biol (Camb) 2013;5(9):1119–29.

[37] Paine MF, Hart HL, Ludington SS, Haining RL, Rettie AE, Zeldin DC. The human intestinal cytochrome P450 "pie". Drug Metab Dispos 2006;34:880–6.

[38] Paine MF, Shen DD, Kunze KL, Perkins JD, Marsh CL, McVicar JP, Barr DM, Gillies BS, Thummel KE. First-pass metabolism of midazolam by the human intestine. Clin Pharmacol Ther 1996;60:14–24.

[39] Thummel KE. Gut instincts: CYP3A4 and intestinal drug metabolism. J Clin Invest 2007;117:3173–6.

[40] Bode C. The nasty surprise of a complex drug–drug interaction. Drug Discov Today 2010;15(9-10):391—395.

[41] US Department of Health and Human Services, FDA Guidance for Industry, Drug metabolism/drug interaction studies in the drug development process: studies *in vitro*; 1999. Available from: http://www.fda.gov/downloads/Drugs/

[42] Available from: http://www.GuidanceComplianceRegulatoryInformation/Guidances/ucm072104.pdf

[43] Guengerich FP. Cytochrome p450 and chemical toxicology. Chem Res Toxicol 2008;21:70–83.

[44] Clark SE, Jones BC. Human cytochromes P450 and their role in metabolism-based drug–drug interactions. In: David Rodrigues A, editor. Drug–drug interactions. CRC Press; 2001. Chapter 3, p. 55–88.

[45] Li AP. Screening for human ADME/Tox drug properties in drug discovery. Drug Discov Today 2001;6:357–66.

[46] Li AP. *In vitro* approaches to evaluate ADMET drug properties. Curr Top Med Chem 2004;4(7):701–6.

[47] Li AP, Jurima-Romet M. Overview: pharmacokinetic drug–drug interactions. Adv Pharmacol 1997;43:1–6.

[48] Li AP, Hartman NR, Lu C, Collins JM, Strong JM. Effects of cytochrome P450 inducers on 17α-ethinyloestradiol (EE2) conjugation by primary human hepatocytes. Br J Clin Pharmacol 1999;48(5):733–42.

[49] Shitara Y, Itoh T, Sato H, Li AP, Sugiyama Y. Inhibition of transporter-mediated hepatic uptake as a mechanism for drug–drug interaction between cerivastatin and cyclosporin A. J Pharmacol Exp Ther 2003;304:610–6.

[50] Li AP, Kato Y, Lu C, Ito K, Itoh T, Sugiyama Y. Function of uptake transporters for taurocholate and estradiol 17 betaD-glucuronide in cryopreserved human hepatocytes. Drug Metab Pharmacokinet 2003;18:33–41.

[51] He XM, Carter DC. Atomic structure and chemistry of human serum albumin. Nature 1992;358:209–15.

[52] Otagiri M. A molecular functional study on the interactions of drugs with plasma proteins. Drug Metab Pharmacokinet 2005;20:309–23.

[53] Sheppard GS, Wang J, Kawai M, Fidanze SD, BaMaung NY, Erickson SA, Barnes DM, Tedrow JS, Kolaczkowski L, Vasudevan A, Park DC, Wang GT, Sanders WJ, Mantei RA, Palazzo F, Tucker-Garcia L, Lou P, Zhang Q, Park CH, Kim KH, Petros A, Olejniczak E, Nettesheim D, Hajduk P, Henkin J, Lesniewski R, Davidsen SK, Bell RL. Discovery and optimization of anthranilic acid sulfonamides as inhibitors of methionine aminopeptidase-2: a structural basis for the reduction of albumin binding. J Med Chem 2006;49:3832–49.

[54] Wendt MD, Shen W, Kunzer A, McClellan WJ, Bruncko M, Oost TK, Ding H, Joseph MK, Zhang H, Nimmer PM, Ng SC, Shoemaker AR, Petros AM, Oleksijew A, Marsh K, Bauch J, Oltersdorf T, Belli BA, Martineau D, Fesik SW, Rosenberg SH, Elmore SW. Discovery and structure–activity relationship of antagonists of B-cell lymphoma 2 family proteins with chemopotentiation activity *in vitro* and *in vivo*. J Med Chem 2006;49:1165–81.

[55] Lombardo F, Obach RS, Dicapua FM, Bakken GA, Lu J, Potter DM, Gao F, Miller MD, Zhang Y. A hybrid mixture discriminant analysis-random forest computational model for the prediction of volume of distribution of drugs in human. J Med Chem 2006;49:2262–7.

[56] Pajeva I, Wiese M. Application of *in silico* methods to study ABC transporters involved in multidrug resistance. In: Miteva MA, editor. Silico Lead Discovery. Bentham Science Publishers; 2011. Chapter 8, p. 144–62.

[57] Masereeuw R, Russel FG. Mechanisms and clinical implications of renal drug excretion. Drug Metab Rev 2001;33:299–351.

[58] Syvänen S, Lindhe O, Palner M, Kornum BR, Rahman O, Långström B, Knudsen GM, Hammarlund-Udenaes M. Species differences in blood-brain barrier transport of three positron emission tomography radioligands with emphasis on P-glycoprotein transport. Drug Metab Dispos 2009;37(3):635–43.

[59] Shen H, Yang Z, Mintier G, Han YH, Chen C, Balimane P, Jemal M, Zhao W, Zhang R, Kallipatti S, Selvam S, Sukrutharaj S, Krishnamurthy P, Marathe P, Rodrigues AD. Cynomolgus monkey as a potential model to assess drug interactions involving hepatic organic anion transporting polypeptides (OATPs), *in vitro, in vivo* and *in vitro*-to-*in vivo* extrapolation. J Pharmacol Exp Ther 2013;344:673–85.

[60] Williams JA, et al. Drug–drug interactions for UDP-glucuronosyltransferase substrates: a pharmacokinetic explanation for typically observed low exposure (AUCi/AUC) ratios. Drug Metab Dispos 2004;32:1201–8.

[61] Safa AR. Identification and characterization of the binding sites of Pglycoprotein for multidrug resistance-related drugs and modulators. Curr Med Chem Anticancer Agents 2004;4:1–17.

[62] Barros TP, Alderton WK, Reynolds HM, Roach AG, Berghmans S. Zebrafish: an emerging technology for *in vivo* pharmacological assessment to identify potential safety liabilities in early drug discovery. Br J Pharmacol 2008;54(7):1400–13.

[63] Smith AC, Raimondi AR, Salthouse CD, Ignatius MS, Blackburn JS, Mizgirev IV, Storer NY, de Jong JL, Chen AT, Zhou Y, Revskoy S, Zon LI, Langenau DM. High-throughput cell transplantation establishes that tumor-initiating cells are abundant in zebrafish T-cell acute lymphoblastic leukemia. Blood 2010;115:3296–303.

[64] Park SW, Davison JM, Rhee J, Hruban RH, Maitra A, Leach SD. KRAS induces progenitor cell expansion and malignant transformation in zebrafish exocrine pancreas. Gastroenterol Oncogen 2008;134:2080–90.

[65] Sabaawy HE, Azuma M, Embree LJ, Tsai HJ, Starost MF, Hickstein DD. TEL-AML1 transgenic zebrafish model of precursor B cell acute lymphoblastic leukemia. Proc Natl Acad Sci USA 2006;103:15166–71.

[66] Rudner LA, et al. Shared acquired genomic changes in zebrafish and human T-ALL. Oncogene 2011;30:4289–96.

[67] Langenau DM, Traver D, Ferrando AA, Kutok JL, Aster JC, Kanki JP, Lin S, Prochownik E, Trede NS, Zon LI, Look AT. Myc-induced T cell leukemia in transgenic zebrafish. Science 2003;299:887–90.

[68] Marques IJ, Weiss FU, Vlecken DH, Nitsche C, Bakkers J, Lagendijk AK, Partecke LI, Heidecke CD, Lerch MM, Bagowski CP. Metastatic behaviour of primary human tumours in a zebrafish xenotransplantation model. BMC Cancer 2009;9:128.

[69] Eguiara A, Holgado O, Beloqui I, Abalde L, Sanchez Y, Callol C, Martin AG. Xenografts in zebrafish embryos as a rapid functional assay for breast cancer stem-like cell identification. Cell Cycle 2011;10:3751–7.

[70] Nguyen AT, Emelyanov A, Koh CH, Spitsbergen JM, Parinov S, Gong Z. An inducible krasV12 transgenic zebrafish model for liver tumorigenesis and chemical drug screening. Dis Model Mech 2012;5(1):63–72.

[71] Zon LI, Peterson RT. *In vivo* drug discovery in the zebrafish. Nat Rev Drug Discov 2005;4:35–44.

[72] Lukianova-Hleb EY, Santiago C, Wagner DS, Hafner JH, Lapotko DO. Generation and detection of plasmonic nanobubbles in zebrafish. Nanotechnology 2010;21(22):225102.

[73] Wagner DS, Delk NA, Lukianova-Hleb EY, Hafner JH, Farach-Carson MC, Lapotko DO. The *in vivo* performance of plasmonic nanobubbles as cell theranostic agents in zebrafish hosting prostate cancer xenografts. Biomaterials 2010;31(29):7567–74.

CHAPTER 7

Animal Utilization in Drug Development: Clinical, Legal, and Ethical Dimensions

Odilia Osakwe

Contents

7.1 Introduction	150
7.2 The Scientific Value of Animal Studies: Pharmacology Objectives	150
7.3 Laboratory Animals Model in the Frontiers of Drug Discovery	151
7.4 Relationships in Animal Taxonomy and Implications in Pharmaceutical Research and Development	152
7.5 The Effect of Species Differences on Study Results	154
7.5.1 Pain Cognition/Recognition or Expression	154
7.5.2 Effect of Dosage Regimen	155
7.5.3 Effects of Genetic Modification	155
7.5.4 Cytochrome P450 (CYP)-Mediated Drug Metabolism and Inhibition	155
7.6 How Reliable is the Animal Toxicity Information Generated Across the Animal Species?	157
7.6.1 Extrapolation of Animal Data to Humans	158
7.7 Landmarks in Preclinical Development: Species Selection and Rationale	158
7.7.1 Animal Models of Depressions: Minipig and Beagle Animal Models	159
7.7.2 Animal Models of Cancer	159
7.7.3 Animal Models of Alzheimer's Disease in Drug Development	159
7.7.4 Insect Models: The Fruit Fly	160
7.8 Animal Models in the Development of Biopharmaceuticals: the Exceptional Use of Nonhuman Primates	161
7.9 Legal Accommodations on the Use of Animals in Pharmaceutical Research and Development	161
7.9.1 United States	161
7.9.2 Canada	162
7.9.3 Europe	162
7.10 Animal Alternatives in Drug Development: Replacing, Reducing, and Refinement of Animals	163
7.10.1 Replacement	163
7.10.2 Reduction	164
7.10.3 Refinement	165
References	165

Social Aspects of Drug Discovery, Development and Commercialization   Copyright © 2016 Elsevier Inc.
http://dx.doi.org/10.1016/B978-0-12-802220-7.00007-7   All rights reserved.

7.1 INTRODUCTION

The cellular and molecular effects of a therapeutic agent could be predicted using *in vitro* systems and the usefulness cannot be underemphasized as it allows high throughput rapid screening of candidate compounds. However, a proper understanding of the complex physiological response needs a whole organism that could exhibit the signs and symptoms of diseases. Thus, animal studies have been introduced as a subset of test systems employed at the preclinical stage of drug development for the prediction of clinical effectiveness in humans. This has been possible due to the ability to correlate data generated from animal studies to humans [1,2].

As detailed in Chapter 5, the compound selection steps of the drug optimization studies that mostly involve the *in silico* approaches also assess the risks using deductive estimation of risk from existing knowledge, bioavailability studies, safety pharmacological studies, and pharmaceutical development. The very essence of animal testing is underscored by the global regulatory constraints, requiring very well-defined animal testing strategies to be integrated into the drug development process, to increase the probability of success in the entire drug discovery program. Demonstrating efficacy of new drug entities is expected to be achieved in targeted preclinical models that show adequate similarity with the human disease to enable the estimation of dose levels, regimens, and drug combinations that are subsequently used for clinical trials. Even though these have been well conducted, the feasibility of providing the ultimate proof of concept for efficacy and safety strictly depends on whether it can be translated into humans. Thus, animal use has been fiercely defended due to its liabilities and relevance in the discovery of drugs [3]. The following discussions will embrace the typical cases of the utility of animals in preclinical drug development, reflecting the opportunities and challenges. This chapter gives general perspectives of the utility and role of animal models.

7.2 THE SCIENTIFIC VALUE OF ANIMAL STUDIES: PHARMACOLOGY OBJECTIVES

Pharmacology objectives could be primary, secondary, and safety related. Primary pharmacology has been defined as investigation of the mode of action and effects on its desired therapeutic target. Secondary pharmacology is unrelated to its desired therapeutic target. Safety pharmacology is concerned with the undesirable pharmacodynamics (PD) effects of a substance on physiological functions when a drug is exposed to a therapeutic range and above [4].

These studies determine the undesirable pathophysiological effects, the mechanisms, and adverse PD effects on the major organ systems like cardiovascular, respiratory, and CNS. Toxicity studies are usually executed using rodent and nonrodent species. This is because of the need of species of distant phylogenic relationship to offer the best chances of detecting adverse effects, a primary or secondary pharmacological effect.

Genotoxicity assays are performed using bacteria and somatic cells for assessing the possibility of mutations or chromosomal abnormality that could arise due to the use of candidate drugs. According to [5] "Good practice guidelines – the selection of nonrodent species for pharmaceutical toxicology," animal studies documentation would have to be satisfied on rodent and one nonrodent and 6–9 months of repeat dosing was recommended as sufficient to provide adequate information on toxicity.

Preliminary studies are usually focused on distribution, metabolism, and pharmacokinetics (DMPK) toxicology and safety pharmacology. DMPK involves exposing different species to clinical candidate drugs in order to understand the varying metabolic profiles of the species, which allows the selection and determination of their drug–drug interactions. They are usually initiated by the use of a single dose but this has changed to dose-range finding and maximal tolerated dose studies performed in rodents and nonrodents (rats and dogs), mostly centered on the cardiovascular systems. For subchronic and chronic toxicity studies, the repeat dose is intended to evaluate the no observed effect level (NOEL), which is instrumental in critical decisions made at this phase. Reproductive and developmental toxicological studies enable determination of further effects on fertility, developmental teratology, or newborn. Mutagenicity studies deal with effects of gene mutations. Carcinogenicity studies identify tumorigenic possibilities and risk in humans. Other special studies are immunotoxicity, mechanistic toxicity, and sensitization or phototoxicity studies.

7.3 LABORATORY ANIMALS MODEL IN THE FRONTIERS OF DRUG DISCOVERY

Rats, mice, dogs, (nonhuman) primates, rabbits, hamsters, cats, guinea pigs, farm pigs, miniature swine, and goats are among the most common species used for preclinical and nonclinical evaluation. Laboratory mice are predominantly used in research when compared to other animals. It is estimated that nearly 20 million rodents are bred for research annually. Mice, plus other rodents such as rats and hamsters, make up more than 90% of the total number of animals used. Other animal species, including dogs, cats, rabbits, farm animals, fish, frogs, birds, nonhuman primates, and many others, make up the remaining 10% of animals used in research. Any animal selected as a disease model is expected to recapitulate all the aspects of the disease in humans. This requires a proper understanding of both the animal model and the human disease to be able to effectively replicate the human symptoms and to enhance the chances of a breakthrough predictive power.

Rodents are the most commonly used animal models due to their short lifecycle and lifespan. These offer complementary benefits of cost and time savings as they can reproduce quickly, yielding faster results. However, large animals live longer, thus allowing for longitudinal studies, and they are more similar in size to humans providing an opportunity to address issues related to scaling up to human therapy. Dogs and nonhuman primates are typical representatives of the nonrodent species but certain experimental needs would require minipigs and rabbits. Selection of species is mostly based on closeness to the physiologic or pathological mechanisms and the nature of response to the adverse effects of drugs. The issue of animal maintenance also influences the selection of species and has become is a major limitation to accuracy of results. This is due to the pattern of handling of animals in housing or in isolation, which could lead to stress and other pathological factors. It could alter what is known about the animals and in particular their physiology, which is a major factor examined in animal studies. Certain variations among the species, even at a minimal level, tend to introduce variables in the generated data. A report compiled by David Salsburg of Pfizer Central Research describes that out of 19 chemicals known to cause cancer in humans only 37% of these chemicals induced cancer in rats and mice.

7.4 RELATIONSHIPS IN ANIMAL TAXONOMY AND IMPLICATIONS IN PHARMACEUTICAL RESEARCH AND DEVELOPMENT

Genes often targeted for diseases of human origin have counterparts in the rat and mice genome, which are evolutionarily conserved, having passed through the lineage relatively unaltered. This is a major reason why rat and mice are a prime choice in biomedical research. Between rat and mice, there are genomic differences even though physical similarities exist. Some of the genes in the rat that are not present in the mouse are involved in metabolism, immunity, and reproduction. The primate lineage is close to that of humans as the chromosomal reorganization in these species is relatively minimal. A stark similarity across the species is the skeletal muscular systems, so that no major differences are expected between species for the bioavailability of intramuscularly administered drugs, when compared on a weight-normalized basis. Physiological parameters, such as body temperature (36–38°C), hematocrit (40–45%), and serum albumin concentration (30–40 g/L) are relatively conserved among animals and which are independent of animal size [6].

The physiological characteristics of different animal species lead to evolutionary adaptations that are necessary for survival within their ecosystem. One exception is the cat, which possesses less genetic diversity due to domestication. The phylogenetic factors have been expressed in physiological functions such as digestive functions involved in drug absorption. Differences between species and genders affect the toxicology, pharmacokinetics (PK), pharmacodynamics (PD), dosing, and biological predictivity. A known fact is that the variable sizes and shapes of organisms relate to their biology, including the metabolic rate, which is partly contributed to by differing surface area to volume ratio. Interspecies difference in drug metabolism is significantly less in terms of drug action as it shows less interspecies disparity but only in special cases.

The dog is the first species employed in the evaluation of candidate drugs that are substrates of P-glycoprotein 1 (Pgp) [7]. Beagle dogs are model animals in preclinical trials used for estimating initial drug dosage regimen but have shown variations among differing strains in PK and PD [8].

There are numerous causes of interspecies differences in drug disposition or PK and exposure – absorption, distribution, metabolism, and excretion (ADME) profiles. Differences in drug action and effect, that is, of PD, are connected to differences in target functions (anatomy, physiology, and pathology) and/or target receptors including pathogenic microorganisms. Attempts have been made to extrapolate PK as well as PD parameters between species in order to ensure data uniformity. The influence of body size on the numerical values of PK or PD parameters has been taken into consideration. This phenomenon is called allometry and has been used as a tool in estimating the first-in-human dose based on a valid quantifiable value but is not applicable in all cases [9].

Physiologically-based pharmacokinetic (PBPK) modeling is a widespread approach for extrapolating data from one species to another. PBPK models consist of compartments, connected by the circulating blood system. The compartments correspond to various tissues in the body and are defined by a tissue volume (or weight) and tissue blood flow rate, which is specific to the species of interest. These parameters are used to calculate the effective half-life or residence time of the drug. In a preclinical setting, PK parameters from different *in vivo* studies enable the ranking of compounds and can be linked to physicochemical, *in vitro*, or structural properties to guide optimization of the PK properties of drug candidates.

Certain factors limit the extrapolation of data generated from animal studies to humans. These are anatomical and physiological variation; tolerance and enzyme induction; PK variations between animals and humans; pathological conditions in humans that are not found in animals and idiosyncratic adverse events in humans that could not be developed in animals; inability of animals to orally communicate responses; ineffective correlation of drugs and metabolites with the underlying disease; and sensitivity of certain pharmacological activities to selective clinical routes of drug administration.

7.5 THE EFFECT OF SPECIES DIFFERENCES ON STUDY RESULTS

Animal models have been applied in the study of the anatomical, physiological, and biochemical differences in the gastrointestinal (GI) tract of humans. However, interspecies differences significantly influence the interpretation and accuracy of the results [10].

The following are typical cases.

7.5.1 Pain Cognition/Recognition or Expression

The level of pain tolerance or pain threshold varies across the various animal species. Those that are more resilient express pain at higher thresholds. Horses have low thresholds for pain when compared to a resilient ass with a high threshold [11]. Intuitively, data from these animal species are not comparable and have been taken less seriously. Dogs have been classified as resilient and as such were not given analgesics after major surgery. But the passing of the Laboratory Animal Welfare Act of 1966, P.L. 89-544 stimulated the acceptance and administering of pain relieving medications for dogs [12]. The study of conditions such as colic can proceed to advanced irreversible stages before they are detected. Due to lack of a clear indicator of pain in fish, the effect of pain relieving drugs is judged by the ease of handling of fish [13]. The proposals concerning the use or theories that are fundamental to the handling of fish have not been scientifically justified. There is a belief that fish have fewer C fibers (pain sensors) than mammals, which are thought to transmit longer signals due to injury. This proposition has led to a conclusion that the aquatic adaptation would respond differently to pain when compared to other mammals [14,15].

7.5.2 Effect of Dosage Regimen

Doses expressed by body weight could result in marked variation in dosage between species. For example, the dosage for aspirin is approximately 40 times higher in cattle than in cats, whereas the effective dose for morphine is 10-fold lower in cats than in dogs. A depolarizing neuromuscular blocker, named suxamethonium (succinylcholine), is 40 times lower in cattle than in cats. As a consequence, extra caution is expected when interspecies comparison is made. Genetic variation in similar mouse models leads to a subtle divergence in physical and physiological traits.

7.5.3 Effects of Genetic Modification

Intraspecies variation, referred to as variation within the same species, is present in genetically modified animals. Intraspecies genetic manipulation could lead to variable phenotypes as there are reasonable differences in the genetic makeup. Certain phenotypic changes resulting from genetic modification are indirect effects and these might not be easily determined. For example, certain physical and physiological (or phenotypic) traits could surface due to genetic manipulation, which are not the same in their human counterparts. A tumor gene knockout could lead to a separate range of tumors in comparison to that of humans [16,17].

7.5.4 Cytochrome P450 (CYP)-Mediated Drug Metabolism and Inhibition

Cytochrome P450 (CYP) enzymes are widely recognized due to their role as drug metabolizing enzymes. They act by binding two atoms of oxygen resulting in the formation of a water molecule and a metabolite with a higher polarity than the parent drug. There are subtle differences in amino acid composition and sequence arrangement, which contribute to differences in function of the CYP isoforms and, consequently, differences in drug metabolism for the highly metabolized drugs. For drugs that are not metabolized at all, interspecies differences are minimal and could be extrapolated to another species through allometry scaling.

In comparison to humans, rat and mouse genomes possess higher numbers of Phase I metabolism genes while other model organisms have relatively similar numbers [18,19].

Out of the 57 human cytochrome P450 genes, 23 are associated with ADMET, whereas the minipig and Duroc pig contain 19 and 18 ADMET-related CYPs, respectively, with minipigs showing a comparable level of abundance and activity of drug metabolizing enzymes as humans [20], but total P450 activity is lower for beagles relative to humans.

Body weight plays a major role in the abundance of hepatic enzymes. For instance, CYP/gram body weight is higher in small animals than in humans [21]. It also directly correlates with the metabolic rate; higher in small animals than in humans. There are variable CYP expression patterns in humans, rats, mice, dogs, and monkeys. CYP1A1 and -1A2 are strongly conserved among the species but CYP1A1 is minimally expressed in the liver of all species. In human and animal species, CYP1B1 is the only gene product of the CYP1B subfamily. In humans and rodents, CYP2A is expressed in liver and extrahepatic tissues. The substrate specificity of human CYP2A6 and CYP2A enzymes in animals are different. CYP2C is the largest and most complicated subfamily across the laboratory animal models, such as, rat and mouse; and humans. CYP2C is present in the liver of rodent and nonrodent species, and its expression in extrahepatic tissue is isoform specific but human forms have different substrate specificities. The CYP2D family displays a genetic polymorphism that plays a role in human drug metabolism. In addition such a trait was observed in rats [22,23]. CYP2E1 is expressed in the liver and in many extrahepatic tissues of numerous animal species. CYP2E1 is only involved in the metabolism of a handful of drugs. A remarkable degree of conservation suggests success in the extrapolation between species. The rat shows superiority as a potential animal model for humans for CYP2E1. CYP3A is the isoform most commonly known to exist in the species; however, various CYP3A isoforms expressed show differing substrate specificities making their suitability for extrapolation to humans impracticable. No animal species possesses all the qualities of a perfect laboratory model for drug development. Thus, *in vitro* studies with liver microsomes and hepatocytes should inform the selection of animals to be used in each case [24].

Similarities in the CYP isoforms are important when choosing animal models for preclinical studies. In the model animal, a candidate drug should show an acceptable range of bioavailability, a comparable metabolic profile (similarity of the cytochrome P450), and systematic exposure more than that of humans. Also the distribution and elimination mechanism should be sufficiently similar. It is important that the phylogenetic status in relation to humans is often backed up with justifiable physiological processes.

7.6 HOW RELIABLE IS THE ANIMAL TOXICITY INFORMATION GENERATED ACROSS THE ANIMAL SPECIES?

One of the major endearing quality of any drug is that it is safe in humans and thus toxicology studies are essential as they provide information that enables scheduling of dose and effect of extended exposure to the drug. Toxicology is concerned with identification of hazards to human health, and it is applied to the varied methods that address drug safety. These studies focus on adverse effects in select animal species and describe the dose–effect relationship over other ranges of doses. It is also a necessary condition required by the regulators in order to progress to clinical trials. To satisfy the regulatory demand, toxicology studies must be conducted in two animal species, a rodent and a larger nonrodent. Rats/beagle and dogs/monkeys fall into these categories and are the most common species of choice for most of the preclinical studies. They are exposed to drugs in a stepwise increment until a toxic level is achieved. This becomes obvious upon manifestation of typical signs of toxicity, which include weight loss and lethargy. Biochemical analysis is provided to determine systemic toxicity and also the body tissues are examined for these effects. The results help determine dosing for humans, which is one-tenth of the maximum tolerated dose in the more sensitive of the two species used in the toxicology studies. These studies are used to confirm the unsafe dose level if it is below the expected efficacy dose, or delayed toxicity (toxicity at a period of time after the last dose is taken), or idiosyncratic toxicity (toxicity that is irreversible or unpredictable). Good judgment chiefly relies on the interpretation proficiency of the toxicologist who makes determinations that are applied for the next step, which is clinical trial.

Certain problems, particularly those associated with reproducibility, number of study subjects, uncommon adverse effects, ruggedness or interlaboratory interpretation of generated data, could limit the effectiveness of animal toxicology results. Even though the guidelines are followed, data have to be well validated and verifiable and this is not always certain. One experimental discrepancy could be mismatching the number of study subjects between humans and animals. Certain drugs are judged differently with respect to their use in humans because of interpretation of toxicity outcomes (or how it is weighted in animals) leading to rejection of certain experimental compounds that have not been efficiently demonstrated to pose a safety issue. Drug toxicity is managed differently by different animals leading to variable mortality rates in response to toxicity, which also amounts to errors in interpretation and translation to humans. It raises certain concerns as it could yield false positive or false negative conclusions as well. Certain drugs that are highly toxic in animals do not reach the stage of being tested in humans and could not be studied retrospectively due to preferential selectivity for those exhibiting favorable safety profiles. Extrapolated data have resulted in both positive and negative results. Species differences in physiology structure and function result in differences in metabolism of toxins, chemical and drug absorption, and mechanisms of DNA repair. These variables account for the incorrect application of animal data to human diseases and drug responses.

The starting and subsequent dose schemes are identified in nonclinical toxicology studies. Reversibility of toxicology is identified in target organs and serum is used for reducing risk. Risk level evaluation is dependent on disease severity, public understanding, and acceptance. Acceptance of risk is also dependent of disease indication. For diseases like cancer higher risk levels are accepted. Risk assessment is based on risk and hazard identification, characterization, and exposure assessment. Risk is evaluated in animal and *in vitro* studies while exposure is characterized in dose-response relationships and mechanisms, assessed through determining the C_{max} and area under the curve. Risk is then defined by acceptability and level of exposure within the safety margin, which altogether depend on the drug usage.

7.6.1 Extrapolation of Animal Data to Humans

The primary objective for understanding animal studies is to extrapolate the findings to humans. In order to achieve this objective, animals are exposed to high doses that are above the human safety range. Moreover, the nonclinical studies do not exactly complement the clinical trials as only healthy animals are used in nonclinical whereas, the clinical trials involves patients. Also, a wider variety of animals species are used in nonclinical safety studies. This has drawn conflicting interests and concerns that question the integrity of animal studies in nonclinical pharmaceutical research.

7.7 LANDMARKS IN PRECLINICAL DEVELOPMENT: SPECIES SELECTION AND RATIONALE

Multiple models, species, and experimental strategies have been used to create a "signature" for a given mechanism so as to narrow the applicability of one model where its use is most effective [25].

7.7.1 Animal Models of Depressions: Minipig and Beagle Animal Models

Minipig and beagle animal model genomes are the ideal choice in pharmaceutical discovery and development. The beagle is a commonly used animal species in preclinical studies even though the genomes are distinct from other key model organisms [26]. The beagle dog has been very useful in cardiovascular safety pharmacology testing. Over time, the minipig has found a niche application in cardiovascular, skin, and renal studies.

7.7.2 Animal Models of Cancer

Cancer disease is a generic term as the word "cancer" covers a multiplicity of disparate biological characteristics and associated pathways. Animal models of cancer are essential in understanding the pathophysiology of the cancer disease for identifying new targets and therapeutic agents. Homogeneity and rapid development are the principal characteristics of the mouse that makes it most suitable as an animal model of cancer. Even though not exactly a perfect fit for use, suitable experimental design and evaluation could enhance the predictive power as cancer models.

Carcinogen-induced models enable the evaluation of time-dependent progression of tumor pathogenesis due to external influences or carcinogens [27]. These same types of models are expected to be useful in determining dose–response relationships, which are needed to understand the tumor PK/PD effects and the potential effect of therapy on tumor progression when exposed to the drug [28]. Genetically engineered mouse models have been limited by time of development of tumor – tumor development does follow the same timing as that of the transgenic host. In addition, they do not often express the clinical symptoms and irregularities in tumor frequency and growth properties [29].

7.7.3 Animal Models of Alzheimer's Disease in Drug Development

The etiology of Alzheimer's disease has not been well established and for this reason "amyloid hypothesis" only provides a working principle used as a premise for developing therapy and experimental modalities [30]. Animal models of Alzheimer's disease are used to study the effect of therapeutic agents on the neuropathological indicators like β-amyloid plaques (Aβ) and neuronal and synaptic loss in brain regions of the disease. Identification of activity is based on certain clinical signs like the cognitive function in animal model even though it lacks definitive information about the effect in humans. Selection of animal is based on the phylogenic proximity to humans and its ability to recapitulate the Alzheimer's neuropathology [31]. Several aging diseases develop in the same way in rhesus monkeys and humans, and this has led to the choice of rhesus monkeys as the most widely accepted model because diagnosis has been possible and they are well suited for development of safe medicines for these disorders. The small prosimian primate is highly recommended due to age-related changes that simulate those of humans. This primate, with a lifespan of 8–10 years, is a prime asset for studying age-related disease [32]. Dogs have been used because the amino acid sequence of the Aβ is similar to that of humans. Mouse lemurs also show the disease patterns.

The transgenic species were created by transferring the amyloid precursor protein to the animal model. The mouse transgenic models are able to reproduce the patterns of Aβ-induced neuropathological manifestations leading to the observed the clinical symptoms like Aβ-production, deposition, and clearance [33] to rapid progression with respect to humans. Mouse lemurs are good models as they develop to full blown at 5 years and older. Certain undesirable effects have been associated with the pattern of distribution of amyloid plaques in the mouse lemur. In humans, it is initiated at the hippocampus while that of the mouse lemur begins at the cortical regions. Since only about 20% of the adult mouse lemur will develop the associated symptoms, a diagnostic-based selection is needed. However, there are no such tools available [34]. There is biochemical composition mismatch between the mouse model and the Alzheimer's disease brain, which has contributed to failure in developing an important pathological signature of Alzheimer's – the neurofibrillary tangles [35]. Even though no single animal has been a true representative model for Alzheimer's disease, certain aspects of the disease have been well represented in certain models, which has been a great utility in understanding and supporting the research objective. Thus, a major hurdle is to find the model that could be used to serve as an experimental model for the underrepresented aspects of the disease. Experimental parameters may need to be modified to create a condition that more closely mimics aspects of the disease.

7.7.4 Insect Models: The Fruit Fly

The fruit fly, even though it has only a portion of human brain cells due to its miniaturized scale, has similarities in the basic cell biology activities and it possesses an excellent brain organization. This is the principal reason why it is an extensively characterized insect model [36]. An interesting quality of the fruit fly is its cuticle – a transparent cuticle facilitates the study of disease progression in unmodified models, which has not been achieved in animals [37,38].

7.8 ANIMAL MODELS IN THE DEVELOPMENT OF BIOPHARMACEUTICALS: THE EXCEPTIONAL USE OF NONHUMAN PRIMATES

Biopharmaceuticals are complex therapeutic molecules derived from microorganisms, blood or blood components, somatic cells, nucleic acids, tissues, recombinant therapeutic protein, and living cells. In stark contrast to small molecule therapeutics (SMs), biopharmaceuticals are characterized by their high selectivity and specificity toward their target [39]. However, biopharmaceuticals elicit severe adverse effect profiles superior to that of SMs[40,41].Biotechnology-derivedproductssuchashormonesandantibodies are regulated differently and require preferential choice of animal models for preclinical studies. Antibodies to the biopharmaceuticals can confound experimental findings and the predictive power of animal models [42,43]. Therefore, nonhuman primate animal models are the only viable animal model that can be used for preclinical studies for monoclonal antibodies-based therapeutics. They are often considered the only species that mirror human-like adverse effects. Certain ethical, practical, and financial roadblocks affect their utility [43,44]. The target drug dynamics are more complicated, as results could be exaggerated, and therefore, the selection of models has been strictly based on relevance.

7.9 LEGAL ACCOMMODATIONS ON THE USE OF ANIMALS IN PHARMACEUTICAL RESEARCH AND DEVELOPMENT

7.9.1 United States

The US Animal Welfare Act (AWA) is a federal law that was established in 1966 and is responsible for research activities that involve the use of animals. Under AWA is the American Association for Laboratory Animal Science, which regulates animal use at the institutional level and oversees the housing welfare procedures, protocols, emergencies, and reports pertaining to animal care and use. Facilities that use vertebrate animals are funded by the Public Health Service and are expected to comply with the Guide for the Care and Use of Laboratory Animals established by the Institute for Laboratory Animal Research. The Association for Assessment and Accreditation of Laboratory Animal Care International is a privately funded organization that recommends the use of appropriate guidelines for the use and care of laboratory animals. The International Conference on Harmonisation, a harmonization guideline for safety pharmacology testing, is applicable in the United States, the European Union, Japan, and other countries. Scientific information is needed and facilitates a decision on selection availability and other constraints.

The Food and Drug Administration (FDA) requires that safety standards be met with data from either animal studies or validated alternatives. Thus, it recommends that alternatives be used when possible. The FDA is working in partnership with the Mandatory Alternatives Petition toward putting together policy guidelines that further emphasize the need for validated alternatives in biomedical research. Sometimes pharmaceutical companies may be hesitant in implementing of new polices and resort to traditional animal testing methods that are well developed as an easier way to regulatory approval.

7.9.2 Canada

The Canadian Council on Animal Care (CCAC) is an independent body and a nonprofit organization created in 1968 to oversee the ethical use of animals in research, teaching, and testing in science in Canada. The CCAC is funded by the Canadian Institutes of Health Research and the Natural Sciences and Engineering Research Council of Canada; other contributions from federal science-based departments and agencies and private institutions participate in its programs. The CCAC policy statement Ethics of Animal Investigation, 1989 says that "Animals must not be subjected to unnecessary pain or distress. The experimental design must offer them every practicable safeguard, whether in research, in teaching, or in testing procedures; ..."

7.9.3 Europe

Animal protection and welfare is covered under EU Directive 2010/63/EU, which was adopted in 2010 and took effect on January 1, 2013. The 1986 Directive 86/609/EEC on the protection of animals used for biomedical research strengthens the principle of the Three Rs (3Rs), to replace, reduce, and refine the use of animals.

The INFRAFRONTIER partners and their national regulations are comprised of various institutes from European nationalities and the Toronto Centre of phenogenomics, Canada, who are subject to policies on animal use. These policies are concerned with the design of procedures, the appropriate use of species, the principles of the 3Rs (reduction, refinement, and replacement), minimization of discomfort, distress and pain, use of appropriate analgesia or anesthetics, and animal husbandry.

7.10 ANIMAL ALTERNATIVES IN DRUG DEVELOPMENT: REPLACING, REDUCING, AND REFINEMENT OF ANIMALS

Laboratory animal husbandry has been around since 1959, when the approach to experimental techniques involving animal handling was revisited, requiring more caution and a humane approach to the use of animals. Major Charles Hume, Founder of the Universities Federation for Animal Welfare, requested a publication on the application of ethical conduct in the use of animals in laboratory experiments. This was followed by two great scientists of the time: William Russell, a zoologist, psychologist, and classical scholar, and Rex Burch, a microbiologist, who subsequently published the 1959 Principles of Humane Experimental Techniques, which emphasized the principles of replacement, reduction, and refinement (the 3Rs) that are actively applied globally today.

7.10.1 Replacement

The depleted ecology, which includes animals that have been completely lost and extinct, is a possible impact of use of animals. Replacement alternatives require the use of other options where possible to minimize the use of animals. These involve the use of tissue cultures including embryonic and adult stem cells, and *in vitro* assays using mammalian or human cell cultures for a wide range of toxic and other endpoints. Modern cell culture techniques have been greatly improved due to emergent models that more closely mimic the *in vivo* milieu as explained in Chapter 5.

Microarray technology allows the assessment of large numbers of genes simultaneously, to permit expression profiling of genes that are activated or suppressed in response to examined molecular pathways or biological activities. These are probed on a chip instead of the animal. Scientists and engineers at Harvard University have created "organs-on-a-chip," including the "lung-on-a-chip" and "gut-on-a-chip." These tiny devices contain human cells in a three-dimensional system that mimics human organs. Structure–activity relationships have enabled prediction of biological activity (e.g., toxicity) of drug compounds, which is based on the molecular structure and other *in silico* modeling activities. These strategies enable a "replacement" of animals as they are highly effective in disease research, drug testing, and toxicity testing.

In silico modeling is a computerized platform that utilizes known rules for predicting the related biological outcomes like metabolic fate, and these rules are mostly about factors affecting toxicity, physicochemical characteristics, and more. Typically, a range of chemical compounds undergo high-throughput screening (HTS) for a drug target or disease model prior to finding the preliminary "hits," or active and functional motifs. These are involved in recognition and targeting activities that are well differentiated from other functional properties of the molecule in which they occur for the generation of cluster, potency, and factors like ligand efficiency or predefined toxicological factors.

7.10.1.1 Virtual Animals and Human Models

Computerized models of complex human biology attempt to reduce animal testing and increase the speed of the drug discovery process. For example, a computerized model, PhysioLab®, is a product of a Californian biotechnology company Entelos. It is a precise algorithm, platform model with equations that describe the biological pathways that are adjusted to the existing information or client proprietary data. This is subsequently adapted to particular biological processes or pathways of interest. Its utility has been reported as an aid to target and biomarker selection, species translation, patient stratification, and clinical trial design. The PhysioLab model has been applied to type 2 diabetes, rheumatoid arthritis, hypertension, and cardiovascular disease modeling (http://www.entelos.com/). The computerized models might present their own pitfalls as no single human model exists due to human genetic diversity. Also, these models are based on certain generalizations based on the most dominant genotypes and phenotypes. This might not be applicable in certain real-time cases and thus might not have a widespread application.

These valued fast-track technology-based accomplishments are the reason for modern-day HTS candidate drug screening, which takes place in a test tube and is subject to automation – a microscale representation of a human disease process. This understanding has been disputed based on the notion that a simplified model is not a true representative of complex human biology and its networks.

7.10.2 Reduction

Animal reduction strategies have been performed through improvement in experimental design and statistical analysis, compound prescreening (HTS), smaller focused studies, pilot tests that enable to properly calculate sample sizes, improvement in education and staff training, policies of recycling of animals, and interim kills. The extent of invasiveness versus potential benefit derived from animal usage is taken into consideration prior to the decision on the number of animal subjects utilized in laboratory experiments. Certain ethical, scientific, and practical considerations enhance the feasibility and predictivity of the animal model chosen.

7.10.3 Refinement

Refinement alternatives refine animal care, focusing on procedures that minimize pain and distress through the use of noninvasive imaging, other convenient devices to avoid surgical trauma, and better blood sampling techniques like venipuncture. Positive reinforcement techniques have been widely applied, especially in primates.

The animal replacement strategies have not yet been entirely possible particularly due to the inadequacy of *in silico* technologies. However, numerous animal reduction strategies have led to clinical success.

REFERENCES

[1] Hondeghem LM, Lu HR, Van Rossem K, De Clerck F. Detection of proarrhythmia in the female rabbit heart: blinded validation. J Cardiovasc Electrophysiol 2003;14(3):287–94.

[2] Huskey SE, Dean BJ, Bakhtiar R, Sanchez RI, Tattersall FD, Rycroft W, Hargreaves R, Watt AP, Chicchi GG, Keohane C, Hora DF, Chiu SH. Brain penetration of aprepitant, a substance P receptor antagonist, in ferrets. Drug Metab Dispos 2003;31(6):785–91.

[3] Cimons M, Getlin J, Maugh, T. Cancer Drugs Face Long Road From Mice to Men. Los Angeles Times, A1. 1998.

[4] Anon, ICH S7A: safety pharmacology studies for human pharmaceuticals, CPMP/ICH/539/00, London, November 16, 2000. Available from: http://www. Emea.eu.int/pdfs/human/ich/05300en,pdf

[5] Hubrecht R, Smith D. Good practice guidelines –The selection of Non-rodent species for Pharmaceutical Toxicology. Laboratory Animal Association. Series3/Issue 1-october 2001. Available from: Emea.eu.int/pdfs/human/ich/05300en,pdf

[6] Davies B, Morris T. Physiological parameters in laboratory animals and humans. Pharm Res 1993;10:1093–5.

[7] Mealey KL. Pharmacogenomics. In: Riviere JE, Papich MG, editors. Veterinary pharmacology and therapeutics. 9th ed. Wiley-Blackwell; 2009. p. 1313–22.

[8] Engel L, Reitz B, Bolten S, Burton EG, Maziasz TJ, Yan B, Schoenhard GL. Evidence for polymorphism in the canine metabolism of the cyclooxygenase 2 inhibitor, celecoxib. Drug Metab Dispos 1999;27:1133–42.

[9] Riviere JE, Martin-Jimenez T, Sundlof SF, Craigmill AL. Interspecies allometric analysis of the comparative pharmacokinetics of 44 drugs across veterinary and laboratory animal species. J Vet Pharmacol Ther 1997;20:453–63.

[10] Hengstler JG, Van der Burg B, Steinberg P, Oesch F., Interspecies differences in cancer susceptibility and toxicity, Drug Metab Rev 1999; 31(4):917-970.

[11] Ashley FH, Waterman-Pearson AE, Whay HR. Behavioural assessment of pain in horses and donkeys: application to clinical practice and future studies. Equine Vet J 2005;37:565–75.

[12] Hansen BD. Assessment of pain in dogs: veterinary clinical studies. ILAR J 2003; 44:197–205.

[13] Anil SS, Anil L, Deen J. Challenges of pain assessment in domestic animals. J Am Vet Med Assoc 2002;220(3):313–9.

[14] Roques JA, Abbink W, Geurds F, van de Vis H, Flik G. Tailfin clipping, a painful procedure: studies on Nile tilapia and common carp. Physiol Behav 2010;101(4):533–40.

[15] Rose D, Arlinghaus R, Cooke SJ, Diggles BK, Sawynok W, Stevens ED, Wynne CDL. Can fish really feel pain? Fish and Fisheries 2014;15(1):97–133.

[16] Crusio WE. Flanking gene and genetic background problems in genetically manipulated mice. Biol Psychiatry 2004;56(6):381–5.

[17] Bothe GW, Bolivar VJ, Vedder MJ, Geistfeld JG. Genetic and behavioral differences among five inbred mouse strains commonly used in the production of transgenic and knockout mice. Genes Brain Behav 2004;3(3):149–57.

[18] Caenepeel S, Charydczak G, Sudarsanam S, Hunter T, Manning G. The mouse kinome: discovery and comparative genomics of all mouse protein kinases. Proc Natl Acad Sci USA 2004;101(32):11707–21112.

[19] Niimura Y, Nei M. Extensive gains and losses of olfactory receptor genes in mammalian evolution. PLoS One 2007;2:e708.

[20] Anzenbacher P, Soucek P, Anzenbacherová E, Gut I, Hruby K, Svoboda Z, Kvetina J. Presence and activity of cytochrome P450 isoforms in minipig liver microsomes. Drug Metab Dispos 1998;26:56–9.

[21] Stevens JC, Shipley LA, Cashman JR, Vandenbranden M, Wrighton SA. Comparison of human and rhesus monkey in vitro phase I and phase II hepatic drug metabolism activities. Drug Metab Dispos 1993;21:753–60.

[22] Yamamoto Y, Tasaki T, Nakamura A, Iwata H, Kazusaka A, Gonzalez FJ, Fujita S. Molecular basis of the Dark Agouti rat drug oxidation polymorphism: importance of CYP2D1 and CYP2D2. Pharmacogenetics 1998;8(1):73–82.

[23] Paulson SK, Engel L, Reitz B, Bolten S, Burton EG, Maziasz TJ, Yan B, Schoenhard GL. Evidence for polymorphism in the canine metabolism of the cyclooxygenase 2 inhibitor, celecoxib. Drug Metab Dispos 1999;27(10):1133–42.

[24] Singh M, Johnson L. Using genetically engineered mouse models of cancer to aid drug development: an industry perspective. Clin Cancer Res 2006;12:5312–28.

[25] Garth T, Whiteside A, James D, Pomonis B, Jeffrey D, Kennedy C. An industry perspective on the role and utility of animal models of pain in drug discovery. Neurosci Lett 2013;557:65–72.

[26] Vamathevan JJ, Hall MD, Hasan S, Woollard PM, Xu M, Yang Y, Li X, Wang X, Kenny S, Brown JR, Huxley-Jones J, Lyon J, Haselden J, Min J, Sanseau P. Minipig and beagle animal model genomes aid species selection in pharmaceutical discovery and development. Toxicol Appl Pharmacol 2013;270(2):149–57.

[27] Bibby MC. Orthotopic models of cancer for preclinical drug evaluation: advantages and disadvantages. Eur J Cancer 2004;40:852–7.

[28] Ruggeri BA, Camp F, Miknyoczki S. Pre-clinical animal models of cancer and their applications and utility in drug discovery. Biochem Pharmacol 2014;87:150–61.

[29] Olive KP, Tuveson DA. The use of targeted mouse models for pre-clinical testing of novel cancer therapeutics. Clin Cancer Res 2006;12:5277–87.

[30] Mattson MP. Pathways towards and away from Alzheimer's disease. Nature 2004; 430:631–9.

[31] Van Dam D, De Deyn PP. Animal models in the drug discovery pipeline for Alzheimer's disease. Br J Pharmacol 2011;164(4):1285–300.

[32] Languille S, Blanc S, Blin O, Canale CI, Dal-Pan A, Devau G, Dhenain M, Dorieux O, Epelbaum J, Gomez D, Hardy I, Henry PY, Irving EA, Marchal J, Mestre-Francés N, Perret M, Picq JL, Pifferi F, Rahman A, Schenker E, Terrien J, Théry M, Verdier JM, Aujard F. The grey mouse lemur: a non-human primate model for ageing studies. Ageing Res Rev 2012;11(1):150–62.

[33] Games D, Adams D, Alessandrini R, Barbour R, Berthelette P, Blackwell C, Carr T, Clemens J, Donaldson T, Gillespie F. Alzheimer-type neuropathology in transgenic mice overexpressing V717F beta-amyloid precursor protein. Nature 1995;373(6514):523–7.

[34] Laurijssens B, Aujard F, Rahman A. Animal models of Alzheimer's disease and drug development. Drug Discov Today Technol 2013;10(3):e319–27.

[35] Goedert M, Klug A, Crowther RA. Tau protein, the paired helical filament and Alzheimer's disease. J Alzheimers Dis 2006;9(3 Suppl.):195–207.

[36] Iijima K, Iijima-Ando K. Drosophila models of Alzheimer's amyloidosis: the challenge of dissecting the complex mechanisms of toxicity of amyloid-beta. J Alzheimers Dis 2008;15(4):523–40.

[37] Sang TK, Jackson GR. Drosophila models of neurodegenerative disease. NeuroRx 2005;2:438–46.

[38] Sinadinos C, Burbidge-King T, Soh D, Thompson LM, Marsh JL, Wyttenbach A, Mudher AK. Live axonal transport disruption by mutant huntingtin fragments in Drosophila motor neuron axons. Neurobiol Dis 2009;34(2):389–95.

[39] Crommelin DJ, Storm G, Verrijk R, De Leede L, Jiskoot W, Hennink WE. Shifting paradigms: biopharmaceuticals versus low molecular weight drugs. Int J Pharm 2003; 266(1-2):3–16.

[40] Baldrick P. Safety evaluation of biological drugs: what are toxicology studies in primates telling us? Regul Toxicol Pharmacol 2011;59(2):227–36.

[41] Hansel TT, Kropshofer H, Singer T, Mitchell JA, George AJ. The safety and side effects of monoclonal antibodies. Nat Rev Drug Discov 2010;9(4):325–38.

[42] Bailey J. Non-human primates in medical research and drug development: a critical review. Biogenic Amines 2005;19(4–6):235–55.

[43] Aggarwal S. What's fueling the biotech engine – 2009-2010. Nat Biotechnol 2010;28(11):1165–71.

[44] Bailey J, Capaldo T, Conlee K, Thew M, Pippin J. Experimental use of nonhuman primates is not a simple problem. Nat Med 2008;14(10):1011–2.

CHAPTER 8

Pharmaceutical Formulation and Manufacturing Development: Strategies and Issues

Odilia Osakwe

Contents

8.1 Introduction	169
8.2 Regulatory Aspects of Pharmaceutical Development	171
8.2.1 Overview	171
8.2.2 The International Conference on Harmonisation Technical Documents for Pharmaceutical Development	172
8.3 Formulation and Manufacturing in Pharmaceutical Development	173
8.3.1 Formulation Development	174
8.3.2 Manufacturing Development	174
8.3.3 Issues Pertaining to Drug Formulations and Public Health Impact : Manufacturing Quality Problems	175
8.4 Clinical Trials Materials	175
8.4.1 Phase I	175
8.4.2 Phase II	176
8.4.3 Phase III	177
8.5 Concepts Used in Pharmaceutical Development	177
8.6 Drug Shortages	179
8.7 Manufacturing Problems Leading to Drug Shortages	180
8.7.1 Impurities in Manufacturing Development	180
8.7.2 Impurity in Drug Formulation	181
8.7.3 Genotoxic Impurities in Developing Drugs	182
8.7.4 Issues of Repetitive Cycle in Drug Manufacturing	183
8.7.5 Sterility Issues	183
8.8 Addressing Drug Shortages: Strategies	184
References	185

8.1 INTRODUCTION

Pharmaceutical development is concerned with developing drug formulations, which, in simple terms, is the combination of the active ingredient and the excipients into a drug with acceptable quality, safety, and efficacy characteristics intended for clinical application. This involves development of analytical methods, the process of manufacture and scale-up, new product transfers, infrastructure, and all the associated materials; production (including packaging and labeling), quality control, and assurance; and the process of distribution. In order to satisfy these manufacturing needs, all these steps have to conform to the applicable regulations to satisfy the ultimate regulatory mandate of quality [1–4].

Chemistry, manufacturing and control refers to all the operations under pharmaceutical development, concerned with the drug substance and product that are critical to safety and delivery of accurate doses with the potency required for adequate therapeutic effect in the human system. The first aspect of pharmaceutical manufacturing in the drug discovery lifecycle is research into the physical properties of the drug components for stability, compatibility, and other qualities that might influence formulation into the desired dosage forms. Complete understanding of the preformulation properties permit specific formulation to be designed and evaluated. In the manufacturing stage, the developing drug compound or new drug entity (NDE) becomes the active pharmaceutical ingredient (API). First, the API is synthesized along with development of the procedure for the manufacturing process followed by formulation into a drug product. Chemical synthesis is a continuous process that parallels the NDE maturity across the development stage of the drug discovery program. The overall aim is to formulate API and excipients into a dosage form of interest based on medical indication, half-life, and frequency of need. Oral drugs are the most compliant and would be a first choice in pharmaceutical development. Oral drugs are usually formulated as suspensions, solutions, capsules, or tablets. Excipients that are acceptable by the US Food and Drug Administration (FDA) are known as "Generally Recognized As Safe" – the first priority in determining the right substances to be used in formulations.

In the manufacturing stage, the extent of API supply is critical and requires significant quantities in order for development activities to begin. Through scale-up, laboratory quantities are increased with special caution so as not to alter the original optimized properties. Sometimes other problems influence the ability to scale up from laboratory size to commercial size. This is the reason for repeating production runs of the original synthesis, done in a manner to demonstrate reproducibility and to generate sufficient quantities with acceptable clinical standards. Limited and measured quantities are dispatched for clinical trials, for package design, and for other application measures for technology transfer for scale-up and commercialization

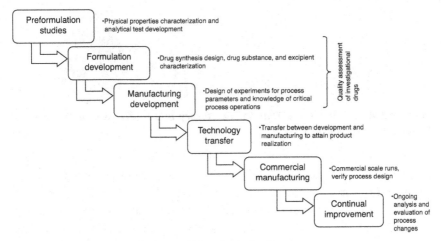

Figure 8.1 *Product Formulation and Manufacturing Process.*

(Figure 7.1). All these activities are rooted in the International Conference on Harmonisation (ICH) guidelines that must be followed for the investigational new drug (IND) to be deemed qualified to progress to the next stage (Figure 8.1).

8.2 REGULATORY ASPECTS OF PHARMACEUTICAL DEVELOPMENT

8.2.1 Overview

Federal regulations strictly control the processes that develop a new drug entity into a drug product to assure "the proper identification, quality, purity and strength of the investigational drug." This means the structure must be proven and kept consistent (identity); assay of the drug substance and drug product should demonstrate stability and potency that is devoid of impurity and degrades (quality), with adequate chemical and microbial purity; and strength of the investigational drug (purity) must be maintained. In order to maintain the regulatory standards, the pharmaceutical industry adopts the culture of quality in all areas of drug manufacturing (Figure 7.2). These demand proper accommodation of all the best practices, especially for manufacturing, good manufacturing practice (GMP); documentation, good documentation practices; and other related activities. GMP is a rudimentary aspect of the pharmaceutical quality system (PQS), which is binding for every drug manufacturer (Figure 8.2).

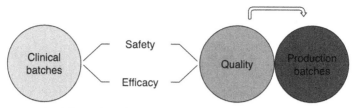

Figure 8.2 *A Crucial Need is That Safety, Efficacy and Quality will be Reproduced Throughout the Product Lifecycle.*

In the manufacturing facility, there is control and consistency in all the operations from receiving of raw materials through to the release and distribution of final product. Systematic changes, both the anticipated and unanticipated, are handled with extreme caution. Only qualified personnel with specific expertise in the assigned roles are employed and must follow written procedures for all equipment used; the layout of the premises must be approved before pharmaceutical operations resume in such facilities. Sterilization processes and cleaning processes must be validated, verified, and monitored continuously for changes. Collection of information, analysis, evaluation, implementation, and monitoring are carried out by trained personnel.

8.2.2 The International Conference on Harmonisation Technical Documents for Pharmaceutical Development

ICH was established in 1990 in a joint industry and regulatory endeavor to strengthen the efficiency of the process for developing and registering new drugs. Generally, ICH Q8, 9, and 10 are a combination of technical requirements that must be strictly followed to cover all the processes involved in pharmaceutical development and manufacturing. ICH Q8 guidelines recommend the principles of Quality by Design (QbD), which means "building quality in" and "right at first time." QbD must be adopted according to regulatory standards as outlined in the Q8 document. ICH Q9 is concerned with identifying risks and analysis, and also the potentials of risky events and evaluation activities involved in addressing these risks. It is expected that drug developers proactively address these issues by incorporating risk assessment during product development to be able to clearly discriminate between critical and noncritical parameters and attributes. ICH Q10 is a harmonized pharmaceutical quality system implemented throughout different stages of a product lifecycle. Application of Q10 is expected to eliminate inconsistencies for robustness and effectiveness. While

PQS covers the entire product lifecycle, the elements are applied vigorously to continually determine areas of future improvement, requiring a complete compliance to be based on application of the three most important ICH Qs, Q8, Q9, and Q10. These guidelines are harmonized among the concerned countries of which the major regulatory powers are the United States, Europe, and Japan.

A major requirement by the federal regulatory authorities is that all the information that supports the proposed manufacturing formulation process be submitted and contains all the information about the product that is critical to product quality. The Pharmaceutical Analytical Technology initiative was introduced by the FDA in 2004 to improve the production processes through implementation of new monitoring and control technology that could enhance the manufacturing processes. This has received wide recognition and acceptance by the industry and other regulatory authorities nationwide. Further discussions explore aspects of pharmaceutical development with factors that affect development productivity.

8.3 FORMULATION AND MANUFACTURING IN PHARMACEUTICAL DEVELOPMENT

The specific goal of the manufacturing program is to develop a drug that meets the regulatory acceptance criteria as shown in Table 8.1.

Table 8.1 Drug product specifications

Attribute	Acceptance criteria (typical values)	Analytical procedure (for example)
Identity	Matches standard	IR or HPLC/UV
Appearance	Color, imprint	Visual
Assay	90–110%	HPLC
Dose uniformity	Statistical criterion (USP)	HPLC or weight
Release from dosage form	80% in 15 or 30 min	Stirred aqueous vessel
Impurities (related substances)	<1% to few percent	HPLC
Microbial limits or sterility	# of total aerobes and fungi per gram pathogen (−)	Growth in special media
Water content	Few %	Chemical or weight loss
Preservative content	NLT 75% of initial	HPLC

Source: Ref. [5].

8.3.1 Formulation Development

The physicochemical characteristics of the API are critical to formulation development. They enable identification of the stability status or any type of changes that may occur during the process. The preformulations are evaluated in terms of technical feasibility, dissolution behavior, stability, and maximum strength for further optimization. The stability studies are conducted under the long-term storage condition specifications (250°C/60% RH), and are needed to obtain the registration data during the market phase (upon approval), and are performed by manufacturers for continuous quality check of products to ensure consistency in quality. Stability provides evidence on how the quality of a drug substance or drug product varies with time under the influence of a variety of environmental factors such as temperature, humidity, and light to recommend storage conditions. The results are used as the basis for defining the recommended storage conditions and the type of protection (e.g., packaging). Quantities in the range of hundreds of grams of drug substance are usually required [6]. The chemical development of drug substance is sensitive to changes in impurity profile for the various types of studies for which its use is directed. These activities are usually completed within 1–2 years prior to resubmitting applications for New Drug Application/New Drug Submission. A validated methodology is essential for testing the drug substance used in clinical manufacturing. Validation must demonstrate accuracy, precision, specificity, reproducibility, sensitivity, ruggedness, and linearity, conducted according to the ICH guidelines. The decision tree approach is needed to maximize the use of time in development and manufacture of drug formulations for the first-in-human oral dose [7]. Accurately documented information derived from the early formulation is utilized toward optimization and preparation for the scale-up and commercial quantities. These procedures require more rigorous analytical control assays and synthetic steps.

8.3.2 Manufacturing Development

The main objective of pharmaceutical manufacturing is continuous supply of API of consistent quality. The API process consists of a series of stages: chemical transformations or purifications that may require isolated or non-isolated intermediates. These comprise numerous unit operations, which are executed according to set limits. They are concerned with the synthetic route selection for the drug substance and product, mechanism of API impurities formation, and the suitability of the optimization studies. All activities are constantly monitored during the laboratory pilot scale to commercial scale. In-process testing cross-verifies a specific condition that has been achieved prior to the next step in the process [8]. It identifies the critical process parameters and control strategies for all of the individual steps, unit operations, and the ranges; in-process controls and specifications constitute the API process. Critical process parameters exist for each step or stage of the manufacturing process and are optimized according to requirements. These are executed according to ICH Q11. Validated test methods are used to detect differences in stability, content, and purity of the API in the clinical samples to be included in the submission dossier for IND.

8.3.3 Issues Pertaining to Drug Formulations and Public Health Impact: Manufacturing Quality Problems

8.3.3.1 Case I: Inconsistency in Drug Quality of Metoprolol ER, Made by Ethex, Based in Missouri

A 57-year-old male received a diagnosis of atrial fibrillation in 2001, which was kept under therapeutic control with Toprol XL. However, in early 2008, about a month after switching to Ethex's version, he developed nasal congestion, breathlessness, and irregular heart rhythm, which led to the diagnosis of atrial flutter. A therapeutic regimen consisted of some evasive procedures; several ablation procedures and multiple antiarrhythmic drugs. The deputy director of the Office of Compliance in the FDA's Center for Drug Evaluation and Research called the recalls "precautionary." It was pointed out that inconsistency in tablet sizes leading to variability in dose proportions (apparent appearance of thick and standard sizes) would have subjected the patient to harm [9].

8.4 CLINICAL TRIALS MATERIALS

Obstacles relating to clinical trial supplies are getting in the way of attaining the critical milestones for the drug manufacturing industries. Effective supply strategies have been a daunting challenge as clinical trials are becoming increasingly more complex. Adequate supply of drugs is needed for both the preclinical and clinical drug development programs for efficacy, GLP toxicology studies, and early formulation studies. Thus, clinical trial materials (CTM) are prepared according to the phase of clinical trials as follows.

8.4.1 Phase I

Phase I clinical trial materials are developed toward the end of the preclinical studies, Phase I of the clinical trials. It follows the "formulated capsule" approach, which is the use of knowledge derived from preformulation and compatibility studies to generate a formulated capsule with scale-up potentials. Several hundreds of grams of drug substance are required in order to develop the formulated capsulated product. Critical processing steps and parameters must be defined in the pilot phase, to enable the validation of the production process. Progressively increasing amounts of API are synthesized depending on the stage of the drug development process, and the demand becomes more crucial with the approach of safety studies (toxicology in animal species). Substantial amounts are also required for development into suitable dosage forms and testing in human beings (clinical Phases I–III). Inconsistencies in development and delivery of standardized API would amount to delayed time to marketing. These are undertaken under strict regulation and control of the processes including the facility for drug manufacture. During formulation, the pilot plant must be qualified prior to in-process activities and any technical problems that exist are linked to its critical processing steps and parameters. In process optimization, the pilot batches are necessary for the long-term studies (Phase III) for marketing application purposes. This process brings the compound into a galenic form to serve the purpose of human consumption for clinical studies, produced in a laboratory scale. Pilot scale levels are not fully optimized prior to IND application and the Phase I clinical studies. For example, for oral formulations, definite quantities are prepared and placed in gelatin capsules for these studies; these may be scaled up to increments of 50 g to allow all possible combinations as required by the clinical study protocol.

8.4.2 Phase II

Phase II studies are a little scaled up from medium-to-large scale, requiring dosage strengths of about 100,000 units or more. Sometimes companies might utilize the Phase II CTM with slight modification on product properties to formulate Phase III but a biopharmaceutical evaluation is usually made to understand the potential impact of such changes on systemic exposure using data from the early clinical formulations as a standard for these later changes. The appearance of these dosage forms is necessary to incorporate the factors needed or to tailor it to the clinical trial protocol and the type of study executed at the time. For example, the double blind studies need no color coding in order to prevent prior identification.

A compatibility test, performed during early formulation studies, attempts to address compatibility with the packaging, excipients, and API. The data generated provide the rationale for selection of the final formulation components. Information about the preliminary manufacturing process, composition, and test results of all preformulation batches and changes to formulations, processes, and specifications during development must be scientifically justified. Thus, all changes to master formulae and processing instructions follow an already established standard operation procedure. Stability and bioequivalence are crucial elements that are seriously considered in any situation. The manufacturing of the Phase III samples can be conducted concurrently with Phase III clinical trials. A more robust approach is utilized in Phase III while reducing the scale-up risk.

8.4.3 Phase III

Considering the Phase III clinical trial objective, which is for safety and efficacy, the formulations are designed with stark similarity in all respects to the commercial sample and with the same container closure system marked for marketing. The pilot scale is about one-tenth of the production scale, which is further scaled up to production scale. Scale-up from the laboratory to the pilot scale usually accompanies lots of changes. Any change in these activities is accompanied by a systematic change control process, which must be approved by the appropriate official of the unit. These changes are reflected in the appropriate documentation. Here, a higher degree of automation greatly contributes to the reproducibility and safety of the process even though certain unanticipated issues could arise during transport. Issues associated with pipes or tubes, shear forces acting on the conveyed substance subjecting them to abrasion, powder agglomeration, phase separation, or air separation could create problems.

8.5 CONCEPTS USED IN PHARMACEUTICAL DEVELOPMENT

Active pharmaceutical ingredient (API): defined as "any substance or mixture of substances intended to be used in the manufacture of a drug (medicinal) product and that, when used in the production of a drug, becomes and active ingredient of the drug product. Such substances are intended to furnish pharmacological activity or other direct effect in the diagnosis, cure, mitigation, treatment, or prevention of disease or to affect the structure and function of the body" (21 CFR 314.3).

API and drug substance are used interchangeably but have the same meaning according to FDA Guidance for Industry CGMP for Phase 1 Investigational Drugs (2008) and ICH document Q7: Good Manufacturing Practice Guide for Active Pharmaceutical Ingredients (2000).

Drug product: A finished dosage form (e.g., tablet, capsule, or solution) that contains a drug substance, generally but not necessarily in association with one or more other ingredients.

Chemical synthesis: A sequence of chemical transformations that modify the chemical structure or the quality attributes of an intermediate or API.

Critical impurity: Impurity or precursor to an impurity that alters the purity profile of an API.

Critical quality attribute (CQA): A quality attribute that when it exceeds the standard limits, alters the quality, safety, and efficacy of the drug product. Examples are the physical state, assay tests, appearance, water content, heavy metals, and impurity profile. The particle size and polymorphism depends on the Q6A decision tree [10].

Critical process parameter (CPP): A process parameter that alters the critical quality attributes of an API and its suitability for use in subsequent steps.

Good manufacturing practice (GMP): Aspects of quality assurance or integrated quality systems that ensure that drugs are produced consistently and controlled as required by quality standards appropriate to their intended use, as required by the marketing authorization.

Quality: The totality of features and characteristics of a product or service that determines its ability to satisfy stated or implied needs.

Quality assurance: The International Organization for Standardization defines quality assurance as the assembly of all planned and systematic actions necessary to provide adequate confidence that a product, process, or service will satisfy given quality requirements.

Validation: The documented act of demonstrating that any procedure, process, and activity will consistently lead to the expected results.

Validation protocol: A written plan of actions stating how process validation will be conducted; it will specify who will conduct the various tasks and define testing parameters; sampling plans, testing methods, and specifications; and will specify product characteristics and equipment to be used. It must specify the minimum number of batches to be used for validation studies; it must specify the acceptance criteria and who will sign/approve/disapprove the conclusions derived from such a scientific study [11–16].

8.6 DRUG SHORTAGES

The FDA defines a drug shortage as "a period of time when the demand or projected demand for the drug within the United States exceeds the supply of the drug." Shortages in drugs and biologics have become a crucial global issue [17,18] as it could result in higher drug costs as well as greater risks to patients. Despite the continuous improvement that has contributed to a number of resolved cases, drug shortages continue to be a societal malaise [19]. Among other potential reasons, quality and specific manufacturing defects have been cited as the major cause of drug shortages in the healthcare system, which has a tremendous impact on patient access, quality of care, and costs of care [20–22]. The consequence is that government and third party payors are financially challenged to cover the costs due to the shortcomings associated with taking poor quality drugs or no drugs (see Chapter 12 for further details). Drug shortages and recalls feed into the overly expensive manufacturing techniques, which charge exorbitantly to compensate for the rigorous time and economic measures required to satisfy regulatory standards. There are both systematic and regulatory problems that hamper manufacturing deficiency. The overall landscape is complex, hindering the maintenance of a culture of quality.

The drug shortage bulletin [23] contains a list of current drug shortages, drugs that have been phased out, not being sold, not commercially available preparations, and resolved shortages. The most frequently encountered areas in this list are cancer drugs, generic sterile injectable drugs, pain medications, heat drugs, and a variety of others [24].

Certain contributing factors undermine manufacturing productivity and some of the frequently cited examples are: lack of innovative techniques implemented, poorly validated techniques, poor evaluation, and audit activities that fail to identify deviations at various manufacturing process activities; lapses in GMP checks, lack of adequate control or monitoring of critical process parameters (indicators of manufacturing performance), poorly documented procedures, poor standard operating procedures for equipment maintenance, and cleaning maintenance; and appropriate API testing (Table 8.2).

Table 8.2 List of shortages on select categories by therapeutic class

Therapeutic class	Number of critical shortages	Percent of critical shortages
Anesthetic and central nervous system drugs	37	17
Anti-infective drugs	34	16
Cardiovascular drugs	27	12
Nutritive drugs	18	8
Endocrine metabolic drugs	16	7
Gastrointestinal drugs	10	5
Oncology drugs	10	5
Diagnostic drugs	9	4
Blood modifier drugs	7	3
Musculoskeletal drugs	7	3
Ophthalmologic drugs	6	3
Respiratory drugs	6	3
Toxicology antidote drugs	6	3
Other*	18	8
Multiple therapeutic classes	8	4
Total	219	101**

From US Government Accountability Office (GAO), University of Utah Drug Information Service and Truven Health Analytics (Red Book). Report from June 2011 to June 2013 [19].
The Red Book is a compendium published by Truven Health Analytics that includes information about the characteristics of drug products.
*Includes other therapeutic classes, such as dermatological drugs and immunological drugs, as well as four drugs whose therapeutic classes were unavailable from the Red Book.
**Total does not sum to 100 due to rounding.

8.7 MANUFACTURING PROBLEMS LEADING TO DRUG SHORTAGES

8.7.1 Impurities in Manufacturing Development

Impurities in pharmaceuticals are the other chemicals or products that are contained within the APIs. New impurities or higher levels of old impurities may surface during process development, scale-up, or storage. These could originate from the synthetic intermediates, during formulation or aging of both API itself or API in the drug product. Those of the key intermediates may or may not convert to other impurities in the APIs. The appearance of impurities in any form or concentration may influence the efficacy and safety of the pharmaceutical products. Impurity profiling (i.e., the identity and quantity of impurity in the pharmaceuticals) is being given a superior consideration in this phase of drug development. Together with the ICH guidelines, the British Pharmacopoeia (BP) and the United States

Pharmacopoeia (USP) specify the guidelines for permissible impurity levels for the APIs or formulations. The impurities in an API that affect the quality and safety of drug products can be process or impact the quality and safety of drug products; they can be process related or environmentally induced (issues of stability). Acceptable impurity levels are very low as specified in the ICH regulatory documents. These could also be related or unrelated impurities. As stated in the ICH guidelines, any impurity at a level of $\geq 0.10\%$ in the API should be identified and addressed accordingly. Typical examples are organic impurities (process and drug related), genotoxic impurities, polymorphic forms, inorganic impurities, residual solvents, and enantiomeric impurities. Initial toxicology studies often determine the status of these impurities and if their levels in tested samples meet the acceptance criteria for qualifying these products [25,26]. Impurity status of drug formulation could change and this has become a daunting challenge in drug development.

8.7.2 Impurity in Drug Formulation

It is critical that the approved dosage form of the API be delivered to the patient, thus the solid state is expected to remain the same and unchanged throughout the drug lifecycle and in the monitoring processes. Approved dosage forms may exist as polymorphs, pseudopolymorphs, salts, cocrystals, and amorphous solids. Different mechanical, thermal, physical, and chemical properties are unique to each of the solid forms. These variations in properties also alter the bioavailability, hygroscopicity, stability, and other performance characteristics of the drug. All this has been given serious consideration as these properties can have a deleterious impact on health if not properly controlled. Data from such studies inform the selection of the most suitable form for drug development. The critical properties of the API are: appearance, solubility, impurities, stability, structure identity (crystalline or polymorphic), counter ions (salts) and crystals, chirality, D enantiomer(s), and other chemical and physical properties. These properties are continuously referenced throughout API scale-up process chemistry and GMP manufacturing.

8.7.2.1 Case II: Crystal Polymorphism in Pharmaceuticals
Ritonavir is the API of Abbott's HIV drug Novir, marketed as an oral liquid and semisolid capsules for the treatment of AIDS, and was launched in 1996. It contains Ritonavir in ethanol/water-based solution, as the solid state did not exhibit the right physical–chemical characteristics to be effective as a drug. Therefore no crystal form control was required [27],

and only one crystal form was formulated, which was devoid of stability problems.

Later in 1998, the new polymorph had less solubility characteristics than the original crystal form. Final product lots failed the dissolution test, and a large portion of the drug substance precipitated out of the final (semisolid) formulated product. This resulted in the suspension of all manufacturing activities and the supply of this life-saving treatment for AIDS, followed by an urgent requirement to reformulate Norvir [28]. Abbott scientists reevaluated and addressed the problem to better control the formation of either Form I or Form II polymorphs, which received FDA approval on reformulated Novir soft gelatin capsules in June 1999. The crystals would not have been found if not for the incidental supersaturation due to the cosolvent, the hydroalcoholic solution.

8.7.3 Genotoxic Impurities in Developing Drugs

Genotoxicity pertains to the ability of the drug to interact with DNA or DNA-associated biomolecules like enzymes and proteins. These can cause point mutations, and induce changes in chromosomal number or in chromosome structure in the form of breaks, deletions, rearrangements, mutations in germlines, and somatic and fetal cells.

8.7.3.1 *Case III: Genotoxic Impurity*

Viracept® (nelfinavir mesylate) is an HIV protease inhibitor marketed in Europe by Roche. Certain critical GMP deficiencies in the manufacturing process led to contamination of the active substance, which seriously threatened safety. A reaction between residual ethanol and methane sulfonic acid (MSA) counter ions resulted in the formation of MSA ethyl ester or ethylmethane sulfonate (EMS), which was found in unexpectedly high levels in the drug product. The marketing authorization holder had identified the presence of the contaminant ethyl mediate in some batches of nelfinavir mesilate (the active substance) in a follow-up investigation when patients complained about a "strange smell" and one adverse drug report of nausea and vomiting. EMS is known to be genotoxic, carcinogenic, and teratogenic in animals. Following investigations, it was discovered that vaporized ethanol was possibly transported through the piping connections of pipes meant for ethanol and nitrogen to the hold tank containing MSA in the final production step. An impurity contained in the MSA named methyl methanesulfonate (MMS) slowly transformed into EMS through a transesterification reaction; this reaction could be accelerated by an excess of ethanol.

The European Medicines Agency (EMA) suspended marketing of the drug in June 2007. But the EU marketing authorization was reinstated in October 2007, when the issue was resolved. Stringent toxicity studies were required to support the safety profile [29]. EMEA later requested evaluation of sulfonic esters in all marketed products (December 2008).

8.7.4 Issues of Repetitive Cycle in Drug Manufacturing

Procedural barriers influence continuous process improvement in manufacturing and this aspect of manufacturing is tightly regulated. Moreover, there are increasing difficulties in altering the regulator-approved procedures that have been validated. Manufacturing techniques that are outdated lead to failed predistribution testing – an inability to separate the "wheat from the chaff". Implementing modernized technology and processes that have been constrained by the FDA regulatory systems is difficult when earlier procedures have been well characterized and validated, and thus there has been series of violations associated with increasing complexity in the hard-to-comply FDA demands. These contribute to major problems in the healthcare system, which include recalls, related contamination events, and drug shortages affecting both brand-name and generic products. Series of recalls are due to manufacturing-related contaminations from equipment, cross-contamination from other drug ingredients, and loose particles form equipment parts. New contaminants or impurities could lead to higher levels of contamination, which could lead to the termination of the entire program. These problems have contributed to drug shortages that have affected the healthcare systems, the patients, society, and even the drug companies themselves. The highly stringent regulatory oversight has also led to the closure of manufacturing plants and drug shortages, all of which account for quality lapses and reduced drug supply. Is the shutdown of a plant a regulatory threat or a win situation for the FDA? Is this a credible threat?

8.7.5 Sterility Issues

Supply disruption is among the most common causes of drug shortage due to manufacturing suspense or delayed production associated with a quality problem, which typically has been connected with bacteria contamination or foreign particles in drug containers or vials. For example, penicillin, an anti-infective drug, is highly sensitizing and could lead to severe allergic reactions even at minimal levels, which might limit the manufacturing lines. Lack of extensive manufacturing lines has a resultant effect of sharing of lines for the manufacture of multiple drugs. This is a possible source

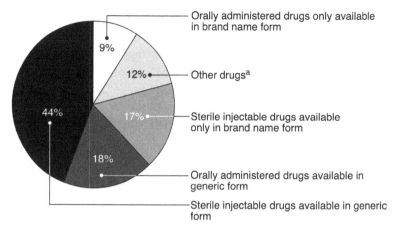

Figure 8.3 *Drug Shortage From January 2011 to June 2013.* [a] Other drugs include those that had other routes of administration such as, nasal, inhalation, topical, ophthalmic, and transdermal methods. In total, there were 18 drugs available through other routes, with 4 available in generic form and the remaining 14 only available in brand-name form. The other drugs category also includes nine additional shortages that had multiple routes of administration or for which either the route of administration or the product type was unavailable from Red Book. *Source: GAO Analysis of FDA Data [19].*

of cross-contamination for companies, which will have to compromise in favor of one drug [19]. Plant closures have been intuitive in response to a warning letter issued by the FDA (Figure 8.3).

8.8 ADDRESSING DRUG SHORTAGES: STRATEGIES

The Healthcare Supply Chain Association (HSCA) and its group purchasing organization (GPO) members have been established for the purpose of addressing the shortage problem to increase supply of needed drugs to the clinics. Their role includes investigating the root cause by investigating the cause of current drug shortages on a case-by-case basis in order to make policy recommendations to facilitate a speedy solution. The GPO negotiates contracts with healthcare manufacturers, distributors, and industry segments involved with the process of supplying drugs to the hospitals for purchase, and there had been ongoing policy dialogues in an effort to strengthen the drug supply chain.

GPO is cooperating with manufacturers and all key players or stakeholders to promote increased performance and innovation in manufacturing, while communicating with the respective stakeholders to improve the flow of drugs among the segments, by improving their marketing portfolio and planning their communication and reporting systems, which include webinars, conferences, newsletters, and electronic systems to alert the appropriate persons of the developments in drug access. Moreover, HSCA has initiated a call to action to address the drug shortage crisis. Strong congressional efforts are in place in an attempt to address the shortage problem with a major focus on certain drugs [30]. The FDA has been advised to permit an accelerated approval process for the listed drugs that are scarce. HSCA and GPO contribute to ongoing policy dialogues on drug shortages to promote savings and efficiencies and to negotiate discounts with manufacturers [31]. Novel scientific discoveries and technologies advance the innovative strategies employed in current drug manufacturing.

Inadequate cross-functional interactions among the different sectors lead to lapses in pharmaceutical research and development (R&D). Thus, reinforcement of the pharmaceutical ecosystem could be materialized through dialogues and adequate communication strategies that establish a common knowledge regarding project progress as there may be overlapping activities among the groups, like preformulation, biopharmaceutics, product design, or optimization groups, to better address certain parameters that could be interpreted differently. Proper communication and cross-interactions could reduce the potential of overlapping activities among the groups allowing even allocation of resources and skills to save costs on extraneous activities.

A collaborative endeavor comprising all the major sectors concerned with drug discovery – the government, industry, and academia – has initiated a series of strategies to improve the drug discovery program. The goal is to modernize and streamline information utility and processes that underpin the accompanying regulatory policies, to promote innovation in clinical evaluations for better patient outcomes. This encourages adoption of novel methods and tools essential for robust product manufacturing to attenuate the impact of failing technology on failure rates. Continuous development of new analytical methods enhances efforts to reduce risk of microbial contamination of products focusing on processes that lead to microbial contamination.

REFERENCES

[1] Available from: http://www.hc-sc.gc.ca/dhp-mps/consultation/drug-medic/qual_ndsands_draft_pdnpadn_ebauche-eng.php#a23 [accessed 20.02.2015].
[2] Available from: http://www.hc-sc.gc.ca/dhp-mps/prodpharma/applic-demande/guide-ld/ctd/draft_ebauche_ctdbe-eng.php#a2 [accessed 20.02.2015].
[3] Available from: http://www.ds-pharma.com/rd/drug_discovery/product.html [accessed 20.02.2015].

[4] Available from: http://www.fda.gov/downloads/Drugs/Guidances/ucm073517.pdf [accessed 20.02.2015].

[5] Matecka D. Quality Issues for Clinical Trial Materials: The Chemistry, Manufacturing and Controls (CMC) Review. Office of New Drug Quality Assessment, CDER. Available from: http://www.fda.gov/downloads/Training/ClinicalInvestigatorTraining Course/UCM340005.pdf [accessed 20.02.2015].

[6] cGMPs for the 21st century: a risk based approach. US Food and Drug Administration. Available from: www.fda.gove/cder/gmp/index.htm [accessed 21.02.2015].

[7] Hariharan M, Ganorkar LD, Amidon GE, Cavallo A, Gatti P, Hageman MJ, Choo I, Miller JL, Shah UJ. Reducing time to develop and manufacture formulations for first oral dose I humans. Pharm Technol 2003;27(10):68.

[8] Ganzer WP, Materna JA, Mitchell MB, Wall LK. Current thoughts on critical process parameters and API SYNTHESIS. Pharm Technol July 2005.

[9] Okie S. Multinational medicines – ensuring drug quality in an era of global manufacturing. N Engl J Med 2009; 361:8. Available from: www.fda.gov/safety/recalls [accessed 22.02.2015].

[10] Q6A Specifications: Test Procedures and Acceptance Criteria for New Drug Substances and New Drug Products: Chemical Substances. International Council for Harmonisation (ICH), 1999. Available from: http://www.ich.org/products/guidelines/quality/quality-single/article/specifications-test-procedures-and-acceptance-criteria-for-new-drug-substances-and-new-drug-produc.html

[11] Guidelines on General Principles of Process Validation. CDER, US-FDA 1987.

[12] Validation Guidelines for Pharmaceutical Dosage Forms (GUI-0029).

[13] Recommendations on validation master plan, Installation and operational qualification, Non-sterile process validation, Cleaning Validation, PIC/S September 2007.

[14] Food drug and cosmetic act, Code of federal regulations (Title 21), 21 CFR 312 (IND content and format), 21 CFR 210 and 211 (CGMP) Guidance FDA ICH Phase 1. Available from: http://bit.ly/IND-Phase-1 [accessed 22.02.2015.].

[15] Available from: http://bit.ly/IND-Phase2-3. Meetings (http://bit.ly/IND-meetings), MaPP 6030.1 (http://bit.ly/IND-MaPP), Exploratory IND (http://bit.ly/Expl-IND), GMP for Phase 1 (http://bit.ly/IND-cGMP). [accessed 20.02.2015.].

[16] Cancer drug shortages hit 83 percent of US oncologists. June 3, 2013. Science Daily. Available from: http://www.sciencedaily.com/releases/2013/06/130603090547.htm. See also "Voluntary drug-shortage reporting adopted despite concerns" CBC News Online. December 28, 2012.

[17] Available from: http://www.cbc.ca/news/health/story/2012/12/27/health-minister-drug-shortageplan-approval.html

[18] Kermani F. Germany's New drug register to help tackle supply shortages, but larger EU problem looms.The Pink Sheet.May 13,2013.Available from:http://www.elsevierbi.com/publications/the-pink-sheet/75/19/germanys-new-drug-registerto-help-tackle-supply-shortages-but-larger-eu-problem-looms

[19] GAO, Drug Shortages, Public Health Threat Continues, Despite Efforts to Help Ensure Product Availability. GAO-14-194. Report to Congressional Addressees. February; 2014.

[20] Premier Inc., Drug shortages 2014: A Premier healthcare alliance update (February 2014). Cancer Drug Shortages Hit 83 Percent of U.S. Oncologists. Penn Medicine News Release, June 3, 2013. Available from: http://www.uphs.upenn.edu/news/News_Releases/2013/06/gogineni/?utm_source=feedburner&utm_medium=feed&utm_campaign=Feed%3A+penn-medicine-news+%28Penn+Medicine+News%29 [accessed 25.02.2015].

[21] Kaakeh R, Sweet BV, Reilly C, Bush C, DeLoach S, Higgins B, Clark AM, Stevenson J. Impact of drug shortages on U.S. health systems. American Journal of Health-System Pharmacy 2011;68:e13–21.

[22] Dr. Peggy Hamburg, FDA Creates Plan To Combat Drug Shortages. Gastroenterology & Endoscopy News. April 2014. Available from: http://www.ajhp.org/site/DrugShortages.pdf?fm_preview=1 [accessed 20.02.2015].

[23] Available from: http://www.ashp.org/menu/DrugShortages/CurrentShortages [accessed 24.02.2015].

[24] Department of Health and Human Services Food and Drug Administration, Report to Congress, First Annual Report on Drug Shortages for Calendar Year 2013. Required by Section 1002 of the Food and Drug Administration Safety and Innovation Act Public Law; 2014;112–144.

[25] Q3A (R) Impurities in New Drug Substances; 2002. International conference on harmonization (ICH) Guidelines.

[26] Guideline Q6A: Specifications: Test Procedures and Acceptance Criteria for New Drug Substances and New Drug Products: Chemical Substances. International Conference on Harmonization, (ICH, Geneva, Switzerland, 1999). Available from: www.ich.org [accessed 24.02.2015].

[27] Berridge J. Proceedings of the Fourth International Conference on Harmonization, Brussels, P.F. D'Arcy, D.W. G. Harron editors Physico-Chemical Characteristics of Drug Substances, Queen's University of Belfast; 1997. p. 66.

[28] Byrn SR, Pfeiffer R, Stowell J. Solid-State Chemistry of Drugs. 2nd ed. West Lafayette, SSCI Inc;1999.

[29] EMEA CHMP Guideline on the Limits of Genotoxic Impurities; 2008.

[30] Six Month Check Up: FDA's Work on Drug Shortages. Available from: http://blogs.fda.gov/fdavoice/index.php/2012/05/six-month-check-up-fdaswork-on-drug-shortages/ [accessed 27.02.2015].

[31] Available from: www.SupplyChainAssociation.org [accessed 27.02.2015].

The Drug Discovery Cycle II: Clinical Development

9. Clinical Development: Ethics and Realities   191
10. Pharmacogenomics in Drug Discovery, Prospects and Clinical Applicability   221

CHAPTER 9

Clinical Development: Ethics and Realities

Odilia Osakwe

Contents

Part I	192
9.1 Introduction	192
9.1.1 General Overview	192
9.1.2 The Clinical Development Pathway	193
9.1.3 The Importance of Clinical Trial	193
Part II Clinical Development of Candidate Drugs	194
9.2 Clinical Trial: Principles and Approach	194
9.2.1 Overview	194
9.2.2 The Phases of a Clinical Trial	195
9.2.3 Pharmacoeconomics: Drug Evaluation	198
9.3 Evaluation Tools in Clinical Trials, Clinical Outcomes, and Relevance	199
9.3.1 Biomarker	199
9.3.2 Study Endpoint	200
9.4 Selected Topics in Clinical Trials	204
9.4.1 Placebo-Controlled Trials	204
9.4.2 Randomized Controlled Trials	204
9.5 Implications of Inappropriate Study Design	205
9.5.1 Inappropriate Gender Selection	205
9.5.2 Ethnic Disparity	206
Part III Clinical Trial Ethics	207
9.6 Ethical Conduct in Clinical Trials	207
9.6.1 Historical Perspective	207
9.6.2 Ethical Principles	208
9.7 Informed Consent	209
9.7.1 How Informed is the Consent?	209
9.8 Conflict of Interest in Clinical Research	210
9.8.1 Primary Conflict of Interest	210
9.8.2 Secondary Conflict of Interest	210
9.8.3 Institutional Conflict of Interest in Biomedical Research	211
9.9 Crucial Cases in Clinical Trials with Implications on Society	211
9.9.1 Case I: Differences in the National Regulatory Authorities	211
9.9.2 Case II: How Ethical are Large Clinical Trials in Rapidly Lethal Diseases?	212
9.9.3 Case III: Clinical Trials in AIDS Research	212

Social Aspects of Drug Discovery, Development and Commercialization Copyright © 2016 Elsevier Inc.
http://dx.doi.org/10.1016/B978-0-12-802220-7.00009-0   All rights reserved.

9.10 International Clinical Trials Across the Globe   213
    9.10.1 Clinical Trials in Canada   213
    9.10.2 Conducting Clinical Trials in Developing Countries   214
    9.10.3 Clinical Trials in China   215
    9.10.4 Case I: Significance of Differences in Patient Diagnosis in
           Multinational Clinical Trials   216
    9.10.5 Case II: The Controversy of Zidovudine (AZT) Trials in African and
           Other Developing Countries   217
References   218

PART I

9.1 INTRODUCTION

9.1.1 General Overview

The realization of drug discovery research objectives could be a daunting challenge. This is due to the growing unanticipated difficulties that build up over the duration of the product lifecycle leading to further challenges in clinical development. The main objective of clinical development is to test efficacy and safety in humans at the first attempt (first-in-human clinical trial) in a novel indication or known clinical indication, to identify a new dose regimen, route of administration, and toxic dose levels. Being the final checkpoint in the lifecycle of a drug product, it is the most regulated, making it financially demanding as it draws the majority of a company's research and development (R&D) budget.

The public depends on drug firms to adopt measures needed to conduct well-controlled and unbiased clinical trials to demonstrate adequacy of therapy by providing medically and statistically meaningful endpoints, using validated biomarkers and selection of the right patient and parameters that address specific objectives in pursuit of the end goal. Increasing safety hurdles encountered in establishing predictive animal models and poor pharmacokinetics (PK) has resulted in failure to adopt results from clinical studies into clinical practice.

In the medical industry, the construction of clinical research ethics is different due to institutional conceptions and mode of understanding. Policies were established to abrogate unjustified use of human subjects in clinical research. Ethical codes that applied in clinical research have diversified the role of the clinical researchers and medical professionals toward patients in the clinics, further complicating the ethical role of the clinical practitioners in their role as clinical researchers. The cumbersome task of addressing all the requirements in clinical development is highly limiting as mounting complexities incrementally slow down the transition of pipeline drugs to the market.

9.1.2 The Clinical Development Pathway

Once the lead drug candidate has passed through discovery screening and has been optimized, it is synthesized in the lab, formulated in a dosage form in pilot scale, and evaluated in animals. Thereafter, the Investigational New Drug/Clinical Trial Authorization application is submitted to the relevant regulatory authority, such as the US Food and Drug Administration (FDA), the European Medicines Agency (EMA), or Health Canada for approval and to obtain the permit to proceed with clinical development as shown in Figure 9.1.

9.1.3 The Importance of Clinical Trial

Clinical trial is referred to as a well-designed, controlled, and thoroughly monitored medical research performed with the consent of healthy patient volunteers with the aim of identifying the potential of risk to the relevant populations, to develop or improve therapies against a disease. It is the most regulated type of research and is subject to national and international regulatory control.

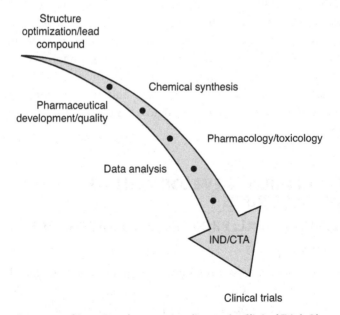

Figure 9.1 *Processes of Drug Development Leading to the Clinical Trials Phase.*

The ultimate goal of a clinical trial is the "4Rs": right patient, finding the required therapy for the patient that needs it most; right time, finding the appropriate time when administration is most effective; right drug, finding the ideal drug; and right dose, which is appropriate to effect a cure devoid of adverse events (AEs) and to determine the dose/dosing regimen that achieves target drug exposures in all relevant populations.

Clinical trial data are highly relevant to drug usage and the information presented in the labeling review is the clinical trial's outcomes. The information displayed on the drug labels discloses critical information regarding the drug being described, as needed by the health professional and the patient. Each statement proposed for drug labeling must be justified by data and results submitted in the New Drug Application (NDA). The Code of Federal Regulations (CFR) describes labeling requirements in 21 CFR Part 201. The major contents of drug labels are: clinical pharmacology, indications and usage, contraindications, precautions, adverse reactions, and drug abuse (related adverse effects when usage is abused).

9.1.3.1 Drug Response in Clinical Trial

The exposure–response relationship of an investigational drug in a clinical trial is critical for regulatory approval as is vital for determining the safety and effectiveness of drugs. Exposure is regarded as the amount of drug entering the body determined from the integrated concentration–time profile in plasma and other biologic fluids expressed as the area under the curve and C_{ss}, C_{max}, and C_{min}. Response is the biologic outcome (physiologic and pathologic processes) and all the effects (endpoints, biomarkers, or survival) of the drug and those related to AEs. Pharmacodynamics effects are generally characterized by an exposure–response relationship of drugs and genetic differences that can lead to changes in the steepness of the exposure–response curve.

PART II CLINICAL DEVELOPMENT OF CANDIDATE DRUGS

9.2 CLINICAL TRIAL: PRINCIPLES AND APPROACH

9.2.1 Overview

Traditionally, clinical development is separated into sequential, distinct phases and each phase is evaluated such that each success is a milestone. An emerging trend incorporates a more integrated approach, which relies on

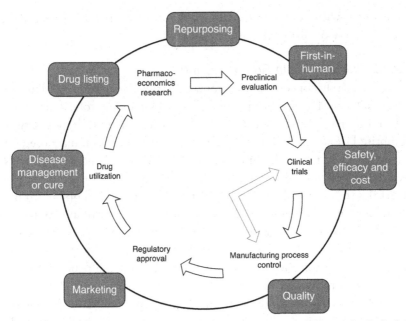

Figure 9.2 *Processes of Clinical Development and Outcomes Leading to the End of the Drug Product Lifecycle.*

accumulated information gained from experience to increase flexibility and to proactively address barriers to effectiveness as shown in Figure 9.2. The inner circle depicts the central activities, and the research results generated during these processes are translated into relevant hypothesis and decision criteria for the outcomes in the outer circles.

9.2.2 The Phases of a Clinical Trial

9.2.2.1 Phase 0: Exploratory Trial

This phase was introduced as an initiating exploratory clinical trial for a faster and more efficient development of drugs [1,2]. Phase 0 permits evaluation of the properties of candidate drugs prior to initiating more traditional Phase I testing. These properties are biologic efficacy; PK, biodistribution, and metabolism. Prior evaluation of these attributes of the drug limits human exposure to drugs since the dose and numbers of participants are minimized. This also lessens the risk of harm. A major challenge encountered in this study is the short duration of trials and limitation in evaluating the psychologic and physiologic benefits to the participant. It could be deduced that the benefit is to others and not the participants, challenging the ethical principle of justice and beneficence. This has drawn controversy with conflicting views over which interest takes precedence, that of society or that of the human subjects [3].

9.2.2.2 Phase I: First-in-Human Testing

Phase I is mainly concerned with human pharmacology conducted in about 20–30 subjects. During this phase, the initial safety and tolerability studies determine the dosage range and identify toxicity. The study population is comprised of normal volunteers or patients that have been diagnosed with a specific illness that is the subject of study. The subjects being tried are selected to reflect the treatment population demographics or any other characteristics that define the target population. As it is focused on determining the toxicity profile in humans, healthy volunteers with no underlying conditions are often chosen so as to abrogate complicated cross-reactions due to disease conditions or unexpected adverse effects that might arise. They are expected to tolerate toxicities in comparison to the patients. Placebos are used to understand the drug-related and nondrug-related AEs. Some minor AEs are nausea, dizziness, headache, and upper respiratory symptoms.

The initial dosing schedule and the safety factors are determined in this stage and are continuously monitored subsequently. Patients' blood and sometimes tissue samples are the study samples that enable establishing of a human PK profile. An important requirement is that doses to be tested should not to be very high but should be within a range significantly lower than that which could cause lethal toxicity. No-observed-adverse-effect-level (NOAEL; the highest experimental point without adverse effect) is usually much lower than the minimum lethal dose. An important consideration is a benefit–risk ratio, which is expected to be high; in other words, showing a minimal net risk. The ethical implication of the dose tolerance studies is that single doses are normally administered at no more than one-tenth of the highest NOAEL dose for the animal safety studies with the highest toxicity. This involves doubling the doses until the unacceptable toxicity is achieved that approximates that which achieves the maximal efficacy. The ethical concern with this is producing significant toxicity in healthy volunteers who have only monetary concerns and thus no clinical conditions.

9.2.2.3 Phase II: Therapeutic Exploratory

Phase II is conducted in about 20–300 subjects. It is concerned with determining dose response and recommendations for further study evaluation. Protocol designs vary even though the end goal is demonstrating drug efficacy in the studied patient. Most importantly, development of protocol design depends on disease or medical condition, stage in development of disease or expected response, and according to the data generated from the preclinical studies. Various trial designs are employed, which can be blinded, placebo-controlled, or open label designs, and the subject data, particularly the patent, are critical to success. A positive result is necessary in defining the scope of a drug's activity in patients with the target condition and leads to further project and determining endpoints for Phase III trials necessary to establish a bargain point for registration to approval of commercialization. In this stage of clinical trials, pharmacoeconomics evaluation is performed, which focuses on population and disease characterization, comorbidities and adverse effects, and regulatory compliance.

9.2.2.4 Phase III: Therapeutic Confirmatory

Therapeutic confirmatory trials are conducted in around 1000–5000 subjects. The purpose is to confirm the efficacy and safety in at least two well-controlled Phase III clinical trials. It is concerned with drug efficacy in a wider population to monitor side effects in comparison to existing treatments, assembling information that is useful for safe use of a drug. Specific statistically significant endpoints for registration trials must be demonstrated for the trial results to be approved. It is mostly an extension of Phase II, intended to expand the scope and number of subjects in order to increase the statistical power and validity of data generated. This study supplements all the necessary information that is needed to meet the regulatory mandate of efficacy and safety in order to seek for approval of a drug for marketing by providing a dossier, called an NDA, for review by regulatory authorities, as discussed in Chapter 1. For certain life-threatening conditions such as cancer, significant efficacy data from a single Phase III trial or even a Phase II trial may be sufficient for regulatory approval of the drug.

Phase III is a critical stage as it is the final checkpoint to drug commercialization, usually conducted after the manufacturing processes, Chemistry, Manufacturing, and Controls (CMC) (Chapter 8). CMC processes scale up drug products to well-validated commercial quantities. Pharmacogenetics in late clinical trials genetically stratifies subjects into subsets of groups depending on tolerance to the drug to avoid adverse drug reactions (ADRs) effects due to noncompliance while targeting the highly responsive population. Certain individuals may show less sensitivity and high efficacy than the others due to genetic factors. This will be fully discussed in Chapter 10.

9.2.2.5 The Integrated Phases

Phase I has been extended from establishing safety and dosing levels, to an increasingly important role of obtaining more data needed to find therapy to maximize the chances of obtaining clinical data to make sound go/no-go decisions. Phases I and IIa are focused on discovering vital aspects of the drug while Phases IIb and III build on the earlier phases to confirm drug performance in the form of efficacy and quality.

9.2.2.6 Phase IV: Pharmacovigilance

Pharmacovigilance refers to evaluation, detection, and prevention of adverse effects of a drug and related problems [4]. It involves collection of data to gain an adequate scientific basis for adverse reactions in patients undergoing treatment and to gain inside information about the world-class use of a drug. The new drug is compared with alternative existing therapies for a more informed comparative analysis, which could not be made prior to marketing, and the research results are used to improve drug labeling and distribute information about unacceptable conditions of use. The possibility of recall due to any new or severe adverse reactions and additional changes that might be needed that would be added to the labeling do occur. All publishable data add to the body of scientific and clinical knowledge.

9.2.3 Pharmacoeconomics: Drug Evaluation

Pharmacoeconomics study is primarily for the purpose of drug listing, competitiveness, pricing, and reimbursement. This type of evaluation encompasses all measurements against the disease being investigated. The judgment is based on quality of life benefit–risk balance, comparative effectiveness, comparators, or other available treatment options over an existing drug and affected population, clinical trial protocol design, therapeutic rationale and need, clinical outcomes, efficacy or effectiveness, safety, and tolerability [5]. Pharmacoeconomics analysis is important for inclusion in formularies or coverage by the drug insurance companies. It assesses therapeutic advantages and disadvantages of the drug and cost-effectiveness of the drug relative to accepted therapy. Only the drugs that show significant difference over existing drugs pass the evaluation criteria needed for listing. Most importantly, those domains that would be most impacted by the treatment, such as quality of life, are given important consideration. Comprehensive assessments outcomes are also needed and required for product labeling or drug promotion. Pharmacoeconomics analysis takes into consideration the stakeholders of the pharmaceutical ecosystem. These are mainly clinical professionals, hospital staff, the payer, the formulary committee, academicians, vendor or clinical research organization (CRO), the patient, the regulator, and the general public. Pharmacoeconomics analysis considers the geographic location due to pricing, for example, hospital charges and insurance services.

9.3 EVALUATION TOOLS IN CLINICAL TRIALS, CLINICAL OUTCOMES, AND RELEVANCE

9.3.1 Biomarker

Biomarker is a laboratory measurement or a physical sign that measures directly how a patient feels, functions, or survives [6]. It is often used as an indicator to determine normal biologic, pathogenic, or pharmacologic process for therapeutic intervention determined retrospectively (before it is done). For example, X lowers blood sugar by 20% when measured against a placebo group. Biomarkers are essential in the diagnosis of a disease, or for predicting or monitoring the response to therapy.

Biomarkers are used to evaluate the target agents that function in the pathway of a disease process in order to discriminate changes in function. These include mechanisms of action of pathway agents, drug metabolism, mutation in enzymes, and transporters. In the early development, biomarkers enabled the exploration of the effects of an investigational drug, which are mostly early sighs of efficacy, toxicity, or off-target effects. The information derived from this study guides the patient recruitment, which is based on established criteria. Biomarkers are not useful in finding the clinically meaningful benefit as there are no proof that there will be a prolongation of survival but could expose disease-related symptoms of death [7,8]. However, new classes of biomarkers help understand disease etiology through the advances in molecular science. Some outstanding achievements include selection of the patient population for trastuzumab by human epidermal growth factor receptor 2 status and a detection for irritable bowel disease to identify patients with Crohn's disease.

These biomarkers are validated and applied to various stages of pharmaceutic R&D for the purpose of predicting the PK properties of developing drugs. Individuals that test positive are further recruited in the clinical trials since they have a marker associated with higher chance of response to the clinical assessment, which enables acceleration of drug development, although this is not applicable for multiple-targeting compounds with an unknown mechanism of action. The use of biomarkers helps to minimize risk to subjects and is the base for surrogate endpoints. Surrogate endpoints are likely to predict the potential for a clinical benefit or morbidity/mortality while clinical endpoints directly measure a therapeutic effect of a drug, which is either a relief or survival. These endpoints are weighed against the risks to enable the determination of overall benefit to patients.

9.3.1.1 Challenges
Development of biomarkers has been challenging. This is due to the hard-to- meet required patient population that is a crucial need in clinical development. Most limitations are interindividual variability caused by variation in a genetic component, disease, environmental exposure, and lifestyle. The advancement in discovery science is further leading to improvement in strategies as it takes into consideration the systems biology approach and also technologic innovations that have revolutionized the discovery of novel clinical biomarkers. Even though a preferred choice, using a single biomarker has not been very practicable due to the prevailing barriers created by studying the complicated human biology.

9.3.2 Study Endpoint
Study endpoint is a symptom, disease, sign, or laboratory abnormality that informs the decision whether to withdraw an individual or entity from the clinical trial (in case of disease exacerbation or survival). For example, a clinical trial investigating the ability of a medication to prevent heart attack might use chest pain as a clinical endpoint.

9.3.2.1 Surrogate Endpoint
Surrogate endpoint is a substitute for a clinically meaningful endpoint that uses a biomarker but which is not a direct measure of the clinical benefit. A validated surrogate endpoint is used for accelerated drug approval based on the intended clinical benefit even though it does not provide sufficient evidence on its own and thus is not solely applicable in approval for marketing. An example is prolonged suppression of HIV viral load in plasma, which reduces morbidity and mortality associated with HIV disease. This enables the prediction of a potential morbidity or mortality effect.

One example is the CD-4 lymphocyte level in blood associated with severity of AIDS; a change in CD-4 concentration is considered an indicator of disease status. This is legally recognized for drug approval in many countries. The effect of a drug on the surrogate is an aspect of the therapeutic mechanism. Surrogate endpoints, when fully validated, predict the clinically meaningful endpoint of a therapy consistently [9]. Surrogate endpoints are very useful in predicting the clinical efficacy of drugs more rapidly and, as such, have been the basis of accelerated approval. Between 2010 and 2012, 45% of 94 new drugs approved by the FDA were based on surrogate endpoints [10]. They are not necessarily accepted for determining a drug's efficacy since their role as valid indicators of clinical benefit has not been empirically demonstrated. The time course of changes in biomarkers more closely approximates that of plasma concentrations and not necessarily changes in clinical endpoint. They are often applied toward making a connection between the preclinical and early clinical exposure–response relationships for establishing a range for the doses in clinical testing. Biomarkers replace the use of clinical endpoints in cases when drug responses could not be obtained and measured quantitatively. In such cases surrogate endpoints become a priority.

9.3.2.2 Quality of Life
The clinical quality of life is the patient's medical health and physical ability and depends on the patient's values, beliefs, and judgments. A psychologist assesses quality of life in terms of social function capabilities while a patient's focus might be the daily impact and quality of life. A common point of interest is disease severity, which is best answered by the physician because judgment is based on clinical measures. The overall measure is tailored to the desired endpoint of analyses. However, the major issue addressed is the extent of impact of a drug on the representative population, when exposed to similar circumstances and conditions, to determine whether it could be extrapolated to the rest of the population. There is a quality of life index for every disease, which has to take into consideration all the relevant factors.

9.3.2.3 Adverse Event
AEs are the major causes of failure in clinical development and drug recalls. An AE is a nonintended injury, caused by medical administration as opposed to the disease process. An AE could be fatal or life threatening requiring hospitalization or ending in disability or incapacity. A life-threatening AE is any event that places the subject at immediate risk of death. Serious AE is that which exposes the patient to hospitalization or persistent disability or incapacity. An unexpected AE is any adverse drug experience that is not common to the investigator brochure or that had been previously observed, and not necessarily "not expected" from the pharmacologic properties of the candidate drug [21 CFR 312.32(a)]. ADRs are referred to as adverse experiences and are undesirable signs that are nonintended.

These could be symptoms or diseases in connection with drug usage, but not judged by the experience from the use of a drug (E6 Good Clinical Practice: Section 1.2). This is experienced in two clinical situations: that associated with healthy volunteers and participating patients in clinical studies of new medicine; and that associated with marketed medicines. The level of severity varies from mild to moderate to severe. Severe cases lead to drug discontinuations but a nonserious or less severe ADR is directly dependent on frequency and of administration and concentration of dose. The benefit–risk evaluation guides the decision process for recommending a drug with ADR issues.

ADR-prone drugs are treated differently depending on the stage of clinical trials: Phase I/II clinical trials utilize less severe ADR-prone drugs for healthy volunteers or patients. This has been supported by nonclinical safety pharmacology studies that enable the prediction of the clinical outcome. If a large number of patients reported an ADR, the use of medicine is minimized. The rare ADRs are mainly due to immunologic reactions, chemical toxicity, and hypersensitivity. Serious ADRs lead to major warnings, precautions, and contraindications in labels and can even lead to regulatory disapproval. A thorough understanding of the mechanisms sheds light on the recommendation on precautions and contraindication on drug labels.

Phase II/III trials require a larger number of patients and enable identification in a larger population spread. ADR complaints are usually observed at varied levels, from mild to severe. The nonserious ones have been associated with mechanism of action, class of drug, or disease. ADRs have been predicted through drug interactions during the pharmacologic evaluation in adult healthy animals. Animal studies have facilitated determination of mechanisms responsible for ADRs, which is the reason for the precautions or contraindications that apply to the drug labels. ADRs are more difficult to track once the drug is licensed and marketed but these are reported by the physicians that care for the affected patients. A large number of deaths associated with ADRs are due to patient-related errors, or clinical error by the clinical professional. Certain ADR causes are related to drug interaction with primary target and nontarget tissues, interaction with secondary targets, and other nonspecific effects. During postmarketing surveillance, or pharmacovigilance, the occurrence of AEs is investigated in large patient populations including reporting systems, interventional or prospective cohort or case studies, and national health insurance. It is a widespread challenge.

9.3.2.3.1 Classification of ADRs

ADRs have been classified into five types:

1. Those that depend on the pharmacologic properties of the drug, which is dose dependent.
2. Those that are due to changes that develop because of long-term exposure of certain drug classes.
3. Those that occur due to chronic conditions like carcinogenicity, but are usually incidental.
4. Those that occur as a result of drug discontinuation known as rebound effects and are specific with certain classes of drugs.
5. Those that are idiosyncratic (nondose related). This has contributed to about 25% of known ADRs. Idiosyncrasy is defined as the uncommon variations in response to certain drugs by a minimal number of individuals that has been attributed to a rare metabolic deficiency.

9.3.2.3.2 Adverse Events: Perspectives

Drugs prescribed by physicians could be single or combinations, and these prescriptions are taken by 64% of the pool of patients that attend hospital [11]. Combination drugs could result to drug interactions and ADRs; there are also other possibilities with combination and single drug prescriptions. Most importantly, the chance of ADR increases with duration of drug usage. Twenty percent of injuries or deaths per year have been attributed to the effect of ADRs [12].

A typical challenge in clinical trials is the ability to properly define a drug's safety profile prior to final approval and commercialization. Most of these studies are conducted with an average of 1500 patient exposures for relatively short periods of time, which intrinsically is not sufficient to identify the low-frequency ADRs that require a wider population for the study. For example, Bromfenac (Duract), a nonsteroidal anti-inflammatory agent, was recalled in 1998 after commercialization. This was due to reports of severe hepatotoxicity, which occurred in 1 out of 20,000 patients that used the drug for over 10 years [13,14]. However, 100,000 was the required number of patient exposures. Considering the time and duration requirement of low-frequency ADR-type drugs, toxicity is only detected following marketing. Safety profile determinations for drugs under development had been a daunting challenge as economic and time factors have constrained clinical trials to such relatively small and homogeneous patient populations. This leads to the conclusion that the safety profile of a drug is never absolute [15,16], as it would be difficult to determine if a drug is responsible for the ADR and if only drugs that have a complete evidence of ADR activity should be reported.

Certain strategies are enabling AE prevention and reduction, which have been implemented through application of computerized medical records and using screening software for early alerts on potentially serious drug interactions [17]. Evolving technologies and new paradigms in drug discovery such as "network medicine," "pharmacologic profiling," or "polypharmacology" are aspects of the modernized integrated models currently being applied in drug discovery programs that have shown promise in identifying multiple drug actions that could potentially lead to AEs during drug usage. Novel computerized databases and cross-functional interactions especially among the healthcare team would represent a collaborative approach in an attempt to combat AE experience.

9.4 SELECTED TOPICS IN CLINICAL TRIALS

9.4.1 Placebo-Controlled Trials

Placebo is regarded as a pill or substance that is given to a patient as a drug but that has no biologic effect on the patient. When a proven treatment is available, the placebo-controlled trials (PCTs) have been questioned. In 1996, the Declaration of Helsinki was revised to clarify the fact that PCTs cannot be justified when there is a well-established standard of care [18]. This was not endorsed by the United States with concerns that it might be too stringent. In 2000, the declaration was revised to permit PCTs, but there must be a "compelling and scientifically sound methodological reason" to use them. PCTs are believed to be reliable if there is valid proof of efficacy. PCTs permit the use of placebos for "minor conditions" on the condition that "the patients who receive placebos are not exposed to an undue risk of serious harm" [19].

9.4.2 Randomized Controlled Trials

Randomized controlled analysis is focused on estimating quantitative differences in predefined outcomes between intervention groups. All intervention group cohorts (cohorts are referred to when identical characteristics are assigned based on some similar characteristics like gender or ethnicity) are treated identically except for experimental treatment, which contains a control and intervention control, which could be placebo-based or treatment-based (already proven). So, each intervention group will have its own control. Participants are normally analyzed within the group to which they were allocated, irrespective of whether they experienced the intended intervention (intention to treat analysis). Random allocation identifies systematic differences between intervention groups caused by an external factor that is a common denominator to both intervention and outcome. Blinded or randomized forms are commonly applied strategies in clinical trial design as they emphasize statistical power and validity. These strategies are very effective when trying a new treatment, as they improve the speed of identification of the most effective therapies. Scientific imperative requires physicians to make right choices among the options, and decide which therapy works best for the patient. Medical treatments of the enrolled patients are often adjusted to suit the research protocol demands. A setback is that this type of trial involves participants that would receive inferior treatment.

9.5 IMPLICATIONS OF INAPPROPRIATE STUDY DESIGN

9.5.1 Inappropriate Gender Selection

Bioequivalence is the property of two dosage forms or active ingredients with similar blood concentration levels that produce the same effect at the site of physiologic activity. Thus, failure to identify the appropriate study population affects the validity of data. Inadequate patient stratification is the reason why the bioequivalence studies in one sex have been extrapolated to the other. Gideon [20] reported a study that did not recognize the female-male gender variability. This study was to determine bioequivalence on drugs that are taken by women but which were conducted in mostly young, healthy, adult male volunteers. The reason provided was that each participant in the study would be administered both types of drug preparations and thus would act as their own control for results comparison and that any difference in the formulations would be noticeable in either of them.

To further refute this claim, a study of bioequivalence on alprazolam was cited [20]. The result did not show huge intrasubject variability in males and, as such, would not need a large number of male participants to demonstrate bioequivalence in men. In stark contrast, the intrasubject variability spiked to sixfold in women requiring a larger number of female participants to demonstrate bioequivalence in women. The study reported that gender differences would have a major effect on the data generated from bioequivalence studies for certain drugs. It also pointed out the fact that varying physiological states of women could alter drug disposition (pregnancy is one of the major factors that influence drug performance and intrapatient variability). For drugs that undergo varying physiologic mechanisms, compliance might be influenced by certain physiologic effects. Absorption mechanisms for oral drugs might be affected by certain factors like food effects, gastric pH, combination of drugs that are metabolized with the same enzymes like CYP450 isoenzymes, drugs with a narrow therapeutic index, and drugs with a potential for resistance.

9.5.2 Ethnic Disparity

Risk for disease is usually variable among ethnic groups or races, which is dependent on both genetic and environmental factors. The outcome of genotype–phenotype associations reveals individual variations that divulge a general pattern of genetic diversity within a population group. Inappropriate racial consideration in studies might taint the quality of research results and in many cases this has not been given adequate consideration. A news report by Moon Chen in the University of California Health System newsletter on "Minority clinical trials participation and analysis still lag 20 years after federal mandate" [21] recommended a revised recruitment or clinical trial protocol design that has been the tradition for the past 20 years, even though Congress had mandated a change before this period that remained ineffective. It reported that less than 5% of trial participants are nonwhite, and less than 2% of clinical cancer research studies focus on nonwhite ethnic or racial groups. In the report, Karen Kelly, a co-author and associate director for clinical research at the University of California Davis Comprehensive Cancer Center, pointed out that an ethnic discriminatory genetic factor, a certain genetic mutation that is essential in determining responsiveness to an oral therapy known as EGFR-TKI, is more frequently found in lung tumors from Asian patients than in their American counterparts. Protocol design that does not adequately factor this issue will generate a misleading result. This finding resulted in a change that reflects in how lung cancer is treated worldwide. Thus, there is "a disproportionate effect of cancer and other diseases on racial and ethnic minorities" [21].

This information has enabled group stratification. Pharmacogenomics is an emerging field that evaluates drug compliance based on genetic factors and which informs assignment of dosage regimen and extent of response to a drug. This has provided information about how the gene of an individual could lead to the level of response or adverse reaction to a drug for proper recommendation of drug usage and dosage within a genetically and metabolically heterogeneous environment. Bias in patient stratification brings a complexity issue often reported by the pharmacovigilance teams as it has affected the stakeholders of the pharmaceutical industry; physicians, government, and society with costs of life to some and financial loss to others. Ethical problems that stem from such population scaling or stratification are due to exclusion of certain populations, which affects the stakeholders of the pharmaceutical industry. Proper understanding of the complexity of human biology at the molecular level would represent a major step on the ladder of success.

The FDA recommendation on clinical trials conducted outside of the United States states that

> To assist in assessing the relevance of foreign study population data to U.S. populations, we recommend that sponsors use the Office of Management and Budget (OMB) standardized categories when collecting data from study participants in clinical trials conducted outside of the United States. However, FDA recognizes that the recommended categories for race and ethnicity were developed in the United States and that these categories may not adequately describe racial and ethnic groups in foreign countries. Therefore, for studies conducted outside the United States, we recommend using more detailed categories to provide sponsors the flexibility to adequately characterize race and ethnicity [22].

PART III CLINICAL TRIAL ETHICS

9.6 ETHICAL CONDUCT IN CLINICAL TRIALS

9.6.1 Historical Perspective

Human exploitation was a part of the Nazi atrocities of World War II (1945–1949) when series of human-inflicted atrocities took place. This attracted a legal prosecution under the Nuremberg Trials [23]. It awakened the entire medical community as it brought attention to the flawed medical practice and international standards on research with human participants. Subsequently, there was a total change in the regulations and all the standards. Thus, toughened regulations with new restrictions were imposed on all drug-manufacturing activities. This reorganization of the pharmaceutical regulatory system includes the incorporation of codes of ethics (Nuremburg Code) as a mandatory requirement for drug manufacturers to guide the pharmaceutical R&D of novel therapeutic agents. Subsequently, the World Medial Association Declaration of Helsinki emerged in 1964, which is basis of the Code of Federal Regulations (CFR) issued by the United States Department of Health and Human Services today, and a major guideline for ethical conduct in biomedical research [24].

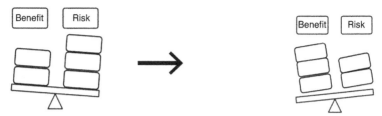

Figure 9.3 *Weighing the Benefit and Risk Ratio.*

The potential risk of harm to clinical trial participants has resulted in a widespread understanding that ethical standards must be observed in clinical research, irrespective of the geographic and economic setting in which it is undertaken. In clinical trials, the expected benefits are expected to outweigh the risks (Figure 9.3).

9.6.2 Ethical Principles

Research ethics is a central theme in medical research, which is premised on the Nuremberg Code, Declaration of Helsinki, and Belmont code.

The ethical principles described by the three ethical codes are based on:
- Respect for Persons: Requires every individual to be treated with courtesy and respect and to protect the person's autonomy. The informed consent must be truthful and conduct no deception.
- Beneficence – Act in the Best Interest: Requires a fostering environment that is free of harm, to maximize benefits while minimizing risks to the research subjects.
- Justice – Treat Me Like I Deserve: Equity and fairness require a fair distribution of costs and benefits to potential research participants.
- Respect for Autonomy – Right to Refuse or Choose: The patient has the right to refuse or choose their treatment.
- Nonmaleficence – Do no Harm: Addressed in clinical research as the disclosure of risks associated with being a participant in a research project.

9.6.2.1 Clinical Equipoise

Clinical equipoise exists when the overall benefit or harm offered by the treatment to a patient is uncertain. Clinical equipoise requires ethical conduct when performing clinical trials that involve assigning patients to different treatment arms. If the outcome of a treatment is known, such a trial has not been encouraged as it could introduce bias. This phenomenon, which is known as "equipoise" in North America, is known as the "uncertainty principle" in Europe. In an ideal situation, the principle of clinical equipoise is recognized, avoiding preferential treatment of one intervention against another. If not followed, it could lead to bias and dilemma in deciding which patient should belong to the arm and which arm of the trial is significantly outperforming the other arm. It is unethical to conduct clinical trials on a drug whose efficacy has been clearly established, as the result cannot be generalized to other populations. There is also ethical impact of uncertainty, which should be justifiable when making a randomized or double-blind selection in trial design. The efficacy of the test drug or the efficacy in a different population should not be known. Documented information suggests that equipoise should be the decision of the physician who determines whether a patient should participate in a clinical trial. Results generated by methodological bias must be supported with a mechanism to reduce the bias, as many trials are known culprits of this unacceptable conduct [25].

9.6.2.2 Dual Role Functions of Clinical Professionals in Clinical Trials: What are the Implications?

The differences in physicians and nurses involved in both medical care and medical research are ethical requirements to allow autonomy and beneficence to their patients. Physicians and nurses participating in medical research have a responsibility to patients according to the medical code of ethics but still follow the mandates in medical research. This is a dual responsibility. Thus, it behoves the researcher to accommodate the interests of society, the pharmaceutical company or sponsor, and humanity by respecting the interests of the participants' need and safety. One example where the medical code is not respected is that, in clinical trials, placebos could be given to those in need of treatment or blood samples could be taken for tests that are not designed to benefit participants directly. Another example is when patients that are challenged with a terminal illness are recruited in a trial that could expose them to a risk of death during the trial.

9.7 INFORMED CONSENT

9.7.1 How Informed is the Consent?

Informed consent is a type of consent or permission given by an individual intentionally and knowingly with a clear awareness of all that applies. It is a means of protecting a patient's right to autonomy. Informed consent introduces the study and its purpose to clarify all that is involved and the risks applicable to the clinical trial procedures, which involves safety issues like physical harm or discomfort, any invasion of privacy threat to dignity, and expected benefits either to the subject or to the scientific institution by gaining new knowledge. It must provide a noncoercive disclaimer, which states that "participation is voluntary and no penalties are involved in refusal to participate." The ability to understand the informed consent depends on literacy level, which contributes to variations in the way the document is interpreted and understood. A presentation is most often preferred as the reader might just glance over the contents and not be well informed. No particular standard has been put forward for determining the literacy level of the participant reading the informed consent. An obvious incompetent patient usually is accompanied by a legally authorized person to give consent.

During recruitment, the principles of ethical conduct are required to be applied effectively to allow the patient the chance to make informed decisions. Decisions could be an issue when the patient is handicapped by illness, flouting the ability to comprehend and the quality of the decision made. A patient's decision could be swayed by emotional need to satisfy the physician as a presumed obligation, which also might affect their willingness to withdraw. The economically disadvantaged are also susceptible to risks as monetary needs could mask the patient's attention to safety necessities. A moral duty of the researchers is to clarify issues for the patients to keep them informed of when they are taking unnecessary steps in their commitment. The uneducated or inappropriately informed are vulnerable to lack of properly informed consent.

9.8 CONFLICT OF INTEREST IN CLINICAL RESEARCH

9.8.1 Primary Conflict of Interest

Primary conflict of interest means that there is more than a single interest, including one that could possibly corrupt the motivation of others. Primary interest refers to the principal goals of activity, such as the integrity of research, the health of patients, and the protection of clients.

9.8.2 Secondary Conflict of Interest

Secondary conflict of interest refers to events that lead to a risk, prompting a judgment or action that aligns with a primary interest that could be dominated by a secondary interest. Secondary interest could be financial gain, promotion, and family and friends advocacy. Conflict of interest rules usually apply to financial relationships because they are relatively more objective and quantifiable.

9.8.3 Institutional Conflict of Interest in Biomedical Research

The main aim of biomedical research is to address the welfare needs of the individual and the public. This is also expected to be reflected in the study design, conduct, and reporting of findings. Relationships between biopharmaceutical, academic research institutions and individual researchers could be strained due to conflict of interest. Academic scientists usually initiate the drug discovery process by identifying novel biologic targets and strategies for disease therapy in a way so as to avoid possible occurrence of AEs. However, bias could be introduced in handling of results and mishandling the participants and other activities with a deliberate purpose of promoting the outcome the data generated. Such occasions often lead to conflict of interest among the parties involved. Also bias could be introduced in clinical design in careful avoidance of financial losses and not necessarily respecting the interest of the patient.

9.9 CRUCIAL CASES IN CLINICAL TRIALS WITH IMPLICATIONS ON SOCIETY

9.9.1 Case I: Differences in the National Regulatory Authorities

Even though policies and regulations influence the breadth of decisions made, decision making is based on available scientific knowledge gained and clinical judgment made in the development processes that permit an evaluation of a drug's effects on the patient populations. A comprehensive understanding of clinical trial outcomes is not limited to the clinical study of effects of drugs on participants but also how drugs are used. This necessitates a consideration of the cognitive and behavioral science aspects of healthcare delivery, which are needed to completely understand the performance of a drug. Differences in judgment among the decision makers might confound regulatory discussions and could result in conflicting recommendations made by different parties. For example, the regulatory tools applied by the three regulatory agencies, the FDA, the EMA, and the Japanese regulatory authorities, that is, the Pharmaceutical and Medical Devices Agency (PMDA) and the Ministry of Health, Labor and Welfare (MHLW), could sometimes differ significantly, and this resulted in differences in the granting of permission for marketing authorization. To patients with life-threatening diseases, the FDA requires results of the early phase of clinical trials to include surrogate endpoints and the proper demonstration of its safety and efficacy, in addition to those obtained by postapproval studies for approval and marketing of the drug. However, the EMA allows conditional approvals if the sponsor demonstrates sound evidence safety and efficacy on a case basis [26]. The FDA and MHLW approve investigational new drugs without randomized controlled trials [27] and postmarketing surveillance is not mandatory [28]. These discrepancies in regulatory oversight affect clinical outcomes and usefulness to society.

9.9.2 Case II: How Ethical are Large Clinical Trials in Rapidly Lethal Diseases?

Horrobin, a clinical trial participant, later died of mantle cell lymphoma after turning in a paper for publication "Are large clinical trials in rapidly lethal diseases ethical" [29] where he shared his experience. In his analysis, he commented that large clinical trials involving patients with fast growing lethal cancers are unethical due to anticipated risks outweighing the benefits, as the large number of this category of patients involved in clinical trials is risky, even though the number is reflective of the need to validate the data or the statistical power to be able to always have an acceptable threshold of population available even when there are dropouts. Unfortunately, this is where the researcher's interest is in conflict with that of the patient since severely ill patients die prior to completion of trials even though the clinical trial guideline of informed consent does clarify this issue proactively. The nature of certain therapeutic agents, which are not patentable and not adequately optimized, is still tested in patients [30]. This dispels the credibility of the requirement of adequate "statistical power" as evidence of a well-conducted trial. Such is an example where a bias is introduced to satisfy the experimental objective rather than accommodating the patient's interest as it restricts the patient to nonconducive circumstances [31]. Furthermore, a recommendation was made for the legislature to allow a minimal number of patients that are already fighting for their lives, in order to reduce costs, increase speed, and save lives. Anthony Mawson asserted that Horrobin's idea could be a misconception as the rapidly lethal clinical trial is a circumstantial issue that is tied to large industry-funded trials that are meant to detect minor differences in patented protected drugs for diseases of this sort [32]. Mawson argues that Horrobin's opinion is more applicable to large clinical trials conducted in developing countries and that the comment was rather premised on his professional experience in oncology trials in countries with the western view [33].

9.9.3 Case III: Clinical Trials in AIDS Research

Clinical development of an AIDS therapeutic agent has often raised several ethical issues due to the type of disease concerned. Certain clinical research designs have led to problems that tend to compromise human rights or ethics. Drugs for AIDS, which are in much demand, would impress sufferers when it shows promise at the early trial stages, but still it has to be certified fit for use according to the regulatory standard. Even though randomization is a widely recommended clinical trial strategy, there are some special considerations that may not quite conform to the objective of applying randomization in the study design for certain drugs for a disease like AIDS [34]. Who would be selected to receive the experimental drugs that are in short supply? This is the dilemma. Soon after the first cases of AIDS were reported in 1981 by Dr Mathilde Krim, the AIDS Medical Foundation (AMF), owned by Krim and the first organization of its kind before it morphed into amfAR, a distinguished national nonorganization, became the voice and brain that publicized and also engaged in active research in developing new therapies for the disease. One of her statements pronounced that "In the case of AIDS, it is immoral to give people nothing at all when there is something that could do them good." A popular topic in AIDS research was in regard to large-scale trials conducted in developing countries on Zidovudine (AZT) treatment for HIV-infected pregnant women to prevent transmission of HIV to the growing fetus. Lurie and Wolfe denounced the idea of denying the patient access to the treatment during clinical trials, particularly those that needed the care [35,36] that have rather been given a placebo based on randomization.

In stark contrast, Harry Schwartz, writer-in-residence at Columbia University College of Physicians and Surgeons, asserted: "The double-blind randomized trial is our best instrument for separating real drug effectiveness from transient, chance phenomena…We should not abandon it when we need its help so much against this terrible killer." This led to speculation that perhaps the research objectives are given superior consideration over those suffering from AIDS. Divided opinions, contradictory remarks, and oppositions continued to emerge. What would be the right judgment? Whose opinion is more ethically correct?

9.10 INTERNATIONAL CLINICAL TRIALS ACROSS THE GLOBE

9.10.1 Clinical Trials in Canada

Socioeconomic status and economic development vary in every country and so does the overall state of affairs. To draw a focus on clinical trials, social dynamics with both public and private sectors play a major role.

Canada is a well-developed economy that supports innovation and scientific maturity, and, importantly, it is a close neighbor to the United States and whose products cost less when in comparison to the United States [37]. The pharmaceutical industry shoulders a high percentage of clinical trials conducted in Canada [38]. In Canada, there is a well-structured federal/ provincial corporate income tax system created for the purpose of elevating its attractiveness to foreign countries to conduct clinical trials in Canada [39]. The recruitment of patients and medical practitioners for clinical trials is done according to the International Conference on Harmonisation guidelines and takes the necessary steps to ensure safety by mobilizing the Research Ethics Boards to scrutinize and approve clinical trials protocol design. Canada partners with the United States to satisfy conditions needed for approval of drugs that have to be approved when reviewed by the FDA. Health Canada compliant drug lifecycle product management is characterized as "point in time," as it focuses on the efficiency of each discrete phase of drug discovery and development, designated as "checkpoints" and uses the knowledge gained to satisfy the long-term goal. The clinical data are scrutinized intensely and almost all institutions prevent research results being commercially driven or publications being influenced. The University of Toronto has specifically taken actions to this effect and these principles guide the negotiation of contracts allowing the investigator to submit manuscript for public within 6 months of sharing the experimental findings.

9.10.2 Conducting Clinical Trials in Developing Countries

The manner with which the ethical principle of justice in clinical research conducted in developing countries is applied has been seriously questioned. The economic development and social–political instability that prevail in these countries is becoming a hallmark problem and unfortunately has seriously hampered the availability of healthcare resources and the quality of healthcare. Language or literacy barriers may contribute to difficulties in interpreting theories, concepts or phrases and may not translate well culturally. Cultural ideologies dominate in these developing countries, which do not have a well-regulated government structure. Male dominance, which is a common social problem in a patriarchal society, has also influenced decisions considered inappropriate for the sponsor. The ardent desire for capital and access to improved healthcare might overcome the motive of clinical trials, as material reward is a major need in a typical underprivileged society. The most uneducated may find it difficult to comprehend the concept of research, clinical trials, and randomization. They would ask, "How would a "doctor" render such care? How could a drug be barred of its healing power and named placebo? Is it possible? – Two tablets, similar in shape and color, but with variable therapeutic potencies?" The doctor's role as a researcher would not be admissible by the uneducated participant. This is a therapeutic misconception.

Lack of resources, which has been associated with inadequate training, may hamper accommodation of the sponsor's standards for ethical review leading to conflicts between the domestic, participating countries and sponsors within a different cultural setting. Disease prevalence and occurrence are more profound in developing countries such that patient recruitment favors the sponsor in terms of cost and time when compared to first world countries. In addition, regulations are less stringent.

A civilian may easily give up rights under duress in poorly regulated developing countries where human rights are not strongly protected. In a survey conducted by Okonta and Rossouw in Nigeria [40], 19.4% of the researchers admitted that they had succumbed to pressure from sponsors to yield to their biased demands [41]. Coercion is frequently used to obtain a participant's consent and it is very simple to achieve this. The selection of published data is often driven by the need to publish all the right data before any other. One example is clinical trials on antidepressants agents acting on serotonin by Melander et al. [42]. It was discovered that out of the 42 clinical trials registered only 25 were published. Out of these 25, 19 documented positive results while six documented negative results.

International clinical trials in developing countries have faced certain major concerns, the question is: what is the medical and social relevance to the host community? How commendable is the standard of care? How informing is the informed consent? How accessible are the interventions following completion of trials [43]?

9.10.3 Clinical Trials in China

Business with a highly populous and economically viable country like China presents a potential growth opportunity for biopharmaceutical companies. In fact, the country is predicted to be the one of the largest prescription drug markets by 2016. There is a well-established tradition of developing medicines from simple natural forms and this has added benefits in formulating modern pharmaceuticals leading to its attractiveness across the globe. China has been ranked as one of the most attractive and low-cost locations for international clinical trials, above India and Russia. The country has been fine-tuning its regulatory landscape trying to harmonize with the international standards. Good clinical practice guidelines were issued by the State Food and Drug Administration (SFDA) in 1999 but have been modified a few times. The SFDA strictly regulates clinical trials, allowing the entire process to be conducted solely by the certified National Institutes of Pharmaceutical Clinical Trials. A large number of clinical trial applications were experienced from 2001 onward, which could mean increasing interest shown by the multinational companies in conducting clinical trials in China. But there are obvious barriers of time, language, maintaining the biologic materials, transportation, and existing regulations that impose restrictions leading to the engagement of the CROs who might be more acquainted with the laws. Sponsors are often exposed to poor language translations during executions and other related activities of the multinational clinical trial as most documents are originally prepared in Chinese. Because it is not a member of the Mutual Recognition Agreement countries, most of the trials are repeated in order to qualify for approval in a foreign country. Phase I studies are required to be conducted in a foreign country as a condition for clinical trial approval. Because the substandard early risk trials have not been well established by the Chinese regulatory authority and Institutional Review Board/Ethical Committee, Phase I and II trials conducted in Korea or Japan are more recognized and believed to operate according to acceptable standards.

One of the largest, randomized, double-blind, placebo-controlled clinical trials, the COMMIT/CCS-2 trial, was conducted into heart disease. It was coordinated by Oxford University, in the United Kingdom, and Fuwai Hospital, the Chinese Academy of Medical Sciences, in China [44], and enrolled about 46,000 patients at 1250 sites in China [45].

9.10.4 Case I: Significance of Differences in Patient Diagnosis in Multinational Clinical Trials

There is a remarkable variation in disease diagnosis in patients from different ethnic groups. This has been linked to varied lifestyles, and economic and social factors that prevail in the different geographic regions. Background genetic factors or predispositions that mask diseases in other countries are due to variants and subtypes, which underlie the fact that certain conditions are prevalent only in certain countries. For example, black Africans are different from those of the Caribbean Islands, which have different cultural values to those that have been raised in North America [46]. This issue has been a challenge to multinational clinical trials particularly as the medical literature has not adequately defined a mechanism to approach diagnosis in patients at different geographic locations [47,48]. Lack of appropriate knowledge about these variations would affect the clinical diagnosis as physicians use various weighing systems in their determinations. Such variations in clinical trials have been made more complicated when laboratory tests are not conducted appropriately or inexperienced clinical professionals have been recruited.

There are economic barriers that limit availability of infrastructure or quality of technology applied in the conduct of clinical trials. Social and cultural values, religion, and education may influence the method of clinical trials that are conducted. Reporting of AEs might vary in different countries as it could occur at different stages in clinical studies of which classification systems are also variable. The efficiency in reporting AEs might be recognized as stigma in certain countries, which may result in suppression of such data to protect integrity. Underdiagnoses of disease also do exist in many countries.

Several barriers to participation of racial and ethnic minorities in clinical research have been identified for both researchers and participants. For researchers, inadequate knowledge about the variation factors among ethnic minorities would hinder operative effectiveness and integrity of research results due to confounding recruitment, enrollment, and retention strategies [49].

These differences affect multinational clinical trials as they have therapeutic implications.

9.10.5 Case II: The Controversy of Zidovudine (AZT) Trials in African and Other Developing Countries

In 1994, the AIDS Clinical Trial Group (ACTG) reported positive outcomes with respect to the use of Zidovudine (AZT) during prenatal treatment to reduce mother-to-child transmission [50]. As such, AZT became the standard of care for HIV positive mothers in the United States and the European Union but not in Africa due to financial considerations. But in later deliberations and approvals, a cause championed by the World Health Organization on clinical trials for the AZT then opened up channels in Africa and Asia. However, the trials involved a placebo control as a replacement to the standard "ACTG 076," a code used to designate the clinical trial samples [51]. The PCTs did not protect the neonates exposed to HIV infection as their mothers did not receive treatment. It violated the principle of beneficence.

REFERENCES

[1] Murgo AJ, Kummar S, Rubinstein L, Gutierrez M, Collins J, Kinders R, Parchment RE, Ji J, Steinberg SM, Yang SX, Hollingshead M, Chen A, Helman L, Wiltrout R, Tomaszewski JE, Doroshow JH. Designing phase 0 cancer clinical trials. Clin Cancer Res 2008;14(12):3675–82.

[2] Twombly R. Slow start to phase 0 as researchers debate value. J Nat Can Inst 2006;98:804–6.

[3] Melnick VL, Dubler NN, Weisbard A, Butler N. Clinical research in senile dementia of the Alzheimer type. J Am Geriatr Soc 1984;32:531–6.

[4] Lazarou J, Pomeranz BH, Corey PN. Incidence of adverse drug reactions in hospitalized patients: a meta-analysis of prospective studies. JAMA 1998;279:1200–5.

[5] Lorgelly PK. Choice of outcome measure in an economic evaluation: a potential role for the capability approach. Pharmacoeconomics 2015;33:849–55.

[6] Temple RJ. A regulatory authority's opinion about surrogate endpoints. In: Nimmo WS, Tucker GT, editors. In clinical measurement in drug evaluation. Indianapolis: Wiley; 1995.

[7] Knepper MA. Common sense approaches to urinary biomarker study design. J Am Soc Nephrol 2009;20:1175–8.

[8] Ginsburg GS, Haga SB. Translating genomic biomarkers into clinically useful diagnostics. Expert Rev Mol Diagn 2006;6(2):179–91.

[9] Lesko LJ, Atkinson AJ Jr. Use of biomarkers and surrogate endpoints in drug development and regulatory decision making: criteria, validation, strategies. Annu Rev Pharmacol Toxicol 2001;41:347–66.

[10] Woodcock J. 21st-Century Cures: Modernizing Clinical Trials and Incorporating the Patient Perspective. Statement of M.D., Director Center for Drug Evaluation and Research, Food and Drug Administration, Department of Health and Human Services, Before the Subcommittee on Health, Committee on Energy and Commerce, US House of Representatives, July 11, 2014.

[11] Schappert SM. Ambulatory care visits to physician offices, hospital outpatient departments, and emergency departments: United States, 1997. National Center for Health Statistics. Vital Health Stat 1999;13(143).

[12] Jacubeit T, Drisch D, Weber E. Risk factors as reflected by an intensive drug monitoring system. Agents Actions 1990;29:117–25.

[13] Lazarou J, Pomeranz B, Corey PN. Incidence of adverse drug reactions in hospitalized patients: A meta-analysis of prospective studies. JAMA 1998;279:1200–5.

[14] Gurwitz JH, Field TS, Avorn J, McCormick D, Jain S, Eckler M, et al. Incidence and preventability of adverse drug events in nursing homes. Am J Med 2000;109(2):87–94.

[15] Friedman MA, Woodcock J, Lumpkin MM, Shuren JE, Hass AE, Thompson LJ. The safety of newly approved medicines: do recent market removals mean there is a problem? JAMA 1999;281(18):1728–34.

[16] Gardiner P1, Sarma DN, Low Dog T, Barrett ML, Chavez ML, Ko R, Mahady GB, Marles RJ, Pellicore LS, Giancaspro GI. The state of dietary supplement adverse event reporting in the United States. Pharmacoepidemiol Drug Saf 2008;17(10):962–70.

[17] Committee on Quality of Health Care in America: Institute of Medicine. To Err is Human: Building a Safer Health System. Washington, DC: National Academy Press; 2000.

[18] Declaration of Helsinki: ethical principles for medical research involving human subjects. Note of clarification on paragraph 29 added by the World Medical Association General Assembly. Washington, DC: World Medical Association; 2002. Available from: http://www.wma.net/e/policy/b3.htm. [accessed 07.04.2015].

[19] National Heart, Lung, & Blood Institute, US Department of Health and Human Services, World Health Organization. Asthma Management and Prevention: A Practical Guide for Public Health Officials and Health Care Professionals, Based on the Global

Strategy for Asthma Management and Prevention NHLBI/WHO Workshop Report. Bethesda (Md): NIH Publication No. 96-3659A; 1995.

[20] Gideon K. Sex dependent pharmacokinetics and bioequivalence – time for change. J Popul Ther Clin Pharmacol 2013;20(3):e358–61.

[21] Chen M. Minority clinical trials participation and analysis still lag 20 years after federal mandate. March 18; 2014. Available from: http://www.ucdmc.ucdavis.edu/publish/news/newsroom/8305 [accessed 10.04.2015].

[22] FDA Guidance Documents on Clinical Trials. Guidance for Industry – Collection of Race and Ethnicity Data in Clinical Trials. III. Collection of Race and Ethnicity Data in Clinical Trials. Available from: http://www.fda.gov/RegulatoryInformation/Guidances/ucm126340.htm#iii [accessed 12.04.2015].

[23] Medical Experiment. Jewish Virtual Library. Retrieved from: March 23, 2008.

[24] The Doctors Trial: The Medical Case of the Subsequent Nuremberg Proceedings'. United States Holocaust Memorial Museum. Retrieved March 23, 2008. Available from: http://www.ushmm.org/information/exhibitions/online-features/special-focus/doctors-trial/nuremberg-code, http://www.wma.net/en/30publications/10policies/b3/ [accessed 07.04.2015].

[25] Cook C, Sheets C. Clinical equipoise and personal equipoise: two necessary ingredients for reducing bias in manual therapy trials. J Man Manip Ther 2011;19(1):55–7.

[26] Boon WP, Moors EH, Meijer A, Schellekens H. Conditional approval and approval under exceptional circumstances as regulatory instruments for stimulating responsible drug innovation in Europe. Clin Pharmacol Ther 2010;88(6):848–53.

[27] Shibuya K, Hashimoto H, Ikegami N, Nishi A, Tanimoto T, Miyata H, Takemi K, Reich MR. Future of Japan's system of good health at low cost with equity: beyond universal coverage. Lancet 2011;378(9798):1265–73.

[28] Richey EA, Lyons EA, Nebeker JR, Shankaran V, McKoy JM, Luu TH, Nonzee N, Trifilio S, Sartor O, Benson AB 3rd, Carson KR, Edwards BJ, Gilchrist-Scott D, Kuzel TM, Raisch DW, Tallman MS, West DP, Hirschfeld S, Grillo-Lopez AJ, Bennett CL. Accelerated approval of cancer drugs: improved access to therapeutic breakthroughs or early release of unsafe and ineffective drugs? J Clin Oncol 2009;27(26):4398–405.

[29] Horrobin DF. Are large clinical trials in rapidly lethal diseases usually unethical? Lancet 2003;361:695–7.

[30] Hennekens CH, Buring JE, Mayrent SL. Epidemiology in medicine. Boston: Little, Brown and Company; 1987. p. 198.

[31] Halpern SD, Karlawish JHT, Berlin JA. The continuing unethical conduct of under-powered clinical trials. JAMA 2002;288:358–62.

[32] Mawson AR. Institute of Epidemiology and Health Services Research, Department of Public Health, School of Allied Health Sciences. Jackson State University, Jackson, MS 39213, USA.

[33] Blend MJ. Can we learn from our patients? Perspect Biol Med 2005;48(1):138–42.

[34] Macklin R, Friedland G. AIDS research: the ethics of clinical trials. Law Med Health Care 1986;14(5–6):273–80.

[35] Lurie P, Wolfe SM. Unethical trials of interventions to reduce perinatal transmission of the human immunodeficiency virus in developing countries. N Engl J Med 1997;337(12):853–6.

[36] Angell M. The ethics of clinical research in the third world. N Engl J Med 1997;337:847–9.

[37] Industry Canada. Canada – Your Innovation Partner in Clinical Trials (2006). Available from: http://scimega.com/downloads/industry-reports/Canada_Innovation_Partner_Clinical-Trials.pdf [accessed 11.04.2015].

[38] Lexchin J. Clinical trials in Canada: whose interests are paramount? Int J Health Services 2008;38(3):525–42.

[39] Warda J. Measuring the Attractiveness of R&D Tax Incentives: Canada and Major Industrial Countries. A report prepared for Foreign Affairs and International Trade Canada, Ontario. Investment Service and Statistics Canada. Statistics Canada, Ottawa, 1999.

[40] Okonta P. Ethics of clinical trials in Nigeria. Nigerian Med J 2014;55(3):188.

[41] Okonta P, Rossouw T. Prevalence of scientific misconduct among a group of researchers in Nigeria. Dev World Bioeth 2013;13:149–57.

[42] Melander H, Ahlqvist-Rastad J, Meijer G, Beermann B. Evidence biased medicine – selective reporting from studies sponsored by pharmaceutical industry: review of studies in new drug applications. BMJ 2003;326:1171–3.

[43] Lorenzo C, Garrafa V, Solbakk JH, Vidal S. Hidden risks associated with clinical trials in developing countries. J Med Ethics 2010;36:111–5.

[44] Paris, France and Princeton. Clopidogrel improved coronary perfusion and reduced mortality in accute heart attack. Available from: http://www.sadofi-aventies.us

[45] Liang K. Clinical Trial Opportunities in China. Appl Clin Trials. Apr 2007; 16, 4; ProQuest p. 58. Applied Clinical Trials on the Web. Available from: www.actmagazine.com

[46] Egede LE. Race, ethnicity, culture, and disparities in health care. J Gen Intern Med 2006;21(6):667–9.

[47] Martins T, Hamilton W, Ukoumunne OC. Ethnic inequalities in time to diagnosis of cancer: a systematic review. BMC Fam Pract 2013;14:197.

[48] Forrest LF, Adams J, Wareham H, Rubin G, White M. Socioeconomic inequalities in lung cancer treatment: systematic review and meta-analysis. PLoS Med 2013;10(2):e1001376.

[49] George S, Duran N, Norris K. A systematic review of barriers and facilitators to minority research participation among African Americans, Latinos, Asian Americans, and Pacific Islanders. Am J Public Health 2014;104(2):e16–31.

[50] Zidovudine for mother, fetus, and child: hope or poison? Lancet 1994;344:207–209 (Authors not listed).

[51] Lurie P, Wolfe SM. Unethical trials of interventions to reduce perinatal transmission of the human immunodeficiency virus in developing countries. N Engl J Med 1997;337:853–6.

CHAPTER 10

Pharmacogenomics in Drug Discovery, Prospects and Clinical Applicability

Odilia Osakwe

The notion of the blockbuster drug that everybody takes is going to change. We will be able to prescribe medications tailored not only to the genetic makeup of the individual, but also to our social, cultural and economic circumstances.

Jeff Balser, MD, PhD, Vice Chancellor for Health Affairs, Vanderbilt Medicine Newsletter, Winter 2011

Contents

10.1	Introduction	222
	10.1.1 Overview	222
	10.1.2 Polymorphism	222
	10.1.3 Pharmacogenomics and Pharmacogenetics	224
	10.1.4 One-Size-Fits-All Approach to Clinical Practice	226
	10.1.5 Personalized Medicine	226
	10.1.6 Biomarkers	226
10.2	Genetic Variations and Implications in Drug Development	227
	10.2.1 Activity of the Cytochrome P450 (CYP) Isoenzymes	227
	10.2.2 Pharmacokinetic Outcomes	229
	10.2.3 Pharmacodynamic Outcomes	230
10.3	The Effectiveness of Clinical Implementation of Pharmacogenomics	230
	10.3.1 In Clinical Trials	230
	10.3.2 In Clinical Practice	231
	10.3.3 In Addressing Adverse Drug Reactions	232
10.4	Promising Outcomes Associated with Clinical Application Pharmacogenomics: Cases	233
	10.4.1 Human Immunodeficiency Virus	233
	10.4.2 Cancer Drugs	234
	10.4.3 Vend (Voriconozole)	234
	10.4.4 LRRTM3 in Alzheimer's Disease	235
	10.4.5 APOE4	235
	10.4.6 Mental Disorders	235

Social Aspects of Drug Discovery, Development and Commercialization Copyright © 2016 Elsevier Inc.
http://dx.doi.org/10.1016/B978-0-12-802220-7.00010-7   All rights reserved.

10.5 Economic and Social Implications of Pharmacogenomics Application   236
    10.5.1 Penetrance   236
    10.5.2 Economic Considerations   236
10.6 National Regulatory Agencies on Pharmacogenomics Implementation   237
    10.6.1 Personalized Medicine Program-University of Florida Health   238
References   239

10.1 INTRODUCTION

10.1.1 Overview

It has been widely recognized that the approach to the understanding, diagnosis, and treatment of disease is evolving. Emerging technologies in genomics, epigenomics, proteomics, molecular diagnostics imaging, and nanotechnology are enabling rapid changes. Previously, the development of drugs has been based on a generalized knowledge that precludes individual genes and effects. This has contributed to attrition rates due to failing clinical trials challenged with variable and unpredictable efficacy and safety outcomes. The fundamental knowledge of the human genome has enabled scrutiny and identification of individual genetic compositions that have been associated with disease susceptibility and responses to therapeutic agents, and the subsequent introduction of the concept of "pharmacogenomics" into healthcare systems [1]. Consequently, there has been a growing need to transform from a one-size-fits-all approach to a more personalized system of predictive, preventive, and precision healthcare that is tailored to a population or an individual.

Pharmacogenomics addresses the genetic underpinnings of pharmacokinetic (PK) anomalies and interindividual variability in clinical response, the effect of genetic polymorphism on the pharmacological variables to understand the effects on drug–drug interactions, and the occurrence of adverse events [2]. The development of genetic analyses and functional genomics (Figure 10.1) has increased along with innovative and high throughput technologies that have hastened the rate of screening of genes that identify the alterations, mutations, and other variations in the genome. Progressively, pharmacogenomics is becoming an integral aspect of drug development, early enough to allow detection of future genetic-based anomalies for an enhanced therapeutic performance.

10.1.2 Polymorphism

In pharmaceutical research and development (R&D), polymorphism is referred to as variations in DNA composition that alter the drug PK leading to variability in clinical efficacy and toxicity of drugs [3,4]. A single nucleotide

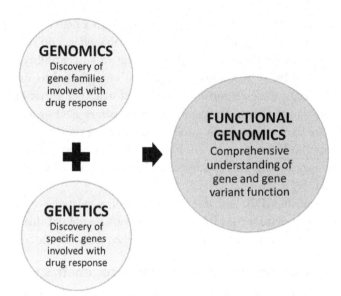

Figure 10.1 *The Genetic and Genomic Strategies in new Drug Discovery.*

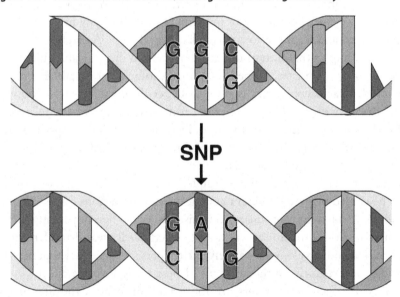

Figure 10.2 *SNPs in Normal and Diseased Condition [8].*

polymorphism (SNP) is the most common form of genetic polymorphism, which is a mutation or change in a single base pair in the DNA molecule (Figure 10.2). It is responsible for individual variations in physical traits, disease phenotype, and other manifestations associated with genetic variations of this type. It can occur at any location in the genome but identifying the genetic loci is essential in associating a disease with a genetic origin. SNPs located in the coding region of genes have variable effects on the expressed protein and accordingly might lead to disease or susceptibility to disease sensitivity and adverse reactions [5]. SNP has contributed to variations in response to drugs, which is mostly the effect of structural variations in drug targets, drug-metabolizing enzymes, and transporters. SNPs found in these structures are used as diagnostic tools for developing therapeutic agents for drug therapy. SNP mapping technology may permit identification of polymorphism associated with a specific drug responsiveness or an adverse drug reaction (ADR) [6,7].

Polymorphism ADR and disease susceptibility-related polymorphisms could overlap and might lead to a simultaneous incidental dual diagnosis. This could present ethical issues that affect privacy and confidentiality.

10.1.3 Pharmacogenomics and Pharmacogenetics

Pharmacogenetics is the study of the contribution of inherited gene variants on interindividual variation in drug response [9]. A single drug may be targeted to a group of numerous individuals with similarity in gene expression pattern and response to a particular drug therapy. As such, a thorough understanding of the biotransformation of certain drugs enables identification of drug candidates, probed for various isoforms of metabolic enzyme involved. Pharmacogenetics is used to target drug therapy to a subset of populations with the highest response to treatment due to the relatedness of certain genetic signatures in the individuals. Series of compounds from combinatorial/parallel chemistry are subjected to high throughput screening against an isolated molecular target in cell-free assays. The picture that emerges is very complex. For example, cancer is not a single disease and can be caused by many different genetic alterations. Various forms of cancer could have different molecular mechanisms in two different patients. Hence, a one-size-fits-all treatment will not be effective. All these drugs have to be discovered and developed separately as they present disparate properties and mechanisms requiring a therapy well adapted for its curative effect.

Pharmacogenomics refers to the study of drug exposure and/or response due to variations in the human genome. According to the International Conference on Harmonisation [10], pharmacogenomics involves genome-wide analysis of the genetic determinants of drug efficacy and toxicity (Figure 10.1). Human genome sequencing and technological sophistication paved the way to synchronous multiple genes analysis, allowing development of drugs that are tailored to specific individuals based on genetic composition – a crucial requirement to creating personalized medicine. Pharmacogenomics is extensive as it is also concerned with the knowledge gained from studying SNPs, proteins, regulatory genes, and metabolites of the cell using holistic approaches. A reductionist approach is technologically reliant and straightforward, which is more aligned to a one-size-fits-all approach. However, pharmacogenomics is well aligned with the systems biology paradigm that takes into consideration all the primary, secondary, and global interactions within the entire organism.

Both pharmacogenetics and pharmacogenomics are identified by genetic SNPs and genomic expression approaches with the aim of developing a personalized drug therapy. Drug exposure refers to the PK profile following administration; drug response refers to the pharmacodynamics (PD) response to the drug, which is all the effects of the drug on any physiologic and pathologic process, in relation to effectiveness and adverse reactions. Pharmacogenomics is focused on differential effects of compounds on the entire expressed genes, which are assessed by pharmacogenomics profiling. Primary candidate genes of interest include those encoding for drug receptors, metabolizing enzymes, and transporters. Selection of optimal drug therapy may involve disease susceptibility genes directly or indirectly affecting drug response. Unlike pharmacogenetics, which is focused on patient variability, pharmacogenomics is focused on compound variability, in a holistic point of view. Pharmacogenomics includes the identification of suitable targets for drug discovery and development.

Clinical trials that incorporate the pharmacogenomics assessment tool identify genetic polymorphisms that are associated with the degree of response (efficacy) or with specific adverse events (safety). *In vitro* studies of metabolism, transport, or drug targets prospectively render the opportunity to integrate pharmacogenomics factors for assessing interindividual variability and its implications for subsequent clinical studies. Genetic expression arrays are used in *in vitro* evaluation to explore associations with clinical outcomes to predict drug response to understand mechanisms of action. This study is also necessary for finding biomarkers of drug response, for determining the effectiveness or toxicity of drugs. With microarray technology, genes in the range of thousands and proteins could be evaluated at the same time. Pharmacogenomics technology is perceived as a milestone among the emerging translational sciences introduced to overcome innovation setbacks that negate pharmaceutical productivity [11]. Patient responses vary with about 30–60% of the population responding to well-known drugs like antidepressants, statins, and antipsychotics [12]. A certain population also experiences ADRs [13]. ADRs are becoming a menace to society due to cost and health effects [14].

10.1.4 One-Size-Fits-All Approach to Clinical Practice

For this approach, drug development relies on cellular mechanism and disease pathway networks that are not specific to any population or individual, leading to patients having the same diagnosis, but who exhibit dramatically different responses to the same drug. Pharmacogenomics is not included in clinical development and thus genetic screening is not included. Drugs are assigned on the basis of a doctor's opinion with a certain degree of guessing. This approach is unfavorable to the patient's health, and a waste of time and resources.

10.1.5 Personalized Medicine

Personalized medicine is increasingly becoming the standard of care due to the pharmacogenomics tool that is currently being used in drug discovery and development, which takes into consideration the individual biological characteristics that influence drug therapy. Preventive or therapeutic interventions are targeted on a predetermined group and not to those who will not benefit from them. The use of biomarkers represents a paradigm shift that has been applied in pharmacogenomics studies in clinical trials and drug discovery programs in general.

10.1.6 Biomarkers

A biomarker is a measurable indicator of a biological process in response to a disease or therapy. Examples are high blood pressure as an indicator of increased risk of stroke or more complex genetic mutation in tumor cells with a unique association to specific forms of cancer. Biomarker application represents a major paradigm shift in biomedical research. It presents useful information about a disease in the form of molecular signatures that are tractable and effective. It could be used to identify the potential risks of diseases, response and method of response, length of progression, patient survival, and length of therapy. For example, genetic tests for gene variants have enabled the improvement of care for patients with metastatic renal cell carcinoma in response to the drug sunitinib [15]. Certain mutations are favorable as they permit prolonged survival from certain diseases when compared to normal genes. For example, in chronic lymphocytic leukemia, certain mutations that affect the immunoglobulin genes provide the chance of longer survival than those lacking the mutations. Biomarkers have been useful in pharmacogenomics as they allow the unraveling of pathways that are important in targeting new investigational agents for the selection of candidates for clinical trials and to assign personalized therapy [16].

Predictive biomarkers enable the selection and recommendation of medical therapy for the most suitable patient population. Knowing the basic biology of diseases enables identification of critical cellular pathways in the progression of the disease. Each disease identifies a biomarker responsive to a treatment and could be used to develop a therapeutic agent effective against that condition [17].

Biomarker discovery has been limited due to specificity in disease pathology per disease, leading to a wide variation of pathways and processes. Thus, biomarkers are expected to be validated in clinical studies for optimal performance and to ensure reliability in generated results. For the heterogeneous population comprising large different patient subtypes, a larger patient pool is required to be able to determine the differences in response in clinical trials to aid identification of the responders and nonresponders. This needs careful interpretation as confounding results are obtainable. Disease phenotypes in individuals harboring certain mutations could be replicated in those without mutations. When there are no standard criteria for identifying the right patients with those who have mutations, additional studies are required for a more effective use of biomarkers in order to access the risk for developing the disease.

Explosive biomedical discoveries are desirable and commendable but still have not proportionately been translated into practical value due to lack of translational tools that could transform concept to usable formats. For example, numerous new and valuable biomarkers have not progressed to practicality as modern clinical trial efforts are still thirsty for astute minds and strategies needed to advance markers into development. Intensive efforts are being directed towards investing in biomarker research to improve its applicability. And, most importantly, to aid the development of novel medicines and to maximize the patient population receiving medical care.

10.2 GENETIC VARIATIONS AND IMPLICATIONS IN DRUG DEVELOPMENT

10.2.1 Activity of the Cytochrome P450 (CYP) Isoenzymes

Drugs that are absorbed through the gastrointestinal tract first travel to the liver for processing before continuing to the heart. In the liver, they are substantially metabolized before reaching general circulation. This is known as the first pass effect. In the liver, various CYP enzymes interact with the drug molecules depending on the molecular nature and transformation to more hydrophilic forms liable for elimination. This is an elimination mechanism as it enables the removal of foreign molecules from the body. The most predominant of the drug-metabolizing enzymes is the cytochrome P450 (CYP) isoenzyme system. There are relatively high incidences of six of the CYPs: CYP1A2, CYP3A4, CYP2A6, CYP2C9, CYPC219, and CYP2D6. Over 20 SNP variants of CYP2D6 have been found and are responsible for the biotransformation of over 500 drugs. Polymorphic existence is the reason why there are three categorizes of metabolizing strengths; poor, intermediate, and extensive metabolizers, which vary among ethnic groups (Figure 10.3).

The rate of enzyme metabolic activities varies in the order of tens (10-fold–100-fold), and has been rated as slow or fast accordingly. It is these variations that account for the PK differences and, consequently, PD. Interindividual variations strongly associate pharmacogenomics with drug metabolism.

10.2.1.1 CYP2D6

The CYP2D6 isoform a is the most common metabolizing form of the CYP enzymes known and which has been associated with approximately 25% of all medicines that are currently prescribed and the popular indications. Over 70 alleles have been identified in CYP2D6, a major contributor to varied levels of responses to a dose of medicine posing a barrier to effective therapy. These considerations have stimulated genotyping and phenotyping screening in clinical trials for drug compounds that are metabolized by these CYP isoforms, a useful mechanism for identifying the ADRs [18].

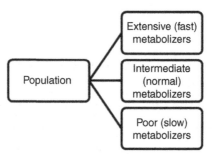

Figure 10.3 *Population Stratification by Response to Drugs.*

Approximately 7% of the Caucasian population has a genetic variant that results in reduced activity of the CYP2D6 enzyme. The CYP2D6 enzyme is regarded as a poor metabolizer. A 2–30% subset metabolize very slowly due to the availability of multiple copies of the CYP2D6 gene. These individuals lack the ability to break down quickly enough by the liver leading to accumulation in the body, which has the possibility of adverse consequences. For certain medicines like codeine, response takes effect following complete enzyme metabolism. This is a limitation to individuals who are deficient in the CYP2D6 enzyme as normal doses are not sufficient. Rapid metabolizers might need a higher concentration of the medicine to achieve the same pharmacological effect as they break down the medicine very quickly. Differences in the metabolism attributed to differences in the CYP2D6 gene have not been followed with pharmacogenetics testing for the relevant variants and have not become the standard of care in clinical practice, although it is slowly gaining ground.

10.2.2 Pharmacokinetic Outcomes

PK describes the absorption and distribution, as well as the chemical changes, of a drug substance in the body (e.g., by metabolic enzymes such as cytochrome P450 or glucuronosyl transferase enzymes), the effects and routes of excretion of the drug metabolites. The uptake of a drug by the body can be disturbed, arising from alterations in biomolecules, mostly drug-metabolizing enzymes and transporters that mediate drug uptake [19]. Activation (metabolism) could lead to the impairment of the function of the enzymes that catalyze such reactions. As a consequence, a drug could be erroneously converted to toxic forms, overprocessed (metabolized), or underprocessed. When important transport proteins become dysfunctional, drugs could be delivered in either too high or too low a concentration to the site of action.

This is a major reason why interindividual variations in the genes that express the enzymes also affect responses and susceptibility to diseases. The genetic differences that are considered very seriously are genes that influence disease susceptibility or progression, genes associated with PK (absorption, distribution, metabolism, and excretion; ADME), genes related to drug targets or other drug's pharmacologic effect, and genes that are not part of the drug's intended therapeutic target that can predispose to toxicities. The mechanism leading to variations in PK profile are mainly related to metabolizing enzymes or transport proteins and genetic polymorphisms.

10.2.3 Pharmacodynamic Outcomes

PD is the study of the exposure/response (E/R) relationship of drugs, and genetic differences can lead to changes in the steepness of the E/R curve. PD is all of the effects of the drug on any physiologic and pathologic process, which is connected to drug efficacy and adverse reactions. Drug response due to its interaction with the intended drug targets is a PD process. These processes are further complicated by intra- and interindividual variability, which are highly frequent and could evolve with time [20]. Genomic effects on PK can seriously alter the optimal dose as it is based on differences in dose– or exposure–response, safety, and efficacy. For example, a known fact is that there are genetic variants in a metabolizing enzyme (CYP2C9). However, genetic variations in warfarin's target (*VKORC1*) significantly affect response and dose requirements [21].

Differences in the structure of drug target receptors associated with normal body function and diseases confound the ability to establish a relationship between drug response and plasma concentrations. For example, asthma patients who carry a specific genotypic variation of the β_2-andrenergic receptor are nonresponsive to most of the available inhaled drug albuterol [22]. Certain abnormal genes expressed in tumors, cancer *BRCA1* and *BRCA2* mutations, are linked to breast cancer. Polymorphism in the G-protein coupled receptor of bradykinin gives rise to a cough, which is a side effect of the ACE inhibitors [23].

10.3 THE EFFECTIVENESS OF CLINICAL IMPLEMENTATION OF PHARMACOGENOMICS

10.3.1 In Clinical Trials

The application of pharmacogenomics approaches during drug development is a continuous process, from discovery to clinical development. Pharmacogenomics approaches are a part of the exploratory and observational studies, as the early-phase data on genomic-dependent dosing may provide leads on the type of patient to be recruited for the later-phase trials and data collection, or inform the strategy for further collection of genetic and related biomarker data in later controlled trials. The plasma concentration–time data generated from drug administration permits the determination of relationships between variants in genes related to metabolic enzymes, the transporters, and the PK properties of the investigational drug. Gene expression profiles help to identify associations with safety and efficacy at a wide range of doses. Administration of larger doses leads to proportionately large adverse effects, enough to establish a link with the genetic variants of drug targets, which could then be conducted on a genomically stratified population for a more personalized and targeted therapy.

In Phase II trials, the candidate-gene approach can be used in conjunction with genotyping to correlate particular polymorphisms with phenotypic differences in efficacy. Phase I/II data are used to generate a genomic hypothesis that may then be tested in prospectively designed Phase III trials. Phase IIb is intended to optimize the dosing but the participant population has not been very permissive in terms of identifying the adverse events or reactions experienced at the postmarketing phase. Hence, adapting Phase IIb trials to an expanded population that targets the responders would enable:

• Identification of specific genetic polymorphisms (mostly SNPs), those are associated with responsiveness to particular drugs.
• Identification of genes to compare the frequency of a given genotype of response or genotype of nonresponse to the drug of interest, to analyze the relationship between genetic alleles and drug–response phenotypes. This will enable determination of differences in the extent of response to a treatment.
• Identification of differences in metabolism or clearance that will affect the PK of a drug to aid in classifying the populations according to metabolic profile, and the extensive, poor, intermediate metabolizers for appropriate assignment of dosage based on absorption, distribution, metabolism, and excretion.

The data generated provide mechanistic support to inform clinical design and for the definitive evidence of safety and effectiveness demonstrated in Phase III. In Phase III trials, pharmacogenomics profiling can be used to distinguish responders from nonresponders. It mostly refines and helps to confirm earlier studies needed to apply therapy to a narrowed or specific subset population to exclude adverse response and optimize clinical efficacy.

10.3.2 In Clinical Practice

The manner of communicating genomic information also contributes to the clinical decision made and has limited the effective translation of pharmacogenomics to clinical practice [24,25]. Thus, the utility of electronic health records (EHR), health information technology, and clinical decision support has been introduced in an attempt to bridge the communication problems encountered in implementing personalized medicine by linking biological material to pharmacotherapy [26]. To date, EHR deployment has played a significant contribution to the advancing clinical research and practice.

The Food and Drug Administration Amendments Act, passed by the US Congress in 2007, suggested increasing postmarket monitoring of drug safety. To this effect, the Food and Drug Administration (FDA) established the "Sentinel Initiative" for the purpose of early and accurate detection of drug safety signals. The real-time monitoring EHRs and medical claims databases contribute to this process. Many cross-institutional networks have been involved in this process (e.g., HMO Research Network, the Pharmacogenomics Research Network, and the eMERGE network). Biomedical informatics platforms are now interrogating a patient's genetic data in the patient's EHR information, which has been a major element in clinical decision making in real time. Thus, EHR technology is well poised to facilitate the clinical actualization of personalized medicine. For example, in Vanderbilt University Medical Centre (VUMC), the patient's EHR is sourced from the PREDICT genetic results database, which is essential to clinical decision making. This information has been made available to patients through VUMC's patient portal, My Health At Vanderbilt, to permit the viewing of personal EHR data and communicate to the provider. This information had a limited utility as in the case of the CYP2C9 analysis where only 2 out of the 13 variants tested could be approved for implementation [27,28]. A well-established EHR system requires collaboration among all the parties involved, mostly the research and clinical trials that are required to work in tandem with healthcare for a better spread of its data and knowledge to enhance the effective incorporation of personalized medicine in the clinics. Funding initiatives have been in place to catalyze this process and the patient advocacy groups are active role players in this process. In addition, society has provided a safe climate to instill confidence in research participants through informed consent, which protects their interests.

10.3.3 In Addressing Adverse Drug Reactions

Eliminating ADRs is one of the major aims of introducing the concept of personalized medicine, which attempts to replace the existing one-size-fits-all application in clinical practice. According to Federal Drug Administration, there have been more than 2 million cases of serious ADRs yearly, contributing to more than 100,000 deaths that have been recorded each year among hospitalized patients in the United States alone. Current research goals have been directed towards bringing this clinical anomaly to an end. This would introduce more personalized parameters in drug prescription rather than one that is based on dosing alone. A tailored-to-fit profile based on a genetic profile is expected to help combat the issue of ADRs among the patient population such that dangerous ADRs and lost revenue to stakeholders and society can be avoided.

Therapeutic drug monitoring (TDM) is a system of monitoring a selected class of drugs with a narrow therapeutic range (drugs that can easily be under- or overdosed) based on the assumption that there is a relationship between plasma drug concentration and therapeutic effect. Certain drug-related toxicity could not be easily detected due to underlying disease symptoms. A typical example is theophylline in chronic obstructive pulmonary disease and in patients with impaired clearance mechanisms like renal failure, which could confound identification of drug accumulation and toxicity upon drug exposure. TDM is aimed at determining the appropriate concentrations of medications that pose a toxicity risk in order to optimize clinical safety. Pharmacogenomic profiling that identifies responsible genes could be used as a new form of TDM as it has a high potential for detecting ADR susceptibility [29]. Early-stage studies would also permit determination of the maximum tolerated doses and the cognate genomic predictors that would result in an increased likelihood of adverse effects in high risk groups susceptible to ADRs.

10.4 PROMISING OUTCOMES ASSOCIATED WITH CLINICAL APPLICATION PHARMACOGENOMICS: CASES

10.4.1 Human Immunodeficiency Virus

HIV is among the few indications that require prescription drugs based on available pharmacogenomic information. A routine genetic test on HIV-infected patients that determines genetic variants and sensitivities has been the criterion for prescribing the antiviral drug abacavir (Ziagen). Abacavir is an inhibitor of HIV type-1 (HIV-1) reverse transcriptase. It is used to treat HIV-1 infection in naive and treatment experienced patients [30]. Patients under treatment normally experience hypersensitivity reactions such as nausea, headache, fever, rash, and other symptoms, which occur within a period of 6 weeks of starting the drug. Upon receiving a second dose, other hypersensitivity reactions set in, resulting in respiratory failure and death [31,32]. For the patients that participated in a clinical study based on abacavir, white participants showed 4.3% hypersensitivity, which is a higher risk rating than black participants. This differential idiosyncratic event was linked genetically and also has been attributed to the presence of the human leukocyte antigen (HLA) B*5701 allele, a risk factor for abacavir hypersensitivity [33,34]. Upon screening, the patients identified with HLA B*5701 allele experience a reduction in the incidence of abacavir hypersensitivity reaction. When they received abacavir-containing antiretroviral therapy, substantial improvement was observed [35,36]. A prospective, double-blind, randomized trial was conducted to validate the use of genetic testing to prevent abacavir hypersensitivity, known as the Prospective Randomized Evaluation of DNA Screening in a Clinical Trial (PREDICT-1) study [37].

10.4.2 Cancer Drugs

Cancer is another very active area of pharmacogenomic research. Studies have found that the chemotherapy drugs gefitinib (Iressa) and erlotinib (Tarceva) work much better in lung cancer patients with a particular genetic biomarker. On the other hand, research has shown that the chemotherapy drugs cetuximab (Erbitux) and panitumumab (Vecitibix) do not work very well in the 40% of colon cancer patients whose tumors have a particular genetic signature. The breast cancer drug trastuzumab (Herceptin) is effective with tumors with a genetic biomarker for overproduction of a protein called HER2, which is a major consideration in the clinics. The FDA also recommends genetic testing prior to administration of the chemotherapy drug mercaptopurine (Purinethol) to patients with acute lymphoblastic leukemia. Certain genetic variants affect drug metabolism, which could result in severe side effects and increased risk of infection, but could be avoided if the standard dose is adjusted according to the patient's genetic composition. Physicians are also expected to perform tests for certain genetic variants in colon cancer patients before administering irinotecan (Camptosar), which is part of a combination chemotherapy regimen. This practice is premised on the notion that one particular variant confers a poor metabolizer predisposition, resulting in severe diarrhea and increased infection risk and thus is prescribed in lower doses.

10.4.3 Vend (Voriconozole)

In vivo studies indicated that an enzyme involved with genetic polymorphism, CYP2C19, is significantly involved in the metabolism of voriconazole. 15%–20% of Asian populations have been identified as poor metabolizers. Among the Caucasian and African subjects tested, 3–5% have been identified as poor metabolizers as well. For a study on Caucasian and Japanese healthy subjects, poor metabolizers have around a fourfold higher coriconazole exposure than their homozygous extensive metabolizer counterparts. For those who are heterozygous, extensive metabolizers have a twofold higher voriconazole exposure when compared with their homozygous counterparts [38,39].

10.4.4 LRRTM3 in Alzheimer's Disease

Substantial research has been focused on unraveling the association between late-onset Alzheimer's disease (AD) and a number of other genes. One example is a SNP in the promoter region and a block of four SNPs in the intron 2 allele of the transmembrane protein LRRTM3, associated with AD. It was reported in a study conducted in two separate groups that out of the case–control data sets from 993 patients and 884 control subjects of the National Institute on Aging Late-Onset Alzheimer's Disease (NIALOAD) group [40], 1 SNP was significantly associated with AD in the NIALOAD data set and 4 SNPs with the Caribbean Hispanic data set (Caribbean Hispanic comprised a cohort data set from 549 patients and 544 control subjects). The controls were without cognitive impairment or dementia [41]. Altogether, this led to the conclusion that variation in the LRRTM3 sequence, expression, and function may influence the development of AD [42].

10.4.5 APOE4

A Phase IIa clinical study of rosiglitazone involved participants that lacked the *APOE4* gene [43,44]. Results from the study showed that no remarkable improvement was found in these patients and supported the speculation that *APOE3/4* or *APOE4/4* genotypes are not very responsive to treatment when compared to those of the *APOE3/3* or *APOE3/2* genotype [45].

10.4.6 Mental Disorders

Pharmacogenomics may also help to quickly identify the best drugs to treat people with certain mental health disorders. For example, while some patients with depression respond to the first drug they are given, many do not, and doctors have to try other drugs. Because each drug takes weeks to take its full effect, patients' depression may grow worse during the time spent searching for a drug that would provide therapy.

10.5 ECONOMIC AND SOCIAL IMPLICATIONS OF PHARMACOGENOMICS APPLICATION

10.5.1 Penetrance

Penetrance in genetics refers to the proportion of individuals with a gene variant (allele or genotype) that also expresses an associated trait (phenotype) [46]. Stratification can be more inclined to individuals treated based on penetrance and not genotype, which could result in bias in choice. Drug administration could be restricted to patients with a particular polymorphism, even though individuals in the larger population might present variable degrees of penetrance. This lends to the unanticipated outcomes of commercialized drugs.

10.5.2 Economic Considerations

Commercial interests have also inspired the utility of pharmacogenomics models in drug discovery and development. In addition, pharmacogenomics testing is needed by policymakers and clinicians to inform the decision made regarding its adoption by the drug manufacturing companies, healthcare systems, and coverage [47]. Hence, quantification of the economic impact of tailor-to-fit medicine as well as cost-effectiveness analyses of the pharmacogenomic models are increasingly becoming an essential consideration for determining its applicability. The comparative value of current genetic testing technologies and the emerging ones can be evaluated through cost-effectiveness analysis for improving the safety and efficacy of drug therapy. Decision makers investigate the comparative clinical and economic effectiveness of pharmacogenomics testing over the existing technologies in order to make informed decisions about its application in a particular case.

What will be the financial costs and societal benefits of integration of pharmacogenomics into healthcare?

Genome-wide SNP scanning arrays have become further simplified, accelerating the screening process to the order of more than a million SNPs, making it increasingly cost-effective [48]. Exome scanning, which sequences all the exons for genes, is being conducted in increasing sample sizes with the prospect that a patient's entire genomes could soon be found in a patient's electronic medical record. Even though these technological novelties are contributing to advancing the field of pharmacogenomics, there are still recurring problems. The value of lowering testing costs could be partially lost by the high cost of new genomically-based therapies [49]. This has resulted in an increasing demand for precision studies that would be restricted to those with greater potential to benefit. Companies might be more selective towards certain category of patients whose genotypes show more promise for marketing their drugs. Patient heterogeneity and the general validity of economic evaluation of the pharmacogenomics models have been highly criticized. However, certain solution pathways have been suggested [37–42,46–52]. Regulatory guidelines have been in place to curtail a trend towards the downsizing market for certain drugs that do not justify development cost.

The so-called "blockbuster" medicines generate substantial revenue as they have been developed based on the one-size-fits-all approach. They are sold to a very large patient population identified as having the symptoms or condition in question. If a paradigm shift results in a stratified population, a company would have to meet the additional expense of developing that medicine when targeted to a subset of the same population. From an economic perspective, it could be argued that the identification of smaller more narrowly defined or targeted groups of patients that show the most promising result would have a negative effect on profitability. Looking at it from the flip side, companies might find utility in the population stratification as they could develop targeted medicines that may otherwise have been rejected during development. The number of patients who would benefit from a medicine could be maximized by using pharmacogenetics information. They could provide pharmacogenetics tests to identify and exclude those at risk of adverse reactions, and also define a specific group of patients in whom the medicine will be particularly effective. The stratification model would exclude side effect and inefficacy susceptibility leading to quality of life enhancement and to rescue of funds lost in the negative effects of drugs.

10.6 NATIONAL REGULATORY AGENCIES ON PHARMACOGENOMICS IMPLEMENTATION

The FDA, European Medicines Agency (EMA), and Japan's Pharmaceuticals and Medical Devices Agency have been the advocates of the implementation of pharmacogenomics in drug development for decades [53]. The US major medical research funding agency, the National Institutes of Health (NIH) and the National Center for Advancing Translational Science are proponents of the utility of pharmacogenetics in clinical practice, for application of individualized therapy [54]. The National Human Genome

Research Institute is focused on integrating genomic medicine into clinical practice such that genetic markers for diseases would enable the understanding of predisposition to disease, provide better treatment strategies, and prevent adverse events [55].

The overall goal of the Canadian Institutes of Health Research – Personalized Medicine Signature is to target therapy by integrating evidence-based medicine and precision diagnostics into clinical practice, which, if well implemented, will be helpful in many areas of health including cancer, metabolic and cardiovascular diseases, infectious diseases, rare diseases, and many others.

Strategies are being implemented in order to:

• Avoid genetic discrimination by employers and healthcare providers.
• Restrict unjustified use in nonmedical applications of genomics.
• Ascertain reimbursement by health insurers: to assess, define, and clarify the criteria for the reimbursement made by health insurance companies for clinical genomics services.

10.6.1 Personalized Medicine Program-University of Florida Health

The University of Florida (UF) Health Personalized Medicine Program is led by faculty in the UF College of Pharmacy and is part of the UF Clinical and Translational Science Institute. This is a huge program with a multidisciplinary team that provides the necessary tools needed to implement genomic medicine. Based on grants from the NIH, it is the lead institute for the NIH Pharmacogenomics Research Network, which collaborates with five other institutions, Vanderbilt University, Mayo Clinic, Ohio State University, University of Maryland, and St. Jude Children's Research Hospital, to collectively gather data on the experience of launching personalized medicine programs.

The Implementing Genomics in Practice (IGNITE) Network is supported by the NIH's National Human Genome Research Institute. IGNITE supports collective projects at Duke University and Mount Sinai. The Pharmacogenomics Research Network is a knowledge resource for providing essential clinical information about the effect of interindividual gene variations on drug response. PharmGKB is a pharmacogenomics knowledge resource that provides all the relevant clinical information including dosing guidelines and drug labels, gene–drug associations with clinical implications, and genotype–phenotype relationships. PharmGKB interprets and distributes knowledge about the impact of human genetic variation on drug responses [56].

REFERENCES

[1] Si SC, Altman RB, Ingelman-Sundberg M. Databases in the area of pharmacogenetics. Hum Mutat 2011;32(5):526–31.

[2] Zineh I, Pacanowski MA. Pharmacogenomics in the assessment of therapeutic risks versus benefits: inside the United States Food and Drug Administration. Pharmacotherapy 2011;31(8):729–35.

[3] Chan A, Pirmohamed M, Comabella M. Pharmacogenomics in neurology: current state and future steps. Ann Neurol 2011;70:684–97.

[4] Li J, Zhang L, Zhou H, Stoneking M, Tang K. Global patterns of genetic diversity and signals of natural selection for human ADME genes. Hum Mol Genet 2011;20(3):528–40.

[5] Davis K. Cracking the Genome: Inside the Race to Unlock Human DNA. New York: Free Press; 2001.

[6] Roses AD. Genome-based pharmacogenetics and the pharmaceutical industry. Nat Rev Drug Discov 2002;1:541–9.

[7] McCarthy A. Pharmacogenetics: implications for drug development, patients and society. New Genetics Soc 2000;19:135–43.

[8] Single nucleotide polymorphism. Available from: http://www.ibbl.lu/personalised-medicine/what-is-personalised-medicine/dna-genes-snps/ [accessed 01.05.2015].

[9] Lindpainter K. Pharmacogenetics and the future of medical practice. Br J Clin Pharmacol 2002;54(2):221–30.

[10] International Conference on Harmonization (ICH) E15 Definitions for Genomic Biomarkers, Pharmacogenomics, Pharmacogenetics, Genomic Data and Sample Coding Categories.

[11] Challenge and opportunity on the critical path of new medical products. FDA White Paper 2004.

[12] Spear BB, Heath-Chiozzi M, Huff J. Clinical application of pharmacogenetics. Trends Mol Med 2001;7:201–4.

[13] Moore TJ, Cohen MR, Furberg CD. Serious adverse drug events reported to the Food and Drug Administration, 1998-2005. Arch Intern Med 2007;167:1752–9.

[14] Eichelbaum M, Ingelman-Sundberg M, Evans WE. Pharmacogenomics and individualized drug therapy. Annu Rev Med 2006;57:119–37.

[15] Diekstra MH, Swen JJ, Boven E, Castellano D, Gelderblom H, Mathijssen RH, Rodríguez-Antona C, García-Donas J, Rini BI, Guchelaar HJ. CYP3A5 and ABCB1 polymorphisms as predictors for sunitinib outcome in metastatic renal cell carcinoma. Eur Urol 2015;S0302-2838(15):00320-6.

[16] Zhang Y, Doshi S, Zhu M. Pharmacokinetics and pharmacodynamics of rilotumumab: a decade of experience in preclinical and clinical cancer research. Br J Clin Pharmacol 2015 Apr 24; [Epub ahead of print].

[17] Mallick A, Januzzi JL Jr. Biomarkers in acute heart failure. Rev Esp Cardiol (Engl Ed) 2015;S1885-5857(15). 00116-4.

[18] Mukherjee G, Lal Gupta P, Jayaram B. Predicting the binding modes and sites of metabolism of xenobiotics. Mol Biosyst 2015 Apr 27; [Epub ahead of print].

[19] Dhoro M, Zvada S, Ngara B, Nhachi C, Kadzirange G, Chonzi P, Masimirembwa C. Body weight and sex are predictors of efavirenz pharmacokinetics and treatment response: population pharmacokinetic modeling in an HIV/AIDS and TB cohort in Zimbabwe. BMC Pharmacol Toxicol 2015;16:4.

[20] Wang XQ, Shen CL, Wang B, Huang XH, Hu ZL, Li J. Genetic polymorphisms of CYP2C19 2 and ABCB1 C3435T affect the pharmacokinetic and pharmacodynamic responses to clopidogrel in 401 patients with acute coronary syndrome. Gene 2015;558(2):200–7.

[21] Yüce GD. Effect of genetic variations on adjusting of warfarin dose. Tuberk Toraks 2014;62(3):236–42.

[22] De Paiva AC, Marson FA, Ribeiro JD, Bertuzzo CS. Asthma: Gln27Glu and Arg16Gly polymorphisms of the beta2-adrenergic receptor gene as risk factors. Allergy Asthma Clin Immunol 2014;10(1):8.

[23] Mukae S, Aoki S, Itoh S, Iwata T, Ueda H, Katagiri T. Bradykinin B2 receptor gene polymorphism is associated with angiotensin-converting enzyme inhibitor-related cough. Hypertension 2000;36:127–31.

[24] Trent RJA. Pathology practice and pharmacogenomics. Pharmacogenomics 2010;11(1): 105–11.

[25] Wilke RA, Xu H, Denny JC, Roden DM, Krauss RM, McCarty CA, Davis RL, Skaar T, Lamba J, Savova G. The emerging role of electronic medical records in pharmacogenomics. Clin Pharmacol Ther 2011;89:379–86.

[26] Peterson JF, Bowton E, Field JR, Beller M, Mitchell J, Schildcrout J, Gregg W, Johnson K, Jirjis JN, Roden DM, Pulley JM, Denny JC. Electronic health record design and implementation for pharmacogenomics: a local perspective. Genet Med 2013;15(10):833–41.

[27] O'Donnell PH, Bush A, Spitz J, Danahey K, Saner D, Das S, Cox NJ, Ratain MJ. The 1200 patients project: creating a new medical model system for clinical implementation of pharmacogenomics. Clin Pharmacol Ther 2012;92(4):446–9.

[28] Johnson JA, Cavallari LH, Beitelshees AL, Lewis JP, Shuldiner AR, Roden DM. Pharmacogenomics: application to the management of cardiovascular disease. Clin Pharmacol Ther 2011;90(4):519–31.

[29] Kager L, Diakos C, Bielack S. Can pharmacogenomics help to improve therapy in patients with high-grade osteosarcoma. Expert Opin Drug Metab Toxicol 2015;16:1–4.

[30] Kuritzkes RD. Pharmacogenomics of abacavir: current clinical implications. MDDisclosures April 12, 2011. Available from: http://www.medscape.com/viewarticle/740288 [accessed 05.05.2015].

[31] Moyle GJ, DeJesus E, Cahn P, Castillo SA, Zhao H, Gordon DN, Craig C, Scott TR. Abacavir once or twice daily combined with once-daily lamivudine and efavirenz for the treatment of antiretroviral-naive HIV-infected adults: results of the Ziagen Once Daily in Antiretroviral Combination Study. J Acquir Immune Defic Syndr 2005;38:417–25.

[32] Staszewski S, Keiser P, Montaner J, Raffi F, Gathe J, Brotas V, Hicks C, Hammer SM, Cooper D, Johnson M, Tortell S, Cutrell A, Thorborn D, Isaacs R, Hetherington S, Steel H, Spreen W. CNAAB3005 International Study Team. Abacavir-lamivudine-zidovudine vs indinavir-lamivudine-zidovudine in antiretroviral-naive HIV-infected adults: a randomized equivalence trial. JAMA 2001;285:1155–63.

[33] Mallal S, Nolan D, Witt C, Masel G, Martin AM, Moore C, Sayer D, Castley A, Mamotte C, Maxwell D, James I, Christiansen FT. Association between presence of HLA-B*5701, HLA-DR7, and HLA-DQ3 and hypersensitivity to HIV-1 reverse-transcriptase inhibitor abacavir. Lancet 2002;359:727–32.

[34] Hetherington S, Hughes AR, Mosteller M, Shortino D, Baker KL, Spreen W, Lai E, Davies K, Handley A, Dow DJ, Fling ME, Stocum M, Bowman C, Thurmond LM, Roses AD. Genetic variations in HLA-B region and hypersensitivity reactions to abacavir. Lancet 2002;359:1121–2.

[35] Rauch A, Nolan D, Martin A, McKinnon E, Almeida C, Mallal S. Prospective genetic screening decreases the incidence of abacavir hypersensitivity reactions in the Western Australian HIV cohort study. Clin Infect Dis 2006;43:99–102.

[36] Zucman D, Truchis P, Majerholc C, Stegman S, Caillat-Zucman S. Prospective screening for human leukocyte antigen-B*5701 avoids abacavir hypersensitivity reaction in the ethnically mixed French HIV population. J Acquir Immune Defic Syndr 2007;45:1–3.

[37] Mallal S, Phillips E, Carosi G, Molina JM, Workman C, Tomazic J, Jägel-Guedes E, Rugina S, Kozyrev O, Cid JF, Hay P, Nolan D, Hughes S, Hughes A, Ryan S, Fitch N, Thorborn D, Benbow A. PREDICT-1 Study Team. HLA-B*5701 screening for hypersensitivity to abacavir. N Engl J Med 2008;358:568–79.

[38] McLeod HL, Krynetski EY, Relling MV, Evans WE. Genetic polymorphism of thiopurine methyltransferase and its clinical relevance for childhood acute lymphoblastic leukemia. Leukemia 2000;14:567–72.
[39] Otterness D, Szumlanski C, Lennard L, Klemetsdal B, Aarbakke J, Park-Hah JO, Iven H, Schmiegelow K, Branum E, O'Brien J, Weinshilboum R. Human thiopurine methyltransferase pharmacogenetics: gene sequence polymorphisms. Clin Pharmacol Ther 1997;62:60–73.
[40] Lee JH, Cheng R, Graff-Radford N, Foroud T, Mayeux R. National Institute on Aging Late-Onset Alzheimer's Disease Family Study Group. Analyses of the National Institute on Aging Late-Onset Alzheimer's Disease Family Study: implication of additional loci. Arch Neurol 2008;65(11):1518–26.
[41] Lee JH, Cheng R, Barral S, Reitz C, Medrano M, Lantigua R, Jiménez-Velazquez IZ, Rogaeva E, St George-Hyslop PH, Mayeux. Identification of novel loci for Alzheimer disease and replication of CLU, PICALM, and BIN1 in Caribbean Hispanic individuals. R Arch Neurol 2011;68(3):320–8.
[42] Reitz C, Conrad C, Roszkowski K, Rogers RS, Mayeux R. Effect of genetic variation in LRRTM3 on risk of Alzheimer disease. Arch Neurol 2012;69(7):894–900.
[43] Risner ME, Saunders AM, Altman JF, Ormandy GC, Craft S, Foley IM, Zvartau-Hind ME, Hosford DA, Roses AD. Rosiglitazone in Alzheimer's Disease Study Group. Efficacy of rosiglitazone in a genetically defined population with mild-to-moderate Alzheimer's disease. Pharmacogenomics J 2006;6(4):246–54.
[44] Lynch TJ, Bell DW, Sordella R, Gurubhagavatula S, Okimoto RA, Brannigan BW, Harris PL, Haserlat SM, Supko JG, Haluska FG, Louis DN, Christiani DC, Settleman J, Haber DA. Activating mutations in the epidermal growth factor receptor underlying responsiveness of non-small-cell lung cancer to gefitinib. N Engl J Med 2004;350(21):2129–39.
[45] Pedersen WA, McMillan PJ, Kulstad JJ, Leverenz JB, Craft S, Haynatzki GR. Rosiglitazone attenuates learning and memory deficits in Tg2576 Alzheimer mice. Exp Neurol 2006;199:265–73.
[46] Cooper DN, Krawczak M, Polychronakos P, Tyler-Smith C, Kehrer-Sawatzki H. Where genotype is not predictive of phenotype: towards an understanding of the molecular basis of reduced penetrance in human inherited disease. Hum Genet 2013;132:1077–130.
[47] Snyder R, Mitropoulou C, Patrinos GP, Williams SM. Economic evaluation of pharmacogenomics: a value-based approach to pragmatic decision making in the face of complexity. Public Health Genomics 2014;17:256–64.
[48] Wilke RA, Xu H, Denny JC, Roden DM, Krauss RM, McCarty CA, Davis RL, Skaar T, Lamba J, Savova G. The emerging role of electronic medical records in pharmacogenomics. Clin Pharmacol Ther 2011;89(3):379–86.
[49] Koelsch C, Przewrocka J, Keeling P. Towards a balanced value business model for personalized medicine: an outlook. Pharmacogenomics 2013;14:89–102.
[50] Annemans L, Redekop K, Payne K. Current methodological issues in the economic assessment of personalized medicine. Value Health 2013;16(Suppl. 6):S20–6.
[51] Buchanan J, Wordsworth S, Schuh A. Issues surrounding the health economic evaluation of genomic technologies. Pharmacogenomics 2013;14:1833–47.
[52] Ramaekers BL, Joore MA, Grutters JP. How should we deal with patient heterogeneity in economic evaluation: a systematic review of national pharmacoeconomic guidelines. Value Health 2013;16:855–62.
[53] Maliepaard M, Nofziger C, Papaluca M, et al. Pharmacogenetics in the evaluation of new drugs: a multiregional regulatory perspective. Nat Rev Drug Discov 2013;12(2):103–15.
[54] Collins FS. Reengineering translational science: the time is right. Sci Transl Med 2011;3:90.
[55] National Human Genome Research Institute (NHGRI). Available from: http://www.genome.gov/17516574 [accessed 05.05.2015].
[56] Personalized Medicine Program-University of Florida Health. Available from: http://personalizedmedicine.ufhealth.org/about-us/our-team/ [accessed 05.05.2015].

The Drug Discovery Cycle III: Authorization and Marketing

11. Patents, Exclusivities, and Evergreening Strategies   245
12. Drug Pricing and Control for Pharmaceutical Drugs   255
13. Direct-to-Consumer Advertising   267

CHAPTER 11

Patents, Exclusivities, and Evergreening Strategies

Syed A.A. Rizvi

Contents

11.1 Introduction: Patents and Exclusive Marketing Rights	245
11.2 US Patent Law Amendments Act of 1984	246
11.2.1 Hatch–Waxman Act of 1984 and Patent Terms	247
11.3 The Interplay of Patents and Exclusivities During the Product Lifecycle	248
11.4 Patents in the Global Pharmaceutical Market Place	249
11.5 Evergreening	250
11.6 Conclusions	252
References	252

11.1 INTRODUCTION: PATENTS AND EXCLUSIVE MARKETING RIGHTS

Drug discovery and development and other innovations in the pharmaceutical industry has brought a tremendous value to society. Besides serving the individual patient, pharmaceutical innovation has helped reduce the cost of healthcare through providing viable therapeutic options with improved efficacy and safety profiles.

Developing and bringing a new drug to market is expensive and time consuming mainly because it is usually subjected to highly stringent regulatory supervision. The cost of bringing a new drug to market has reached $5 billion [1]. It has been noted that for about every 5000 compounds developed and tested, only 5 eventually advance to human testing, which would be further scrutinized for commercialization [2,3]. Due to direct and dramatic effects on human life, the US Food and Drug Administration (FDA) heavily regulates manufacturing and marketing of pharmaceuticals compared to food products and cosmetics [4].

Patents can be defined as a set of exclusive rights granted by eligible authorities in a country to an inventor for a limited period of time. In return for such protection, a patent holder provides full public disclosure of the invention, which becomes immediately available to researchers worldwide. It can

Social Aspects of Drug Discovery, Development and Commercialization Copyright © 2016 Elsevier Inc.
http://dx.doi.org/10.1016/B978-0-12-802220-7.00011-9 All rights reserved. **245**

be a form of intellectual property. Under exclusive patent rights as covered by TRIPS Agreement (Article 28), the government recognizes patents on both products and processes such that the patent holder has the exclusive right to make, use, sell, or import the product in their country for an allotted period of time [5,6]. The process of producing an invention in the pharmaceutical environment could be seen as be the method of producing a drug and/or for the product, the drug itself. A utility patent covers pharmaceuticals since it involves discoveries of chemicals, such as new pharmacologically active molecules, machines, etc. [7]. A pharmaceutical patent requires the details of synthesis and characterization of the drug molecule, its pharmacological properties, formulation, and method of administration. Pharmaceutical patents serve as stimulants for pharmaceutical innovation. When a patent is granted, the patent holder maintains the exclusive rights on the product, and provides complete published disclosure of the product [8].

In the pharmaceutical industry, varied levels of competition exist. Originator drug companies undergo rigorous competition from their "peers" (other originator drugs in the same therapeutic class) for the patent duration prior to expiry when the generic drug companies come into the picture. Generic entry increases the rate at which sales drop upon patent expiration, which further reduces the returns from marketing a new drug.

Patents in the United States are issued by the US Patent and Trademark Office for a period of 20 years. A time investment of about 10–15 years is required to develop a new medicine from the earliest stages of compound discovery through FDA approval. As a result, significant portions of the patent term for a new drug are lost before a drug product launch. Patent life for medicines is estimated to last an average of 11.5 years.

The pharmaceutical industry is subject to much tougher and very different regulatory standards, for the right reasons. The increasing need for better and safer treatment drugs has immensely contributed to the soaring cost of producing new drugs. Since initial cost of investment in pharmaceutical research and development (R&D) is so high, strong patent protection is an important approach to gain monopoly and recovery of investments on new products. Also there are provisions available for extending and limiting patent protections and nonpatent exclusivities.

11.2 US PATENT LAW AMENDMENTS ACT OF 1984

Patent law is based upon the Patent Act of 1952, codified in Title 35 of the United States Code. The first major change amended the patent law to add to the exclusive rights monopoly in importing into the United

States products produced by a patented process. This was intended to prevent competitors of a patent owner from avoiding the patent by practicing the patented process outside the United States and marketing the resulting product in the United States. The second major change prevents copiers who might be avoiding US patents by supplying components of a product patented in the United States, which could eventually be assembled abroad.

The 1984 amendment facilitated generic drug manufacturing through an abbreviated approval mechanism. Prior to 1984, no streamlined FDA process existed for generic drugs approval and companies conducted the lengthy and very expensive clinical trials as the originator drug. Currently, generic drugs are approved based on therapeutic equivalency using an abbreviated new drug application (ANDA). Under an ANDA, the generic drug manufacturer demonstrates that the generic drug is effectively a duplicate of the originator drug, or the reference listed drug – an 80–125% bioequivalence must be shown [9]. This law also allows a balance benefit to the original drug manufacturer and challenging generic drug company. Usually, the original manufacturer or brand company challenges the generic sponsor for patent violation. This will yield a FDA-approved two and half years (30 months) of additional exclusivity to the brand name manufacture and until then, no generic drugs are allowed to be marketed. This in turn provides 6 months' (180 days') exclusivity to the company that initially challenged the patent as the only generic market [9]. During this time, only generic alternatives can reap the full advantage of exclusivity, and usually these drugs are priced lower than their counterparts (80–90% of the brand name product) [10,11]. The generics industry had blossomed in the past 30 years, since the enactment of the Hatch–Waxman Act. In 1984, generic drugs accounted for 19% of US prescriptions, and according to the data collected in 2013 they reached 86% [12].

11.2.1 Hatch–Waxman Act of 1984 and Patent Terms

The Drug Price Competition and Patent Term Restoration Act commonly referred to as the Hatch–Waxman Act [13] outlines the process for pharmaceutical manufacturers to file an ANDA for approval of a generic drug by the FDA. The Act allows generic pharmaceutical manufacturers to duplicate a patented originator drug without undertaking the clinical and nonclinical studies or risking liability for patent infringement damages.

The Hatch–Waxman Act allows certain market exclusivity periods for new drug applicants based on both nonpatent- and patent-based factors. The nonpatent exclusivities are: orphan drug exclusivity, new chemical entity (NCE) exclusivity, new clinical study exclusivity, and pediatric exclusivity.

Orphan drug exclusivity is granted to drugs for a disease that affects fewer than 200,000 people in the United States. For NCE exclusivity, drugs with a new chemical entity that has not been subjected to regulatory approval qualifiy for extension of the patent term. The extension term is estimated to be equivalent to half of the clinical development period, which is usually 6–8 years, which is added to the regulatory review period, which is about 2 years. The extension granted cannot exceed 5 years and the maximum total of patent protection is 14 years from the date of drug approval. This 14-year limit is the reason why the Hatch–Waxman extension is limited to 3 years. The Waxman–Hatch Amendments also allow the companies to obtain an additional 6 months of pediatric exclusivity as an add-on to already existing marketing exclusivity and/or patent protection that may be reaching expiration. A company can file for pediatric exclusivity if new clinical studies are needed to assess safety and efficacy of dosage for the pediatric population [14]. This exclusivity extension is provided under the FDA Modernization Act of 1997, section 505A of the Federal Food, Drug and Cosmetic Act (21 U.S.C. § 355(a)) [15]. For patent exclusivity, originator companies typically obtain patent protection that covers approved drugs and grants a period of exclusivity preventing unlicensed third parties from manufacturing, selling, or importing the patented invention.

The Hatch–Waxman Act has played a role in increasing generic competition and generic market share due to increased numbers of generic manufacturers for a single drug and subsequent drop in prices. The generic manufacturer must only demonstrate bioequivalence to the innovator.

11.3 THE INTERPLAY OF PATENTS AND EXCLUSIVITIES DURING THE PRODUCT LIFECYCLE

The following is a hypothetical example that has been adopted from Seamon's article [16]. It clearly demonstrates how patents and exclusivities play a complementary role in maximizing the lifecycle of a drug and describes how the patent and exclusivity dynamics contribute to extension of the exclusive rights.

Assuming amphotericin B was discovered in 2000, a patent would have been issued on January 1, 2002, and the drug would have commenced human clinical testing in 2008. In 2015, the manufacturer would submit data to the FDA, and the drug would be approved on January 1, 2019. At this time, approval confers 5-years exclusivity with a new chemical/drug. As mentioned earlier, patents last for 20 years. Thus, the drug would be patent protected against generic competition until January 1, 2022. The drug would have exclusive marketing rights with the FDA until January 1, 2024. Suppose a generic company files an ANDA and challenges the patent on the drug on January 1, 2024. The manufacturer of amphotericin B would, in turn, file a suite for infringement and the company would gain 30 months of additional exclusivity that lasts until July 1, 2026. Prior to that date, if the same company submitted a study on pediatrics and gained an additional 6 months that would last until January 1, 2027. Amphotericin B, which would be scheduled to lose patent protection on January 1, 2022, would not face generic competition until 5 years later. The generic company that filed the ANDA would gain approval on January 1, 2027, with 180-day exclusivity as the sole generic. Accordingly, only until around July 1, 2027 patients would see any real cost savings. The manufacturer of amphotericin B could further retain market share through a number of innovative strategies referred to as evergreening.

11.4 PATENTS IN THE GLOBAL PHARMACEUTICAL MARKET PLACE

Intellectual property is the key to innovation and growth in our society, but still, has been streamlined by key advances in science, technology, and arts. This has brought tremendous economic growth and highly priced value to the society. A society devoid of intellectual property/patent laws would incur huge risks and costs in science and technology, which has the potential of deterring innovation and creativity. According to the World Bank report, starting from 1980, developing nations that have been very receptive to foreign technologies and business methods, and have protected the intellectual property rights of their developers, have also been significant contributors to one the world's greatest economic gains. For instance, Japan, South Korea, and Italy have had economic growth due to strong intellectual property protection; in Mexico, R&D investment skyrocketed following the adoption of full intellectual property protection in 1991. Countries with weak intellectual property protections do have minimal direct foreign investment, but the ones in their possessions would be less technologically sophisticated.

The World Trade Organization TRIPS agreement (Trade-Related Aspects of Intellectual Property rights) is one of a series of trade agreements administered by the World Trade Organization World Trade Organization that establishes the rules for intellectual property rights for all the member countries to incorporate into their domestic laws.

Developing countries sometimes face pressures from World Trade Organization property rights rules on patent protections [17]. They were mandated to introduce TRIPS-compliant patent laws as far as a decade ago [17], which in turn impacted the economically compromised countries that would have to pay royalties to those countries that hold patents. Thus, developing countries are paying a high price for the TRIPS agreement. While countries cannot exclude entire fields from patenting (under article 27.1 of TRIPS), they do have the right to determine standards of patentability [18].

The emerging economies of Thailand, India, Brazil, Egypt, and others have tried to address access to drugs by producing cheaper and more generic drugs. South Africa has tried to purchase cheaper generic drugs from where the pricing is the lowest to preclude high dependency on the multinational corporations with high price tags. India dominates the supply of low-cost, generic drugs to developing countries. India supplies 80% of antivirals used to treat HIV/AIDS in low-income countries [18].

TRIPS has led to upward harmonization of patent laws including restricting countries' abilities to exclude entire pharmaceuticals from patentability. It hinders production of patented medicines by other countries, but some exceptions exist where generics could be allowed. TRIPS flexibilities extend the timelines for the required TRIPS compliance and the extent to which the patentability standards are defined such that additional drug modifications or repurposing could be achieved [19]. Such patenting is sometimes characterized as "evergreening," since such patents are often filed late in the product lifecycle and are used to temporarily extend market exclusivity.

11.5 EVERGREENING

The ability of a drug company to retain market share when patents expire is referred to as evergreening [20]. However, it has been noted by Swiss researchers that these tactics are partially responsible for increasing healthcare costs [21]. The following are common evergreening strategies employed by the pharmaceutical industries under such conditions:
- New similar indications
- New formulations
- New routes of administration
- Combination products
- New dosing regimens
- Racemic versus enantiopure drugs
- New polymorphic form

- Pediatric market exclusivity
- Prescription to over-the-counter switches

A pharmaceutical company can in some cases use the same drug for another similar indication. An example is a chemotherapeutic drug prescribed for similar types of cancer. Reformulating existing commercial drugs or repurposing is the easiest and most commonly used trick to continue to hold market share. If the new formulations are suitably close to the original approved product, the drug company can benefit from the associated expedited FDA approval process. Eli Lilly, in order to maintain blockbuster share of the antidepressant drug Prozac, introduced a once weekly, sustained release Fluoxetine formulation and obtained FDA approval. A similar strategy was used by Bristol-Myers Squibb for Glucophage (metformin hydrochloride). The new extended release formulation was sold as Glucophage XR [22]. If a new formulation can also be administered via a new route, this leads to an opportunity for other drug launches, new marketing applications, and market exclusivity. A successful example of this strategy is the 2006 FDA approval of Imitrex for intranasal delivery by GlaxoSmithKline (GSK). The drug Imitrex was originally launched in 1993 for the treatment of migraine with over $1 billion in annual sales [23].

Killing two birds with one stone is a famous expression. When executable, a combination of two or more drugs can be employed to enhance the efficacy of a marketed drug and result in a new FDA approved product. GSK secured regulatory approval of Treximet, a combination of sumatriptan and naproxen with better efficacy than either medicine used individually [24]. Eli Lilly combined olanzapine (Zyprexa) for treating schizophrenia and Fluoxetine (Prozac) for treating depression, and called this combination Symbyax. This resulted in a new patented FDA approved product for the company and generated more than $80 million in annual sales in the United States alone until its patent expired in 2012. Moreover, Eli Lilly continued to market its blockbuster drugs Zyprexa and Prozac (Fluoxetine) [25]. GSK markets azidothymidine (AZT), lamivudane, and abacavir sulfate as individual products under the brand names Retrovir, Epivir, and Ziagen, respectively. In order to gain more market share GSK also markets a combination of AZT and lamivudane (brand name Combivir). Another combination of AZT, lamivudane, and abacavir sulfate has been also marketed as Trizivir. New dosing regimens can be sought for a marketed product to suit a specific population. However, obtaining a patent and ultimately FDA approval has been difficult because dosing variation is considered to be the doctor's choice in clinical practice [26].

The human body is intelligent in terms of detecting stereochemical differences and often enantiomers of the same drugs have exhibited markedly different pharmacological attributes. The majority of racemic drugs have one major enantiomer that would normally possess the desired pharmacological activity (termed eutomer), while the other would have no/less activity (distomer), worse toxicity profiles, or other undesired pharmacological outcomes [27]. Many advantages of a single enantiomeric drug formulation have been noted, which include a selective and less complex pharmacokinetic (PK)/pharmacodynamic (PD) profile and potential for an improved therapeutic index. A prime example is the marketing of the single enantiomer drug Prilosec (omeprazole). AstraZeneca, after the expiration of the patent on Prilosec, introduced the single enantiomer omeprazole, with noticeable superior bioavailability and efficacy. Both of them are proton pump inhibitors for the treatment of gastroesophageal reflux disease. The new single enantiomeric product was marketed as Nexium and is another blockbuster drug for AstraZeneca [28].

Very often, drug molecules exist in more than one crystalline form; this phenomenon is called polymorphism and is considered a doubled-edged sword in the pharmaceutical industry. Polymorphs often show marked differences in aqueous solubility, formulation, and shelf life. Such attributes permit several polymorphs of a drug to be patented. Acetaminophen (APAP) is an analgesic drug and has three known polymorphs. Marketed acetaminophen is a type I form, although this polymorphic form has poor compressibility that leads to poor tableting characteristics. However, the type II form is directly compressible and ideal for tablet manufacturing but it is metastable and can convert into another polymorph eventually.

Furthermore, a brand drug manufacturer can switch the status of a drug from prescription to over-the-counter, thus further enhancing market exclusivity. These companies can market "authorized generics," commonly known as "brands in a bottle." It has been reported that some companies will resort to paying off the competition and not enter the market place [29].

11.6 CONCLUSIONS

The production and commercialization of novel drugs is very rewarding if the goal is successfully attained. But it is also a risky business. Thus, patent protection and marketing exclusivity play a significant role in sustaining the pharmaceutical business. This has also compelled a prolongation of patent duration and the pharmaceutical industries have developed several ways of achieving this goal.

REFERENCES

[1] The cost of creating a new drug now $5 billion, pushing big pharma to change. Available from: http://www.forbes.com/sites/matthewherper/2013/08/11/how-the-staggering-cost-of-inventing-new-drugs-is-shaping-the-future-of-medicine/ [accessed May 2015].

[2] Backgrounder: How New Drugs Move through the Development and Approval Process. Tufts Center for the Study of Drug Development, 2001.

[3] Dickson M, Gagnon JP. Key factors in the rising cost of new drug discovery and development. Nat Rev Drug Discov 2004;3:417–9.

[4] Crimm NJ. A tax proposal to promote pharmacologic research, to encourage conventional prescription drug innovation and improvement, and to reduce product liability claims. 29 Wake Forest L. Rev. 1994;1007:1020–1022.

[5] The Drug Price Competition and Patent Term Restoration Act of 1984, Pub. L. No. 98-417, 98 Stat. 1585; 1984.

[6] US Code § 154 – Contents and term of patent; provisional rights. Available from: http://www.law.cornell.edu/uscode/text/35/154 [accessed 14.09.2014].

[7] Worthen DB. American pharmaceutical patents from a historical perspective. Int J Pharm Compound 2003;7(6):36–41.

[8] Food and Drug Administration. Frequently asked questions on patents and exclusivity. Available from: http://www.fda.gov/Drugs/DevelopmentApprovalProcess/ucm079031.htm [accessed 14.09.2014].

[9] US Department of Health and Human Services. Orange Book: Approved Drug Products with Therapeutic Equivalence Evaluations; 2014.

[10] Food and Drug Administration. Generic competition and drug prices. Available at: http://www.fda.gov/AboutFDA/CentersOffices/CDER/ucm129385.htm. [accessed 28.09.2014].

[11] Pharmaceutical life cycles: patents, exclusivities and evergreening strategies. http://www.cedrugstorenews.com/userapp/September%202011%20Law%20Column.cfm [accessed 13.10.2014].

[12] Thayer AM. 30 years of generics. Available from: http://cen.acs.org/articles/92/i39/30-Years-Generics.html. [accessed 19.01.2015].

[13] Drug Price Competition and Patent Term Restoration Act of 1984. Pub. L. No. 98-417 (21 U.S.C. § 355).

[14] Food and Drug Administration. Frequently asked questions on pediatric exclusivity, the pediatric "rule," and their interaction. Available from: http://www.fda.gov/Drugs/DevelopmentApprovalProcess/DevelopmentResources/ucm077915.htm   [accessed 23.11.2014].

[15] Jenei S. Why a pediatric exclusivity add-on? http://www.patentbaristas.com/archives/2007/03/22/why-a-pediatric-exclusivity-add-on/. [accessed 10.03.2015].

[16] Seamon MJ. Antitrust and the biopharmaceutical industry: lessons from Hatch–Waxman and an early evaluation of the Biologics Price Competition and Innovation Act of 2009. Nova Law Rev 2010;34:629–77.

[17] Deere C. The implementation game. New York: Oxford University Press; 2009.

[18] Carlos C, Matthews D. The Doha Declaration ten years on and its impact on access to medicines and the right to health. UNDP. Available from: www.undp.org/content/dam/undp/library/hivaids/Discussion_Paper_Doha_Declaration_Public_Health.pdf; 2011.

[19] Kapczynski A, Chan P, Bhaven S. Polymorphs and prodrugs and salts (oh my!): an empirical analysis of "secondary" pharmaceutical patents. PLoS One 2012;7(12):e49470.

[20] Gaudry KS. Evergreening: a common practice to protect new drugs. Nat Biotechnol 2011;29:876–8.

[21] Krans B. Pharmaceutical "evergreening" raises drug costs, study says. http://www.healthline.com/health-news/policy-drug-companies-use-evergreening-to-extend-market-share-060413 [accessed 14.04.2015].

[22] Gupta H, Kumar S, Roy SK, Gaud RS. Patent protection strategies. J Pharm Bioallied Sci 2010;(2):2–7.

[23] Drugs.com. FDA approves new formulation of Imitrex Injection. http://www.drugs. com/news/fda-approves-new-formulation-imitrex-1710.html [accessed 14.04.2015].

[24] Brandes JL, Kudrow D, Stark SR, et al. Sumatriptan-naproxen for acute treatment of migraine: a randomized trial. JAMA 2007;297(13):1443–54.

[25] Drugwatch. Symbyax. http://www.drugwatch.com/symbyax/ [accessed 14.04.2015].

[26] Jerry I, Hsiao H, Wang W. Dosage patenting in personalized medicine. http://bciptf. org/wp-content/uploads/2012/06/Dosage_Patenting_in_Personalized_Medicine.pdf [accessed 14.04.2015].

[27] Nguyen LA, He H, Pham-Huy C. Chiral drugs: an overview. Int J Biomed Sci 2006;2(2):85–100.

[28] Drugs.com. Top 10 money-making drugs of 2012. http://www.drugs.com/slideshow/ top-10-money-making-drugs-of-2012-1034 [accessed 14.04.2015].

[29] Hemphill CS, Sampat BN. Evergreening patent challenges, and effective market life in pharmaceuticals. J Health Econ 2012;31(2):327–39.

CHAPTER 12

Drug Pricing and Control for Pharmaceutical Drugs

Odilia Osakwe

Contents

12.1 Introduction	255
12.2 Drug Assessment and Pricing in Various Geographical Locations	256
12.2.1 United States	256
12.2.2 Europe	258
12.2.3 Canada	260
12.3 Pharmaceutical Drug Pricing and Ethics	263
12.4 References	264

12.1 INTRODUCTION

Medicines are essential for the promotion of health and longevity, which are crucial needs in society. The role of medicines in global healthcare systems has advanced along with innovative treatments that have become widely available, increasing efficiency in the delivery of medical solutions to the patient, of which universal health coverage is a driver.

A manufacturer's drug price is a fundamental determinant for listing and reimbursement claims. The major goals needed to be achieved in order to have a balanced pricing policy are lowering prices, adequate drug supply, adherence to rules, and promoting incentives for entry to the market. Drug plans primarily seek to pay the lowest possible price at the threshold of profits for the manufacturer. Formulary committees exert legislative control of addition or withdrawal of drugs from formularies, which reflect the number of approved drugs in the listing.

Due to variations in national economic development and infrastructure availability, level of innovation and regulatory structure, drug prices vary largely because the underlying factors are executed differently and with differing levels of risk. For drug originators, publicity for a drug or creating awareness of new drug availability involves a reasonable amount of outlay as most brand manufacturers are involved in scientific research and development (R&D) of new drug therapies. However, generic drug manufacturers

Social Aspects of Drug Discovery, Development and Commercialization Copyright © 2016 Elsevier Inc.
http://dx.doi.org/10.1016/B978-0-12-802220-7.00012-0   All rights reserved.   **255**

are not involved in research and development as the focus is on finding compounds that could demonstrate bioequivalence with the brand version upon expiration of its patent [1]. Generic drugs promote savings through lowering drug prices relative to the brand version. This improves its accessibility especially for low income populations.

Drug pricing is based on assessment of the extent of cost and therapeutic effectiveness. The cost-effectiveness review considers factors other than safety, efficacy, and quality prior to approving new drugs for marketing or reimbursement [2]. A drug that is not cost-effective might not be needed so much and, as such, a price reduction will make the drug acceptable. Cost-effectiveness requirements can create registration delays and increased costs for manufacturers, which could, in turn, affect the rewards for innovative drugs.

Reference prices are typically applied at market entry and followed up with later revisions. The approach of reference pricing may be based on country or therapeutic class. External referencing is based on prices of identical or comparable products in other countries. In international drug pricing, drug prices are initiated by pricing policies that are country specific. This depends on the product type and country of manufacture, while for others it depends on the purchase price by the pharmacy and the value-added tax rate, which has to fall within the regulated price to allow room for negotiation of drug prices along the distribution chain (which are negotiated in business-to-business transactions) [3]. The approach to calculating the reference price differs among countries and details of algorithms used often remain unclear. For example, in Brazil generic manufacturers may offer discounts of over 50% from list prices, while originators may offer discounts in the range of 10–15%. Cross-national pharmaceutical price comparison lacks standardization due to variation in name, dosage form, strength, and presentation. It is difficult to adjust to per capital income among these countries and other factors mitigate the effectiveness. Price comparison can influence pricing and revenues in another country.

Therapeutic class reference pricing is based on the lowest or average price of other already existing drugs within the same therapeutic class. This allows freedom to choose between similar products in favor of cost.

12.2 DRUG ASSESSMENT AND PRICING IN VARIOUS GEOGRAPHICAL LOCATIONS

12.2.1 United States

The US government healthcare system was introduced through provision of benefits to veterans after the Civil War [4]. In the United States, the federal government has a strong influence on company drug pricing. This is achieved through persuasion for a moderate price increase. In the 1990s when drug prices increased, several initiatives were suggested by President Clinton's health policy advisers for control of prices that had been termed "excessive" [5]. Federal government oversight for premarket testing and proof of drug safety had been around since the late 1930s but did not impose strict regulation on the price of drugs.

This apparent insensitivity eventually changed as demand for drugs increased following increasing cases of long-term chronic diseases. This started in the 1960s [6].

Universal insurance has been highly contested in the United States. Even though universal insurance is not implemented in the United States, it has been reported as the largest prescription drug market [7]. Pharmaceutical revenue per person supersedes that of Europeans. Due to this reason, US policymakers are imposing controls on pharmaceutical spending and prices. Copays reduction allows a relatively modest benefit to the public [8].

The US system is an exception among developed countries as it combines private insurance with public financing of Medicare, which differs from other OECD countries like Canada, which has a state/provincial control or coordinated social insurance systems. In the United States, the external reference pricing system has not been applied [9].

The private health insurance market in the United States constitutes a combination of national, regional, and local insurers. A typical example is the Blue Cross Blue Shield plan, which is an independent, locally operated insurance plan [10]. Healthcare delivery is through private hospitals and independent physicians who are empowered to operate with uncontrollable charges rendered for services. Medicare sets reimbursement levels and private insurers negotiate fee schedules with hospitals and other providers. Private insurance coverage is achieved through employer-managed programs. Physicians take on a fee-for-service pricing, which does not provide many opportunities or financial incentives for long-term preventive care [11].

The US Department of Health and Human Services, through the provision of the Patient Protection and Affordable Care Act, requires insurance companies to offer coverage to young adults up to the age 26 years under family plans and also imposed new rules to protect patients with preexisting conditions or highly costly treatments, so that they could remain in coverage. Every US citizen is expected to carry health insurance; it could be acquired through their employer, government-run Medicare, Medicaid, Veteran's Administration programs, or a private plan. Medicaid is public medical insurance for low-income populations, financed by both the federal government and the states. But the States administration is subject to federal government regulations and the criterion differs by state [12].

Medicare was not allowed to negotiate drug prices with manufacturers; the government paid up to 58% more for the same medicines under Part D than through the Veterans Administration. With minimal incentives available to limit available treatment, US spending has constantly been on the rise, which was not the case with other major OECD countries, whose spending has dropped in the past decade [13]. The Medicare Prescription Drug, Improvement, and Modernization Act of 2005 provided prescription drug insurance to Medicare beneficiaries through a private-market mechanism. According to reports, the program has cut down out-of-pocket spending by just over 18% [14].

The government used other indirect means to stimulate moderation of prices by the drug companies. For example, reducing a drug company's franchise value creates a negative publicity that could lead to a loss, and the affected companies would rather yield to government-imposed demands and avoid the potential loss.

International firms are attracted to the United States due to comparatively higher drug prices than other regions like Europe, Germany or the United Kingdom [15,16]. There is no doubt that pharmaceutical companies earn more revenue per person in the United States than in Europe [17]. Pharmaceutical companies that are based in Europe have seen a need for market authorization in the United States for trade reasons. Policy interventions have been through reduction of both manufacturers' revenues (by fixing market prices) and prices paid by consumers (by fixing manufacturing prices). This is meant to constrain aggressive negotiation of manufacturer prices. Subsidizing copayments for consumers and locking manufacturer prices are ways to achieve this. These policies have been termed "price controls" and "copayment reductions." Average manufacturer price, the average price a wholesaler paid to a manufacturer for drugs distributed to retail pharmacies, was a benchmark created by Congress in 1990 in calculating Medicaid rebates.

12.2.2 Europe

Europe's share of global pharmaceutical sales was 10% less than that of the United States even though it has a higher population and more accommodating insurance coverage. This is because of higher drug prices set by the United States for many of the highly purchased drugs, which are higher than Germany or the United Kingdom [14]. European policymakers incorporate reference-based pricing and thus the member states are mandated to comply with the requirements of Directive 89/105/EEC and the Treaty. This is based on a median cost within a therapeutic class across the comparator EU countries.

National control of the prices of medicinal products restricts the range of medicinal products covered by European national health insurance systems. Germany, Europe's largest pharmaceutical market, currently adopts reference-based pricing as a part of international convergence in price regulation, unlike the United States, which fails to utilize a national approach to drug price negotiations. In Germany, price controls are focused on margin and this has been achieved through reimbursement. It permits manufacturer free pricing of in-patient drugs. The reimbursement decisions are judged based on quality of life metrics common to the countries of United Kingdom [18]. In France, price is controlled indirectly through national pharmaceutical budgets, which requires rebates from manufacturers. France employs negotiations between government and the pharmaceutical industry to determine the price of new and highly valued medicinal products, informed by external reference pricing, which is also the case in Italy and Spain [19]. In Spain, universal coverage is provided for all residents; health services are publicly funded and financed through national taxation. Services are free with nonrefundable copayments mandated for prescription drugs [20]. An external reference pricing policy has been implemented in all European countries. For publicly reimbursed medicines, Austria, Croatia, Czech Republic, Estonia, Finland, France, Germany, Ireland, Italy, Latvia, Lithuania, Malta, Poland, Slovakia, Slovenia, and Switzerland are all involved but with subtle variations in the extent of applications. Bulgaria, Estonia, Cyprus, Germany, Malta, and the United Kingdom have not applied external reference-based pricing substantially [21]. For generics, internal reference pricing has been adopted by Italy and Spain, and price capping by France. The Netherlands uses government-set maximum wholesale prices for all outpatient prescription-only medicines. The prices of nonprescription drugs are not regulated. Therapeutic value is considered a core criterion in all countries, whereas cost-effectiveness or budget impact is taken into account by a smaller number of countries, which include Italy, the Netherlands, and Spain. Profit controls are used in the United Kingdom; it utilizes a profit framework for pricing and which is negotiated periodically between the Department of Health and the pharmaceutical industry (Pharmaceutical Price Regulation Scheme, PPRS) [22].

Re-evaluation of prices could follow the setting of the initial price but the frequency differs among countries. Most of the countries compare prices at an ex-factory level using official public price databases but the pharmacy purchasing price and pharmacy retail price are set through external reference pricing. A common external reference pricing strategy is calculating the average price of reference countries as done in Austria, Belgium, Cyprus, Denmark, Iceland, Ireland, Portugal, Switzerland, and the Netherlands. Another method is to use the lowest price among all the reference countries: Bulgaria, Hungary, Italy, Romania, and Spain. Some countries such as Greece, Norway, Slovakia, and Czech Republic calculate the maximum price using the average of the three or four lowest prices of all countries in the basket. France applies prices that are similar to those in the reference countries [23].

Health technology assessment (HTA) is a decision making criteria for medicines and other health interventions that qualifies for reimbursement by the healthcare system in a particular member state. The European Medicines Agency (EMA) is subject to the HTA standards, which has an influence on the access of novel medicines to patients. Following marketing authorization, HTA bodies carry out their own assessments of medicines by comparison based on relative effectiveness of medicines over the existing ones, utilizing the data from clinical trials and other relevant information generated during drug development. HTA also takes into consideration the cost of medicines as mandated by national legislation. Certain important medicines do not qualify for reimbursement and have prompted a collaborative effort between medicines regulators and HTA bodies with the aim of reducing the drug development expenditure by manufacturers as well as fine-tuning the development program to align with the regulator and HTA standards.

The European Network for Health Technology Assessment (EUnetHTA) is a network of government-appointed organizations from European Union member states, the European Economic Area, other regional agencies, and organizations associated with HTA in Europe. Information on the benefits and risks of a medicine is documented in the European public assessment reports as a way of addressing the needs of HTA bodies. Advice and recommendations made by the Agency and EUnetHTA include improvement on development strategies for specific designated medicines and other disease-specific guidelines.

12.2.3 Canada

In Canada, the federal government's authority over healthcare is constitutionally empowered by taxation, spending, public property, and the criminal law. This allowed the government to fund a national single-payer healthcare system in 1966, which was modified in 1984 with passage of the Canada Health Act.

Canada and United States are federal states. The difference is that the United States has a Constitution with a legal authority at the federal government level, but Canada is provincially controlled. Healthcare is an area of the law that has no distinct authority but an intermix of powers and control exercised at both federal and provincial levels. The Constitution allocates hospital control to the provinces but healthcare is regulated collaboratively by both the federal and provincial governments. The Canadian Constitution grants to the provinces specific control over hospitals and certain powers to make laws that regulate healthcare delivery and health insurance but in compliance with the Canada Health Act, which establishes the compliance standard for receiving federal funding. It ensures that provincial health insurance programs meet certain criteria. Over 90% of hospital and physician care is funded publicly but the government provides funds for less than 50% of all prescription drug expenditures and with a minimal amount on dental and eye care. The provinces are under pressure to reduce costs [23]. However, the Constitution's functions preclude the regulation of healthcare delivery. Typically, it sees that the provincial healthcare insurance system is publicly administered: first, on a nonprofit basis to ascertain that it is comprehensive; second, all insured health services are covered and are universal with services reaching 100% of insured persons; finally, provincial health care insurance system is accessible as it offers terms and conditions that would not hinder access. Enhanced care or services are used to provide private insurance, which cannot be covered under the public (provincial) plans and which cannot pay for services that are already covered under provincial insurance schemes.

The prices of patented drugs are evaluated and regulated at the federal level by the Patented Medicine Prices Review Board (PMPRB). This board ensures that prices are not "excessive." But drugs and medical devices that are covered under provincial health insurance systems must be approved at the provincial level. The PMPRB does not have jurisdiction over prices charged by wholesalers or pharmacies, or over pharmacists' professional fees. The PMPRB's principal goal is to support innovation (R&D) and hence does not cover generics. Lack of control over generics may sometimes disfavor the public health system budgets and reduce access to treatment as it reduces the incentive for pharmaceutical companies to invest in innovation leading to increased costs for care. The Canadian Agency for Drugs and

Technologies in Health (CADTH), an independent nonprofit agency, evaluates the drug portfolio in comparison to an already existing one as a criterion for listing in the formulary. Formularies are used to negotiate deeper price discounts with manufacturers and set cost-sharing levels to influence rate of use and choice of drugs. This is achieved through a "Common Drug Review" process that provides the formulary with recommendations for all provinces except Québec. It uses a reference pricing system, which is based on a median cost within a therapeutic class, or an average price across comparator countries based on quality of life metrics. Thus, the recommendations for listing by CADTH are evidence based, which depends on the effectiveness of drugs and other health technologies. It focuses strongly on cost-effectiveness and issues reports through its HTA and "optimal medication" programs. Decision making often involves comparing a new treatment to standard care by conducting a cost-effectiveness analysis and providing an estimate of the extra cost per extra unit of effect computed as $\Delta C/\Delta E$.

Canada uses the external reference pricing system for the pricing of innovative medicines that have been recognized as breakthrough, significant, or moderate improvement. It was first adopted in 1987 as part of the price regulation process. The peer countries are selected based on extent of economic development, which must be similar to that of Canada. These include the United States, France, Germany, Italy, Sweden, Switzerland, and the United Kingdom. These countries tend to share Canada's goals of encouraging research and innovation in the pharmaceutical sector. Exchange rates are determined based on a 36-month average exchange rate for each country as published on the PMPRB website [24].

In Canada, substitution of generics for brand drugs is generally legally authorized save in specific circumstances detected by the physician. Generic drugs are competitive due to low product prices and this is only applicable in a "pharmacy-driven" market. In contrast, a "physician-driven" market disarms the power of decisions of the pharmacist, as it is controlled by the physicians. The generic drug manufacturer is licensed to market a drug only following an approved notice of compliance after demonstrating bioequivalence to the reference-branded drug. At this time, an application must be approved by the provincial government for a designation of interchangeability with the brand drug. This confers on the pharmacist legal protections against the potential problems associated with generic brand substitution for the brand drug counterpart. Interchangeable generics are usually listed in the drug plan formulary for the provincial government. Pharmacists, however, are given the authority to dispense a choice of interchangeable generic drug unless specifically directed by the physician, which applies for beneficiaries of the public drug plans, in which case a supporting report should include a medical reason for not choosing a generic [25]. In addition to the physician recommendation, generic substitution could also be a personal choice, which may be influenced by the fact that generic drugs are sometimes not as effective as the original brand name drug [26,27].

A choice of branded drug is allowed at extra cost. Generally, brand drugs are more commonly prescribed by the physicians for the recipients in the private plans as there is a much less control in their case [28]. Ontario government formulary lists generic versions of the popular drugs. For the generic manufacturers, price, payment terms, ease and readiness in service, time to marketing, product catalog are some of the factors that influence accessibility and marketing success [29]. Generic drug manufacturer can also gain a competitive advantage by being first to market. Certain attributes of drug such as methods of manufacture, therapeutic indications, and other physical aspects (i.e., the active ingredient, coatings) are a guide to patient's preferential selection and are seriously considered by the manufacturers [30].

12.2.3.1 Drug Plan Reimbursement of Generic Drugs

The amount paid by the public drug plan to the pharmacy for generic drugs is based on a maximum milliliter or another unit. These prices are listed in the government formulary. Many provincial government plans, in turn, use the price set by the Ontario Drug Benefit (ODB) plan, the largest drug plan in Canada. In 1993, the ODB generic reimbursement price was set based on a stated percentage of the interchangeable brand drug, which is at the rate of 75% or less and depends on a number of factors. This allowed pharmacies to be able to purchase generics for less than these reimbursed amounts. The margins earned constituted a substantial share of pharmacy revenues of about $2 billion in Canada in 2005 [31]. In some provinces, governments have mandated that pharmacies lower prices charged to private plans and cash paying customers.

12.3 PHARMACEUTICAL DRUG PRICING AND ETHICS

Certain problems linked to drug manufacturing and pricing heavily impact society. For drug developers whose products help to combat diseases, extreme maximization of profits is not acceptable. A well-known fact is that it could hinder drug accessibility especially for the lower income class.

While new trends in economic research seek to draw more attention to increased access, further research points out that such efforts that increase access through price reduction have given rise to unintended consequences for innovation and clinical utility. Thus, collaborative efforts through cross-disciplinary interaction among economists, ethicists, and physicians could attenuate these rising issues while strengthening healthcare delivery. The pharmaceutical ecosystems need to be nourished in order to achieve robust healthcare systems [31].

REFERENCES

[1] International Federation of Pharmaceutical (IFPMA); 2010. Available from: http://www. ifpma.org/innovation/rd/about-research-development.html [accessed 02.06.2010].
[2] Pharmaceutical Research and Manufacturers Association, Foreign Government Pharmaceutical Price and Access Controls. Federal Register Notice Submission. FR Doc. 04-12205: July 1, 2004; p. 13.
[3] Aitken M, Machine C, Troein P. November, 2014. Understanding the pharmaceutical value chain. Report by the IMS Institute for Healthcare Informatics.
[4] Skocpol T. Protecting Soldiers and Mothers: The Political Origins of Social Policy in the United States. Cambridge: Harvard University Press; 1992. Department of Veterans Affairs, "VA History," www.va.gov. [accessed 03.06.2015].
[5] Pear R., May 19, 1993. Clinton backs off drug price limits. New York Times, as printed by San Jose Mercury News.
[6] Greene J. Prescribing by Numbers: Drugs and the Definition of Disease. Baltimore, MD: Johns Hopkins University Press; 2007.
[7] Daemmrich A., September 14, 2011. U.S. Healthcare Reform and the Pharmaceutical Industry. Harvard Business School, Boston, Massachusetts. Working Paper 12-015.
[8] Lakdawalla D, Goldman DP, Michaud P, Sood N, Lempert R, Cong Z, Vries H, Gutierrez I. U.S. pharmaceutical policy in a global marketplace by OECD. Pharmaceutical pricing policies in a global market. Available from: http://www.oecd.org/fr/els/systemes-sante/pharmaceuticalpricingpoliciesinaglobalmarket.htm [accessed 04.06.2015].
[9] Folland S, Goodman A, Stano M. The Economics of Health and Health Care. 6th ed. Boston: Prentice Hall; 2010. pp. 215–218.
[10] Elhauge E. Why We Should Care About Health Care Fragmentation and How to Fix It. in The Fragmentation of U.S. Health Care. Oxford: Oxford University Press; 2010. p. 1–20.
[11] The Kaiser Commission on Medicaid, Medicaid Facts. Washington, DC: Kaiser Family Foundation; 2009. Available from: www.kff.org/medicaid/upload/7235_03-2.pdf [accessed 01.06.2010].
[12] Lichtenberg FR, Sun SX. The impact of Medicare Part D on prescription drug use by the elderly. Health Affairs 2007;26(6):1735–44.
[13] Daemmrich A., 2010. Cameron E. U.S. Healthcare Reform: International Perspectives. Harvard Business School case 710-040;
[14] Sood N, Vries HD, Gutierrez I, Lakdawalla DN, Goldman DP. The effect of regulation on pharmaceutical revenues: experience in nineteen countries. Health Affairs 2009;(1):129–37.
[15] Danzon PM, Furukawa MF. Prices and availability of biopharmaceuticals: an international comparison. Health Affairs 2006;25(5):1353–62.

[16] Danzon P, Wang Y, Wang L. The impact of price regulation on the launch delay of new drugs: evidence from twenty-five major markets in the 1990s. Health Econ 2005;14:269–92.

[17] Schwermann T, Greiner W, Schulenberg J. Using disease management and market reforms to address the adverse economic effects of drug budgets and price and reimbursement regulations in Germany.Value -Health 2003;6:S20–30.

[18] Puig-Junoy J. Incentives and pharmaceutical reimbursement reforms in Spain. Health Policy 2004;67:149–65.

[19] García-Armesto S, Abadía-Taira M, Durán A, Hernández-Quevedo C, Bernal-Delgado E. Spain: health system review. Health Syst Transit 2010;12(4):1–295.

[20] Mondher T., Rémuzat C.,Vataire A., Urbinati D. External reference pricing of medicinal products: simulation based considerations for cross country coordination. European Commission; 2014.

[21] Kanavos P.,Vandoros S., Irwin R., Nicod E., Casson M. Differences in Costs of and Access to pharmaceutical products in the EU. Brussels: European Parliament, Policy Department Economic and Scientific Policy; 2011.

[22] Canadian Institute for Health Information (CIHI). Exploring the 70/30 split: how Canada's health care system is financed. 2005.

[23] Ruggeri K, Nolte E. Pharmaceutical pricing. The use of external reference pricing. Rand Corporation; 2013.Available from: http://www.rand.org/pubs/research_reports/RR240.html [accessed 04.06.2010].

[24] Substitution Ontario Ministry of Health & Long-Term Care 2011. Ontario Ministry of Health & Long-Term Care. 'Ontario Drug Benefit Formulary search.Available from: https://www.healthinfo.moh.gov.on.ca/formulary [accessed 04.06.2010].

[25] Hakonsen H, Toverud EL. A review of patient perspectives on generics substitution: what are the challenges for optimal drug use. Generics Biosim Initiative J 2012;1(1). Available from: http://gabijournal.net/wp-content/uploads/GaBIJ-2012-1-p28-32-ReviewArticle-HÂƒÂ¥konsen.pdf.

[26] Dylst P,Vulto A, Godman B, Simoens S. Generic medicines: solutions for a sustainable drug market? Appl Health Econ Health Policy 2013;11(5):437–43.

[27] Balaban DY, Dhalla IA, Law MR, Bell CM. Private expenditures on brand name prescription drugs after generic entry.Appl Health Econ Health Policy 2013;11(5):523–9.

[28] Hollis A.The importance of being first: evidence from Canadian generic pharmaceuticals. Health Econ 2002;11(8):723–34.

[29] Kapczynski A, Park C, Sampat B. Polymorphs and prodrugs and salts (oh my!): an empirical analysis of "secondary" pharmaceutical patents. PLoS One 2012;(12):e49470.

[30] Grootendorst P, Rocchi M, Segal H.An Economic Analysis of the Impact of Reductions in Generic Drug Rebateson Community Pharmacy in Canada; Competition Bureau, Canadian Generic Drug Sector Study. November 21, 2008.

[31] Sara PL, Santoro M, Koski G. The ethics and economics of pharmaceutical pricing. Annu Rev Pharmacol Toxicol 2015;55:191–206.

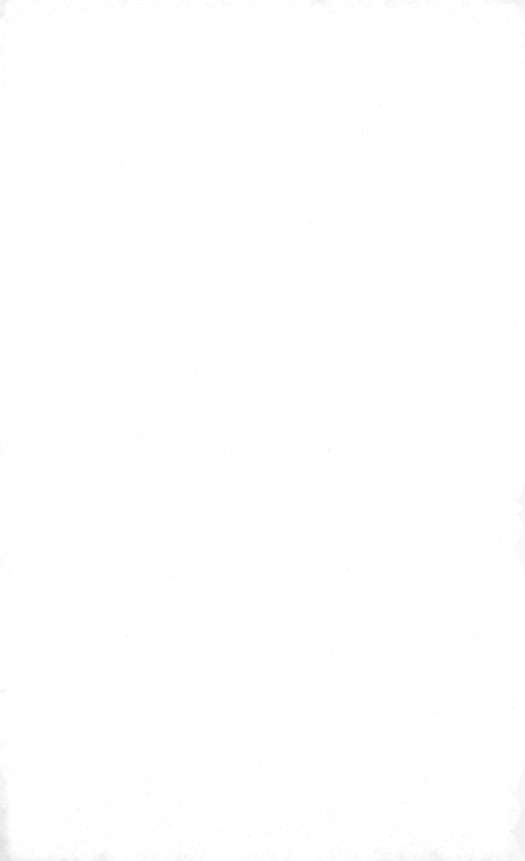

CHAPTER 13

Direct-to-Consumer Advertising

Odilia Osakwe

Contents

13.1 Introduction		267
13.2 Ethics and Relevance of Pharmaceutical Advertising		268
	13.2.1 Guiding Principles of the 2012 IFPMA Code of Practice	271
13.3 Pharmaceutical Advertising and Government Control		272
	13.3.1 United States	272
	13.3.2 Europe	274
	13.3.3 Canada	274
	13.3.4 Developing Nations	275
13.4 Prescription Medicine Advertising Codes		276
13.5 Conclusions		278
References		278

13.1 INTRODUCTION

It costs about $1.5 billion to execute the complicated research and development (R&D) programs required to develop a new drug introduced to the market, as the total investment time has been estimated to reach 15 years, despite the hurdles of investment risks – a common experience in the pharmaceutical enterprise. Pharmaceutical companies that manufacture the originator drugs spend proportionally much more on R&D than firms in other industrial sectors. However, profits tend to be generated by relatively few products in their overall portfolios. Being research based, pharmaceutical companies focus on innovation strategies that promote robust revenues, which also funds the development of novel medical products.

Due to competitive markets, market saturation, generic competition, and related issues, pharmaceutical sales have not always generated the expected returns. Robust sales and increasing profits is a tough terrain for the drug sponsor in the face of an ever-expanding and competitive market. Most of the time, branding differentiation and other strategies have been used as tools for market penetration or out-competing the competitors. The target market profile (TMP) is created at the initial stage of drug discovery before clinical development, which captures all the key information about

Social Aspects of Drug Discovery, Development and Commercialization   Copyright © 2016 Elsevier Inc.
http://dx.doi.org/10.1016/B978-0-12-802220-7.00013-2   All rights reserved.

the market for the proposed drug to ensure that it meets the needs of the market. It focuses on the unmet needs, patient population, and economic cost of disease. However, this is not certain as drug portfolios change along with the development process. TMP is only a vision and must be supported with strategic planning, by determining the value drivers, pricing, patient share, revenue, profitability, R&D investments, cost of goods, licenses, and royalties. In general, competitive assessment entails developing a customized drug portfolio as a premise for attaining a controlled share of the market. Drug companies utilize a variety of means to satisfy this need and advertising is the most utilized.

Direct-to-consumer advertising (DTCA) is a relatively new area of prescription drug promotion, which has evolved through the years from the 1980s when drug companies started to convey drug information to the general public who obtained direct access to the information. From a societal perspective, advertising has been pictured as a strategy to increase profits and not merely reach the patient with the right medication. A quote from a medical writer goes: "Science may be defined as a critical analysis of data from well-designed studies. Advertising, on the other hand, is a self-serving and biased promulgation of data." Joseph Stiglitz, the former World Bank Chief Economist and Nobel Prize winner for economics, declares: "Drug companies spend more on advertising and marketing than on research, more on research on lifestyle drugs than on life saving drugs, and almost nothing on diseases that affect developing countries only" [1]. Quinn et al. reported that influence on the consumer is an integral objective of advertising, which either directly or indirectly takes advantage of the vulnerability of the consumer, the patient, or healthcare provider [2].

13.2 ETHICS AND RELEVANCE OF PHARMACEUTICAL ADVERTISING

A standard goal for the supply of medicines is achieving the best attainable (i.e., optimal) level of health for the population. It is not expected that the same population are primarily targeted for specific corporate goals and/or economic benefits.

According to the World Health Organization, health is "a state of complete physical, mental and social well-being and not merely the absence of disease or infirmity." This definition has been subject to criticism [3–5]. The regulators of health systems measure health and the performance of health systems according to goodness (optimal health) and fairness (noticeable differences among individuals) [6]. Generally, advertising is not expected to merely promote the fairness but also the goodness.

A recent observation is that advertising would help to increase visibility of the product, as it facilitates faster access by the right patient. However, choices may be influenced to increase sales. On the other hand, the influence exerted through advertising might affect a consumer who would have made better alternative choices [7], thus misleading in advertising could be the choices made that bring undesirable consequences.

DTCA has been received in favorable terms. For example, it has been supported in instances where the consumer could gain access to a treatment that otherwise would not have been possible. Advertising in social media is also an easier way for patients to get information about a medicinal product or medical treatment while using known tools. For pharmaceutical companies, advertising in social media can reach more consumers than with any other medium. Posted information is available to a much broader audience and for an indefinite period of time. Promotion has been used as a source of information about new drugs by physicians especially those in private practice or those who have been in practice for some time rather than the emerging ones [8]. DTCA creates awareness of diseases and treatment options, empowers patients with information, and enhances communication. It abrogates underdiagnoses through raising awareness of disease symptoms and treatments thereby prompting patients to seek medical attention [9,10]. Drug samples allow better access to the needed treatment and time to treatment, which is of tremendous value to those that lack the resources to obtain the necessary care. Pharmaceutical marketing to healthcare providers keeps physicians abreast of the current treatment options, risks, and benefits. The current information about medicines facilitates the translation of novel technologies into clinical practice.

Public health experts also highlight the negative impact of DTCA. According to McKenna et al. [11], DTCA constitutes "escalating drug spending, an oversimplified understanding of illness and treatment, a devaluation of preventive health behaviors, and inappropriate hype for drugs that may have incomplete safety profiles." If there is an increased health benefit to an individual patient but not to the general health system, the societal cost of providing a new therapy is unacceptable as it has not been directed to the wider population. This represents an opportunity cost; the lost of a potential gain that would have been possible when a therapeutic choice is directed to the wider population. Generally, promoting highly valued therapies is beneficial to both patients and society when it results in increased level of use that translates into some measure of improvement in health. However, promoting those of a lower value (potentially from being overpriced or because there is too much uncertainty), therapies could eliminate opportunities for health gains for other patients who access the health system, which indirectly is rather an undesirable outcome for patients by wasting healthcare resources [12]. In general terms, if the net health gains, the difference between the level of health achieved in a world with advertising and one with no advertising is a higher number, then the advertising is worth it.

Seventy-four percent of the emergency medicine residents were surveyed by Keim et al. [13]. This work reported that sales representatives had given distorted information in the clinical areas while giving monetary gifts, and conducting studies that were not authorized. These practices are unethical. Promotional information could create an impression for the physician, the consumer or the patient that would change the focus in the wrong direction. It could also influence individuals to produce no change, deleterious or beneficial use of a new therapy, even though they had made the choice with the right goal in mind. Loss of health would be the consequence of inappropriate use, or a therapy that is suboptimal [14]. Approximately 30–50% of American adults are unable to comprehend or interpret basic health information [15]. Adverse effects associated with low health literacy are due to poor health outcomes in individuals and increased healthcare costs nationally [11], due to poorly informed choices [16]. Printed material written in technical terms and unfavorable printing colors and font sizes sometimes might not take into consideration those low literacy levels, the older people, and those with vision issues.

The inverse benefit law states that the patient benefit-to-harm ratio for new drugs varies in contrast to extent of drug marketing [17]. According to the quoted, the benefit-to-harm ratio of drugs tends to vary inversely with the extent of the marketing of drugs. This is a fact because the public has been highly attracted to communications about the product, and tend to belief that the advertised drug would be more effective in all respects than the unadvertised ones. However, drug approval evaluation by US Food and Drug Administration (FDA) precludes drug advertisement. In a report by Brody and Light [18], a minor change in the number of drugs prescribed could lead to a significant improvement in generated revenue by the pharmaceutical company. The report then claimed that, while the scientific professionals have engaged in relentless efforts with the objective of creating the best drugs with optimal therapeutic benefit, the marketing departments publish literature that could be biased and might extrapolate the value estimated by the scientists. Some examples include overstating the efficiency and safety qualities, encouraging and listing unapproved uses, and engaging physicians in advertising. Marketing departments could possibly create bias in physicians about medications, influencing their clinical recommendations. They could even be paid to give company-sponsored educational lectures to their colleagues in order to accommodate company interest. Advertising could exclude less obvious drug risk information such as drug interaction risks. Drug–drug interactions may adversely affect or harm the patient and is an important requirement in DTCA. A research company offers benefits for a researcher's positive results that could represent illegal efforts invested in reporting positive results.

The International Federation of Pharmaceutical Manufacturers and Associations (IFPMA) Code is the foundation for ethical pharmaceutical practices, and encourages equally high standards across healthcare sectors.

13.2.1 Guiding Principles of the 2012 IFPMA Code of Practice

1. The healthcare and well-being of patients are the first priority for pharmaceutical companies.
2. Pharmaceutical companies will conform to high standards of quality, safety, and efficacy as determined by regulatory authorities.
3. Pharmaceutical companies' interactions with stakeholders must at all times be ethical, appropriate, and professional. Nothing should be offered or provided by a company in a manner or on conditions that would have an inappropriate influence.
4. Pharmaceutical companies are responsible for providing accurate, balanced, and scientifically valid data on products.
5. Promotion must be ethical, accurate, balanced, and must not be misleading. Information in promotional materials must support proper assessment of the risks and benefits of the product and its appropriate use.
6. Pharmaceutical companies will respect the privacy and personal information of patients.
7. All clinical trials and scientific research sponsored or supported by companies will be conducted with the intent to develop knowledge that will benefit patients and advance science and medicine. Pharmaceutical companies are committed to the transparency of industry-sponsored clinical trials in patients.
8. Pharmaceutical companies should adhere to applicable industry codes in both the spirit and the letter. To achieve this, pharmaceutical companies will ensure that all relevant personnel are appropriately trained [19].

13.3 PHARMACEUTICAL ADVERTISING AND GOVERNMENT CONTROL

Drug advertisement has been governed by a combination of government and voluntary codes adopted by industry associations and medical organizations. Prescription-only products are primarily restricted due to toxicity susceptibility and limited knowledge about the risks and benefits. Since advertising might lead to greater exposure and increased decision of its usage, laws have been established to restrict companies' marketing and advertising of such drugs. Laws and regulations are enforced by government regulatory bodies although this is not always the case for some emerging countries. The United States and the United Kingdom have dedicated regulatory enforcement units that are responsible for investigating possible violations [20–22]. The US and European regulatory systems are the most significant and are increasing in relative importance in issues regarding drug advertising. Advertising of prescription drugs to the public is generally forbidden in all countries except the United States and New Zealand.

13.3.1 United States

In the United States, DTCA and other forms of pharmaceutical promotion are heavily regulated under statute by the FDA. Its regulatory control over advertising is also associated with its role in drug manufacturing and marketing approval. The federal regulation of drugs began in 1906 but evolved and expanded to incorporate three major pieces of legislation between 1938 and 1962. In 1951, Congress passed the Durham Humphrey Amendments to the Food, Drug, and Cosmetic Act (FDCA), with statutory definition of prescription drugs that emphasized "because of [their] toxicity or other potentiality for harmful effect, or the method of [their] use, or the collateral measures necessary to [their] use, [they are] not safe for use except under the supervision of a practitioner licensed by law to administer such drug[s]" (Public Law 82-215, 65 stat 648).

As an amendment Congress enacted the Kefauver–Harris Amendments to the FDCA in 1962. As mentioned in Chapter 1, this amendment required the testing of new drugs for both effectiveness and safety prior to marketing. Also, the FDA gained the power to control prescription drug advertising. This was controlled by the Federal Trade Commission (FTC), not the FDA; it had the duty to regulate drug advertisements before 1962. Currently, the FTC regulates the advertising of over-the-counter medicines. Companies have been permitted to advertise prescriptive drugs to healthcare providers but not to consumers. Increasingly from the 1980s pharmaceutical companies started DTCA. This was stimulated by an initial 2-year voluntary moratorium on DTCA, a survey that led to a final decision by the FDA to allow drug manufacturers to advertise prescription drugs directly to consumers pursuant to already existing FDA regulations. In 1997, the FDA issued a draft guidance, which was finalized in 1999, on Consumer Directed Broadcast Advertisements for television and radio. The mandatory conditions for advertising were: availability of a toll-free telephone number for consumers for access to product information, a link to current publications that cover the FDA-approved labeling for the product, advice for consumers to consult with their healthcare provider, and internet website addresses that contained product information. The Division of Drug Marketing, Advertising, and Communications (DDMAC), which is a part of the FDA, oversees prescription drug advertising activities. DDMAC ensures that the entire information provided by drug companies that advertise drugs has no component that is fabricated and must remain truthful and authentic. It educates the industry and takes legal action against both advertisements that violate the law and any publication or deceptive promotion that has influenced people's attitude in such a way that facilitates commercialization. US drug advertising has been grouped under three categories: product-claim advertisements, which involve the name of the drug, uses, risks and benefits, and indication; reminder advertisements, which only provide the name of the drug and exclude other information communicated in the product-claim advertisements; and help-seeking advertisements – also known as disease awareness advertisements – which discuss the medical condition without any drug product connection. They can also provide information relative to the disease or health condition and the suggestion to "ask your doctor" [23].

In order to promote authentic drug promotional practices, the FDA's Center for Drug Evaluation and Research (CDER) launched the Bad Ad outreach program in May 2010 that could aid the healthcare professionals in recognizing and reporting untruthful or misleading prescription drug promotion [23]. CDER's Office of Prescription Drug Promotion was formerly the DDMAC. It is dedicated to educating healthcare professionals such that they could be proactive in identifying misleading prescription drug promotion – from both a legal and clinical perspective. The process has been simplified to provide easy reporting of violation suspicions to the FDA. Guidance has been established for the US Department of Health and Human Services, the FDA, CDER, the Center for Biologics Evaluation and

Research, the Center for Veterinary Medicine, and the Center for Devices and Radiological Health to address the use of social media for off-label use and associated risks, which is more specific to its intended purpose. The hazard of off-label promotion through social media is a primary concern since there is a tendency for a company to provide information inconsistent with that required by the authority.

13.3.2 Europe

In the European Union, strict restrictions have been imposed on advertising of drugs, especially prescription drugs. Each member state of the European Union has specified an approach to advertising of medicinal products. The varied interstate regulatory measures exert influence over the internal market. Therefore, the European Parliament and the European Commission have adopted directives for regulating specific medicinal product advertising. The following rules set by the European Union regulate and influence drug advertising. Directive 92/28/EEC of March 1992, Chapters II–V of Council Directive 65/65/EEC of 26 January 1965, and Directive 92/28/EEC, which has been replaced by Directive 2001/83/EC; all pertain to the advertising of medicinal products for human use, and misleading advertising of medicinal products. The directives define advertising of medicinal products as "canvassing and door-to-door activities or extra inducement activities geared toward the promotion of prescription medicines by supply, sale, or consumption". Advertising for off-label use, or certain indications, is allowed for only members of the medical profession, which excludes vaccination campaigns that are performed by the industry and approved by the competent authorities of the member states [24].

13.3.3 Canada

In Canada, prescription drug advertising is prohibited. However, guidelines apply to advertising for nonprescription drugs, including natural health products, in all Canadian media, which include mass print (e.g., magazines, newspapers), radio, television, out-of-home (e.g., transit, billboards), point-of-purchase, direct mail, and internet advertising. The Pharmaceutical Advertising Advisory Board of Canada (PAAB) is charged with the review of advertising and promotional systems for approved pharmaceutical products. It recognizes the importance of product launch timelines, and in this guideline, provides guidance on the procedures for advertising review before the issuing of the notice of compliance. PAAB is mandated to ensure accuracy in product communication for prescription, nonprescription, biological, and natural health products, that communications are balanced and evidence based, and they reflect best practice. Advertising Standards Canada is the only agency delegated by Health Canada to review and preclear broadcast and mass print advertising to consumers for nonprescription drugs including natural health products. It requires that the advertisement must not be misleading as the information provided must include the recommended duration of use and that wording must be consistent with the marketing authorization information. Claims found in the product's Terms of Marketing Authorization may be paraphrased, but must remain consistent with those authorized. The Natural Health Products Directorate established a Compendium of Monographs, which has been used in the evaluation of the safety and efficacy of many commonly used medicinal ingredients contained in natural health products.

13.3.4 Developing Nations

Even though there are well-established legal systems in most developed nations the same type of regulatory systems might not be applicable in all the developing nations, and only a limited portion of prescription medicines might be supplied to some countries. Certain countries as cited later have gained wide attention internationally, increasingly drawing business activities of the international pharmaceutical companies. Some of these have relied on other legal and regulatory mechanisms where there is no applicable mechanism of control or codes of practice.

For drug advertisements in India, a Code for Self-Regulation in Advertising (ASCI Code) controls the commissioning, creation, placement, or publishing of advertisements. This ASCI Code covers all forms of advertisements that are perceived within India regardless of source. Though nonstatutory, the ASCI Code is recognized under various Indian laws. It is established to complement legal controls and to replace medical services. Advertisement for nutritional supplements is regulated under the Food Safety and Standards Act. Over-the-counter and prescription medications are not legally recognized. Prescription-only drugs are those medicines that are listed in Schedules H and X of the Drug and Cosmetics Rules, 1945 [25]. The majority of pharmaceutical companies in India are merely national as they do not operate in other countries. A large number of these companies are represented by national trade associations that are subject to the national codes and that are not bound by the standards and procedures set out by the international IFPMA Code. India-based companies that operate internationally are members of Organization of Pharmaceutical Producers of India (OPPI) and are governed by its advertising code [26].

In South Africa, the local industry associations have produced a joint code [27]: the Marketing Code Authority of South Africa. This is a code of marketing practice (http://ipasa.co.za/) that conforms to the legal provisions in the Medicines Act, which was implemented in 2011. The Marketing Code Authority is an independent enforcement authority that was established under the code to control the certification process for industry professionals.

In China, research-based international pharmaceutical companies are only a handful when compared to the entire pharmaceutical market. The R&D-based Pharmaceutical Association Committee (RDPAC) is a non-profit organization made up of 39 member companies with pharmaceutical R&D capabilities. It was established under the China Association of Enterprises with Foreign Investment. RDPAC represents international pharmaceutical companies in China, and has a code of practice that is generally adapted from the IFPMA Code [27,28]. Nevertheless, these are predominantly controlled by the legal forces and, as such, the status of the voluntary code remains uncertain. Most often, advertisements must be preapproved by the Chinese regulatory authorities for approval before they are communicated [29].

In Mexico, the local and international pharmaceutical industry, healthcare, and government bodies collaborated to a collective mandatory transparency guideline in 2008. Mandatory codes cover good promotional practices, ethics, and interaction with patient organizations and these are operated by Consejo de Ética y Transparencia de la Industria Farmacéutica (CETIFARMA): Codes of the pharmaceutical industry established in Mexico [30].

13.4 PRESCRIPTION MEDICINE ADVERTISING CODES

Advertising of prescription medicines utilizes integrated international and national codes of practice, which are mostly applicable to multinational corporations (Table 13.1). National codes of practice are often operated by a local industry trade association, and are in use by both the developed and in many developing countries [31]. These codes have been revised to strengthen commitment to the high ethical standards in all marketing practices and patient care in the healthcare systems.

Table 13.1 Codes of practice governing the pharmaceutical companies

Organization	International code	Date initiated
World Health Organization	Ethical Criteria for Medicinal Drug Promotion	May 1988
International Federation of Pharmaceutical Manufacturers and Associations	Code of Pharmaceutical Marketing Practices	January 2000
International Federation of Pharmaceutical Manufacturers and Associations	Code of Pharmaceutical Marketing Practices	June 2006
European Federation of Pharmaceutical Industries and Associations	Code of Practice on the Promotion of Medicines	November 2004

National codes

Organization	National code	Date
Association of the British Pharmaceutical Industry, with the Prescription Medicines Code of Practice Authority Constitution and Procedure, United Kingdom	Code of Practice for the Pharmaceutical Industry	January 2006
Health Canada, Pharmaceutical Advertising Advisory Board of Canada (PAAB)	The Canadian Code of Advertising Standards The PAAB code of Acceptance	
Medicines Australia	Australia Code of Conduct Edition 15	December 2006
Stichting Code Geneesmiddelenreclame	The Netherlands Code of Conduct for Pharmaceutical Advertising	2004
Pharmaceutical Association of Malaysia Code of Conduct for Prescription Ethical Products	Pharmaceutical Association of Malaysia Code of Conduct for Prescription Ethical Products	November 2005

13.5 CONCLUSIONS

Significant advances have been made in the regulation of the advertising of prescription medicines. The unified and collaborative codes applicable to different healthcare sectors that have been developed with government and healthcare professional organizations streamline pharmaceutical communication and promotion of pharmaceuticals across the global market place.

REFERENCES

[1] Stiglitz J. Scrooge and intellectual property rights. BMJ 2006;333:1279–80.
[2] Quinn MJ, Goldman E, Nerenberg L, Piazza D. Undue influence: definitions and applications. 2010. Available from: http://www.courts.ca.gov/documents/UndueInfluence. pdf
[3] Callahan D. The WHO definition of health. Hastings Center Studies; 1973:77–87.
[4] Saracci R. The World Health Organization needs to reconsider its definition of health. BMJ 1997;314(7091):1409.
[5] Bircher J. Towards a dynamic definition of health and disease. Med Health Care Philos 2005;8(3):335–41.
[6] World Health Organization. The world health report 2000 – health systems: improving performance. Available from: http://www.who.int/whr/2000/en/ [accessed 20.06.2015].
[7] Competition Bureau – Misleading Advertising Guidelines [Internet]. Available from: http://www.competitionbureau.gc.ca/eic/site/cbbc.nsf/eng/01222.html#a [accessed 20.06.2015].
[8] Norris P., Herxheimer A., Lexchin J., Mansfield P. Drug promotion – what we know, what we have yet to learn. Reviews of materials in the WHO/HAI database on drug promotion.
[9] McGlynn EA, Asch SM, Adams J, Keesey J, Hicks J, DeCristofaro A, Kerr EA. The quality of health care delivered to adults in the United States. N Engl J Med 2003;348(26):2635–45.
[10] Weissman JS, Blumenthal D, Silk AJ, Newman M, Zapert K, Leitman R, Feibelmann S. Physicians report on patient encounters involving direct-to-consumer advertising. Health Aff (Millwood) 2004; Suppl Web Exclusives:W4-219-233.
[11] McKenna C, Chalabi Z, Epstein D, Claxton K. Budgetary policies and available actions: a generalisation of decision rules for allocation and research decisions. J Health Econ 2010;29(1):170–81.
[12] Mackert M, Guadagno MG, Amanda M, Lindsay C. DTC drug advertising ethics: laboratory for medical marketing. Int J Pharm Healthcare Market 2013;7(4):374–90.
[13] Keim SM, Sanders AB, Witzke DB, Dyne P, Fulginiti JW. Beliefs and practices of emergency medicine faculty and residents regarding professional interactions with the biomedical industry. Ann Emerg Med 1993;22(10):1576–81.
[14] Chen HD, Carroll NV. Consumer responses to direct to consumer prescription drug advertising. Int J Pharm Healthcare Market 2007;1(4):276–89.
[15] Van der Heide I, Wang J, Droomers M, Spreeuwenberg P, Rademakers J, Uiters E. The relationship between health, education, and health literacy: results from the Dutch Adult Literacy and Life Skills Survey. J Health Commun 2013;18(Suppl. 1):172–84.
[16] Ashida S, Schafer EJ. Family health information sharing among older adults: reaching more family members. J Comm Genet 2015;6(1):17–27.
[17] Scien HB. Direct-to-consumer drug advertising. Am J Nurs 2015;115(1):11.

[18] Brody H, Light DW. Efforts to undermine public health the inverse benefit law: how drug marketing undermines patient safety and public health. Health Policy Ethics 2011;101(3):399–404.

[19] Francer J, Izquierdo JZ, Music T, Narsai K, Nikidis C, Simmonds H, Woods P. Ethical pharmaceutical promotion and communications worldwide: codes and regulations. Philos Ethics Humanit Med 2014;9:7.

[20] Egilman D, Druar NM. Spin your science into gold: direct to consumer marketing within social media platforms. Work 2012;41(Suppl. 1):4494–502.

[21] US Food and Drug Administration: The Office of Prescription Drug Promotion (OPDP). Available from: http://www.fda.gov/AboutFDA/CentersOffices/Officeof-MedicalProductsandTobacco/CDER/ucm090142.htm [accessed 21.06.2015].

[22] Medicines and Healthcare Products Regulatory Agency: Advertising of medicines. Available from: http://www.mhra.gov.uk/Howweregulate/Medicines/Advertisingof-medicines/index.htm [accessed 21.06.2015].

[23] Smirniotopoulos A. Bad medicine: prescription drugs, preemption, and the potential for a no-fault fix. Rev Law Soc Change 2012;35(4):793–862.

[24] Auton F. Pharmaceuticals and government policy: direct-to-consumer advertising (DTCA) of pharmaceuticals: an updated review of the literature and debate since 2003. Econ Aff 2006;26(3):24–32.

[25] Banerjee S, Dash KS. Effectiveness of disease awareness advertising in emerging economy: views of health care professionals of India. J Med Market 2013;13(4):231–41.

[26] Organization of Pharmaceutical Producers of India: OPPI Code of Pharmaceutical Practices 2012. Mumbai: OPPI; 2012 [http://www.indiaoppi.com] which is closely linked to the IFPMA Code.

[27] Marketing Code Authority of South Africa: Code of Marketing Practice. Available from: http://ipasa.co.za/

[28] China Association of Enterprises with Foreign Investment, R&D-Based Pharmaceutical Association Committee: RDPAC Code of Practice on the Promotion of Pharmaceutical Products. Beijing: RDPAC; 2012. Available from: http://www.ifpma.org/fileadmin/content/About%20us/2%20Members/Associations/Code-China/RD-PAC_Code_of_Practice_2012_print_final_web.pdf

[29] China Food and Drug Regulatory Information Network: Provisions for drug advertisement examination. Available from: http://former.sfda.gov.cn/cmsweb/webportal/W45649037/A48335975.html

[30] Consejo de Ética y Transparencia de la Industria Farmacéutica (CETIFARMA): Codes of the pharmaceutical industry established in Mexico.

[31] IFPMA: Member Association Codes. Available from: http://www.ifpma.org/about-ifpma/members/associations.html [accessed 22.06.2015].

INDEX

A

Abacavir, 233
Abbreviated New Drug Application
(ANDA), 15, 247
Absorption, distribution, metabolism, and
excretion (ADME) profiles,
130, 153
PK studies
human drug toxicity, prediction, 135
relevance of, 133–135
Absorption, distribution, metabolism,
elimination, and toxicity
(ADMET)
properties, 113
proteins, 121
screens, 135
Academic professionals, 64
Acetaminophen (APAP), 252
Acinetobacter baumannii, 45
Act/Enabling Act, 5
Activation, 229
Active pharmaceutical ingredient (API),
19, 170
impurities formation, 174
AD. *See* Alzheimer's disease (AD)
ADME profiles. *See* Absorption,
distribution, metabolism, and
excretion (ADME) profiles
ADRs. *See* Adverse drug reactions (ADRs)
Advancing Regulatory Science Initiative
(ARS), 23
Adverse drug reactions (ADRs), 11,
43, 197
classification of, 203
prone drugs, 202
Adverse effects, 270
Adverse events (AEs), 194
prevention, strategies, 204
AIDS Clinical Trial Group (ACTG), 217
AIDS Medical Foundation (AMF), 212
AIDS therapeutic agent, clinical
development, 212
Aldehyde oxidase (AO), 136

Alzheimer's disease (AD), 39, 46, 48,
159, 235
animal models, 159
brain, 160
Amgen, 66
Amphotericin B, 248
Analgesic signature, 158
ANDA. *See* Abbreviated New Drug
Application (ANDA)
Animal models
of Alzheimer's disease, 159
of cancer, 159
cytochrome P450 (CYP)-mediated drug
metabolism, 155
of depressions, 159
dosage regimen, effect of, 155
genetic modification, effects of, 155
legal accommodations, 161
Canada, 162
Europe, 162
United States, 161
pain cognition/recognition/expression,
154
reduction, 164
refinement, 165
replacement, 163
virtual animals and human models,
164
study results, differences effect, 154
Animal reduction strategies, 164
Animal studies-pharmacology
distribution, metabolism, and
pharmacokinetics (DMPK)
toxicology, 151
objectives, scientific value of, 150–151
Animal taxonomy, implications in
pharmaceutical research, 152–154
Animal toxicity
animal data to humans
extrapolation of, 158
animal species, information, 157
Antimicrobial drug discovery, challenges
case studies, 45

APOE4 gene, 235
ASCI Code, 275
Aspirin, 99
AstraZeneca, 30
Axitinib, 44

B
β_2-andrenergic receptor, 230
Benefit–harm effect, 11, 12
Big pharmas, 30, 90
Biochemical assays, 113
Bioequivalence, 205
Biological assays, 112
Biologic and Genetic Therapies Directorate
        (BGTD), 8
Biomarkers, 39, 132, 199, 227
    clinical trial, evaluation tools, 199
Biomedical informatics platforms, 232
Biopharmaceuticals
    nonhuman primates, animal models in
            development, 161
    organizations, 104
    research & development, 91
Biotechnology-derived products, 161
Biotechnology incubators, 72
Bipolar disease, 46
Blockbuster medicines, 237
Blue Cross Blue Shield plan, 257
Bradykinin, G-protein coupled receptor
        of, 230
Brazil, Russia, India, and China (BRIC)
        economies, 32
Bristol-Myers Squibb's candidate drug, 44
British Pharmacopoeia (BP), 180
Bromfenac, 40
Brookhaven National Laboratory and the
        Defense Advanced Research
        Projects Agency (DARPA), 74

C
Caco-2 cells, 137
CADD. *See* Computer-aided drug design
        (CADD)
Canada and EU Comprehensive Economic
        and Trade Agreement (CETA), 17
Canada Health Act, 261
Canada–United States regulatory
        systems, 18

Canadian Agency for Drugs and
        Technologies in Health
        (CADTH), 261
Canadian Council on Animal Care
        (CCAC), 162
Canadian Innovation Commercialization
        Program, 75
Canadian Institutes of Health Research –
        Personalized Medicine Signature,
        238
Canadian linkage regulations, 17
Cancer disease, animal models, 159
Candidate drugs, part II clinical
        development, 194
Carcinogenicity studies, 151
Carcinogen-induced models, 159
Casablanca, 49
Cash flow, 78
    financially stability, 78
    return on investment, 78
CD-4 lymphocyte, 200
Cell-based assays, 113
Cell culture systems, 135, 139
Cells grown, as monolayers, 136
Cellular disease models, 138
Center for Devices and Radiological
        Health (CDRH), 7
Center for Drug Evaluation and Research
        (CDER), 35, 273
Centers for Therapeutic Innovation
        laboratory, 71
Centre for Biologics Evaluation and
        Research (CBER), 7
Centre for Drug Evaluation and Research
        (CDER), 7
Centre for Drug Research and
        Development, 79
Certificates of Analysis (COA), 22
Chemistry, Manufacturing, and Controls
        (CMC), 197
Chemotherapy drugs cetuximab, 234
Chemotherapy drugs gefitinib, 234
ChemSpider, 36
China's population explosion, 21
Chromosomal reorganization, 152
Class B G-protein-coupled receptors, 112
Clinical and Translational Science Awards
        program, 73

Clinical development pathway, 193
Clinical equipoise, 208
Clinical research organization (CRO), 198
Clinical trial application (CTA), 13
Clinical trial materials (CTM), 175
Clinical trials
  AIDS therapeutic agent, 212
  drug response, 194
  ethical conduct, 207
  evaluation tools, 199
  exploratory trial, 195
  FDA recommendation, 207
  first-in-human testing, 196
  importance of, 193
  integrated phases, 198
  pharmacoeconomics – drug evaluation, 198
  pharmacovigilance, 198
  phases of, 195
  principles and approach, 194
  processes of drug development, 193
  selected topics, 204
    placebo-controlled trials (PCTs), 204
    randomized controlled trials, 204
  study endpoint, 200
    adverse event, 201
      ADRs, classification of, 203
      perspectives, 203
    quality of life, 201
    surrogate endpoint, 200
  therapeutic confirmatory, 197
  therapeutic exploratory, 196
Clinton's health policy, 256
Close-knit interactive framework, 60
Code of Federal Regulations (CFR), 5, 194
Collaborative drug discovery (CDD), 36
Combinatorial chemistry, 124
COMMIT/CCS-2 trial, 216
Committee on Safety of Drugs, 4
Common Drug Review process, 261
Common Technical Document (CTD), 16
Compartmentalization-based applications, 138
Computational chemistry algorithms, 117
Computational tools, 117
Computer-aided drug design (CADD), 116
  approach, 117
  structure-based, 118

Computer simulations, 96
Computer technology, 122
Conflict of interest rules, 210
Consejo de Ética y Transparencia de la Industria Farmacéutica (CETIFARMA), 276
Consumer Directed Broadcast Advertisements for television and radio, 272
Contract research organizations (CROs), 67
Cost-effectiveness requirements, 256
Critical Path Initiative (CPI), 22
Cross-national pharmaceutical price, 256
Crucial cases
  clinical trials, with society implications, 211
  national regulatory authorities, differences, 211
Current Good Manufacturing Practices (cGMP), 47
Cyclosporin, 143
CYP. *See* Cytochrome P450 (CYP)
CYP2A enzymes, 156
CYP3A isoforms, 156
CYP3A4 metabolizes, 140
CYP2C9 analysis, 232
CYP2D6 enzyme, 229
CYP2D6 inhibitor, 141
CYP450 isoenzymes, 205
Cytochrome P450 (CYP), 136
  enzymes, 155–156
  isoenzyme system, 227
  isoforms, 156
Cytotoxicity, 137

D

Data mining, computation platforms, 36
Data reduction, 94
Decision-making process, 13, 236
Depolarizing neuromuscular blocker, 155
Depressions, animal models, 159
Derisking, 78
Direct-to-consumer advertising (DTCA), 6, 267–269
  defined, 268
  government control, 272
    Canada, 274
    developing nations, 275–276
    Europe, 274
    United States, 272

Direct-to-consumer advertising (DTCA)
(*cont.*)
medicine advertising codes. *See*
Prescription medicine advertising
codes
pharmaceutical advertising, ethics/
relevance of, 268–271
2012 IFPMA Code, guiding principles
of, 271
research and development (R&D)
programs, 267
target market profile (TMP), 267
Disease mapping techniques, 96
Disease phenotype, 89
Distribution, metabolism, and
pharmacokinetics (DMPK)
toxicology, 151
Dizziness, 196
DNA-associated biomolecules, 182
Doctor–patient responses, 42
Dose–response evaluation, 44
Drug advertisements, 275
Drug assessment
geographical locations, 256
Canada, 260–263
Europe, 258–260
United States, 256–258
pharmaceutical drug, pricing and
ethics, 263
Drug, benefit-risk profile, 16
Drug/Clinical Trial Authorization
application, 193
Drug development, pitfall in, 65
Drug discovery, 92
complex drug interactions, model of, 96
current challenges, 101
network–system biology, limitations
of, 103
pharmaceutical ecosystem, impact of,
104
setbacks in identification and selection,
101–103
size/capability, effect of, 104
cycle, 64
disease mapping techniques, 96
genome-wide association studies
(GWAS), 97
in pharmacogenomics, 98

extracellular RNA (exRNA)
communication, 91
modern trends, 91
multiple transporters drug targeting, 101
network-based drug discovery, 95
omics technology, 93
definitions, 94
perturbations, in human disease, 86
polypharmacological profiling, 98
for polypharmacology, 100–101
realization of, 192
systems biology, applicability of, 92–93
target-based drug discovery, 88
Drug discovery projects, 104
Drug discovery researchers, 92
Drug–drug interactions, 222, 270
assays, 142
Drug eliminating agents
drug–drug interactions, 141
plasma binding proteins, 142
types of, 141
and mechanisms, 139
metabolizing enzymes–CYPs (P450),
140
assays used, in evaluating drug
metabolism, 140
transporters, 143
UDP-glucuronosyltransferases
(UGTs), 144
Drug interactions, 134
Drug limits human exposure, 195
Drug molecules, 119
Drug-one-target, 98
Drug originators, 255
Drug plan reimbursement, of generic
drugs, 263
Drug pricing/control, 255, 256
geographical locations, 256
Canada, 260–263
Europe, 258–260
United States, 256–258
Drug product lifecycle
clinical development and outcomes, 195
Drug-related toxicity, 233
Drug response, 230
Drug shortages, 179
bulletin, 179
Case II–crystal polymorphism, 181

Case III: genotoxic impurity, 182
Case I inconsistency in drug quality of
     metoprolol ER, 175
categories by therapeutic class, 180
genotoxic impurities, 182
from January 2011 to June 2013, 184
manufacturing problems, 180
     impurities, 180, 181
repetitive cycle in drug manufacturing,
     183
sterility issues, 183
strategies, 184–185
Drug's ligands, 142
Drug Submissions Policy, 15
Drug substance, 170
Drug therapies, 85
Drug toxicity, 157
DTCA. See Direct-to-consumer advertising
     (DTCA)

E

ECDC/EMEA Joint Technical Report, 24
Economic barriers, 217
Economic growth, 36
Electronic Code of Federal Regulations
     (eCFR), 7
Electronic health records (EHR), 231
EMA Benefit–Risk Methodology
     Project, 12
eMolecules, 36
Enterobacter species, 45
Enterococcus faecium, 45
Epigenomics, 95
ESKAPE pathogens, 45
Ethical codes, 192
Ethical conduct
     in clinical trials, 207
          historical perspective, 207
          weighing, benefit/risk ratio, 208
Ethical principles, 208
     clinical equipoise, 208
     clinical professionals, dual role functions
          of, 209
     pharmaceutical drug pricing, 263
Ethical problems, 206
Ethics, clinical trial, 207
Ethnic factors, guideline, 21
Ethyl-methane sulfonate (EMS), 182

EudraLex. See European Drug Regulatory
     Legislation (EudraLex)
European Clinical Trials Directive, 10
European Commission's regulatory
     authority, 17
European Community (EC) system, 9
European Drug Regulatory Legislation
     (EudraLex), 10
European Free Trade Association, 19
European Medicines Agency (EMA), 6, 9,
     183, 193
European Medicines Evaluation Agency
     (EMEA), 10
European Network for Health Technology
     Assessment (EUnetHTA), 260
Exposure–response relationships, 133
exRNA. See Extracellular RNA
     (exRNA)
Extracellular RNA (exRNA)
     communication, 91
     processes, 91

F

Federal Food and Drugs Act, 4
Federal Food, Drug, and Cosmetic Act
     (FD&C Act), 4
Federal Register and the Government
     Printing Office, 7
Federal regulation of drugs, 272
Federal-sponsored subsidiaries, 74
Federal Trade Commission (FTC), 272
Figitumumab, 44
First-in-human clinical trial, 192
Fluoxetine, 251
Food and Drug Regulations (FDR) of
     Canada, 5
Food and Drugs Act, 8
     of Canada, 5
Food and Drug Administration (FDA), 162
     approval process, 60
Formulated capsule, 175
Fruit fly, insect models, 160
Funding models, 74
     Canada, case for, 75
     Canadian financing models, 75
     nongovernment. See Nongovernmental
          funding models
     US financing models, 74

G

Gastrointestinal stromal tumors, 37
Gastrointestinal (GI) tract, 154
GenBank's submission program, 123
Gene expression profiles, 230
Gene manipulation, 85
Genentech, 70
Generally Recognized As Safe, 170
Generic drugs, 262
    drug plan reimbursement, 263
Generic manufacturers
    Brazil, 256
Gene therapy, 85
Gene Therapy Institute of Florida, 70
Genome Project era, 85
Genome-wide association studies (GWAS),
    97, 98
    SNP scanning arrays, 236
Genomics sequencing, 94
Genotoxicity, 182
    assays, 151
Genotype–phenotype associations, 206
Genzyme, 66
Germinal-center B cell-like, 93
GlaxoSmithKline (GSK), 30, 251
    azidothymidine (AZT), 251
Globalization, 18
Global pharmaceutical business
    (GPB), 30
Global pharmaceutical industry-
        harmonization and partnerships, 18
    government regulations, prospects for
        multinational clinical trials, 21
    Pharmaceutical Regulations in Asia, 21
international conference on
    harmonisation
    scope, 19–21
Global pharmaceutical sales, 258
Global pharmaceutical systems,
        modernization, 22
    combating NTDs in Africa, 25
    critical path initiative (CPI), 22
    European Medicines Agency's
        Roadma, 23
    Global Initiatives, 24
    Health Canada
        Progressive Licensing Model
            (PLM), 24
    world health partnerships, 25

GMP. *See* Good manufacturing practice
    (GMP)
Good manufacturing practice (GMP),
    4, 171
    checks, 179
Government intervention, in drug
    discovery, 71
Government investments, 74
Group purchasing organization (GPO)
    members, 184
Gulf Cooperation Council, 20
Gut-on-a-chip, 163
GWAS. *See* Genome-wide association
    studies (GWAS)

H

Harmonization, 18
Hatch-Waxman Act, 16, 247
Headache, 196
Heads of Medicines Agencies, 10
Health Canada (HC), 6, 8, 274
Healthcare Supply Chain Association
    (HSCA), 184
Health technology assessment (HTA), 260
Hepatitis C, 44
Herbalomics, 95
High throughput screening (HTS), 110,
    164
    sound performance, 112
    technology, 137
HIV/AIDS disease, 37, 46
HIV fusion, 100
HIV type-1 (HIV-1), 233
HLA B*5701 allele, 233
HTS. *See* High throughput
    screening (HTS)
Human-based experimental systems, 130
Human disease biology, models, 88
    phenotypic drug discovery, 89–90
    target-based drug discovery, 88–89
Human exploitation, 207
Human Genome Project, 85, 88
Human genome sequencing, 224
Human immunodeficiency virus/acquired
        immunodeficiency syndrome
        (HIV/AIDS), 46
Human leukocyte antigen (HLA), 233
Human pharmacokinetics, 133
Hypertension, 46

I

Immunity, 152
Implementing Genomics in Practice
    (IGNITE) Network, 238
Inappropriate study design, implications
    of, 205
    clinical trials, FDA recommendation, 207
    ethnic disparity, 206
    gender selection, 205
Infectious Diseases Society of America
    (IDSA), 45
Informatics technology, 110
Informed consent, 209
    biomedical research
        institutional conflict of interest, 211
    in clinical research, 210
    interest, primary conflict of, 210
    interest, secondary conflict of, 210
INFRAFRONTIER partners, 162
Innovation failure
    drug repositioning/repurposing, 51
    mergers, acquisitions, and outsourcing, 48
    new avenues of personalized medicine, 51
    pharmaceutical ecosystem, building, 52
    pharmaceutical research and
        development (R&D), 50
    regulatory approach, 47
    strategies/approaches to addressing, 47
Innovation setback, consequence of, 46
Innovative Medicines Initiative (IMI), 79
Insect models, fruit fly, 160
In silico toxicology prediction, 121
Intellectual property (IP), 245
International clinical trials, 215
    across globe, 213
    Canada, clinical trials, 213
    clinical trials in China, 215
    conducting clinical trials, in developing
        countries, 214
    multinational clinical trials, patient
        diagnosis, 216
    zidovudine (AZT) trials in African, 217
International Conference on
        Harmonisation (ICH) guidelines,
        6, 100, 133, 170, 174, 180
    S7A guidelines, 100
International Federation of Pharmaceutical
        Manufacturers and Associations
        (IFPMA) Code, 271

International Federation of Pharmaceutical
        Manufacturers & Associations, 24
International Organization for
        Standardization (ISO), 18
Intracellular-level preclinical evaluation,
        131
Investigational medicinal product dossier
        (IMPD), 13
Investigational new drug (IND), 13, 170
    application, 13
    organism animal models for, 144
Investment decision-making tool, product
        valuation, 59–60
IP/patent laws, 249

K

Kefauver–Harris Amendment, 4
Kefauver–Harris recommendations, 4
Klebsiella pneumoniae, 45
Knowledge-based economy (KBE), 30
Knowledge-based screening, 115

L

Laboratory animals model
    in frontiers of drug discovery, 151–152
Laboratory Animal Welfare Act of 1966,
        154
Legal accommodations
    Canada, animal models, 162
    Europe, animal models, 162
    United States, animal models, 161
Legal instruments, 5
    Act/Enabling Act, 5
    guidelines, 6
    regulations, 5
Lethal diseases, rapidly
    clinical trials, ethical, 212
Lilly-sponsored Phenotypic Drug
        Discovery (PD2), 90
Lipitor, 35
LRRTM3 sequence, 235
Lung-on-a-chip, 163

M

Malaria, 46
Marketing-associated risks, 13
Marketing Authorization (MAA), 15
Marketing Code Authority, 276

Market recalls, 40
Medical milestones of 2014, 37
Medicare, 258
Medicines Act, 276
Mekinist, 51
Metabolic proteins, 86
Metabolic stability, 140
Metabolism, 152
Metabolomics, 95
Methane sulfonic acid (MSA), 182
Methyl methanesulfonate (MMS), 182
Microarray technology, 163
Millennium Development Goals, 37
Ministry of Health, Labour, and Welfare
        (MHLW), 6, 211
Model plasma binding proteins, 142
Molecular Libraries program, 79
Molecular modeling software packages, 118
Monoamine oxidases (MAO), 136
Morocco, 49
mRNA levels, 101
Multicomponent analysis, 93
Multidrug resistance protein 1, 143
Multinational enterprises (MNEs), 70
Mutual Recognition Agreement countries,
        215
Mutual recognition agreements (MRAs), 9
Mutual recognition procedure (MRP), 9
Myriad development activities, preclinical
        development, 129

N
National Cancer Institute, 37
National Center for Advancing
        Translational Sciences (NCATS),
        73
    Strategic Alliances Office, 78
National Institute on Aging Late-Onset
        Alzheimer's Disease (NIALOAD)
        group, 235
National Institutes of Health (NIH), 37, 64,
        91, 237
National Institutes of Pharmaceutical
        Clinical Trials, 215
National regulatory authority (NRA), 6
    European Medicines Agency (EMA), 9
    European Drug Regulatory
        Legislation, 10

FD&C Act, 7
    drug laws, evolution, 8
Food and Drug Administration (FDA),
        6, 7
    Health Canada (HC), 8
    Canadian Food and Drugs Act, 9
    Pharmaceuticals and Medical Devices
        Agency (PMDA, KIKO), 10
    Pharmaceutical Affairs Act of Japan, 11
National Research Council's Industrial
        Research Assistance Program, 75
Nausea, 196
Neglected and tropical diseases (NTDs), 24
    case report, 25
    HIV/AIDS, malaria, and TB, 26
Net present value (NPV), 78
Network analysis, 95
Network-based biological computational
        tools, 114
Network-based drug discovery, 95
Network Target-based Identification of
        Multicomponent Synergy model,
        114
New chemical entity (NCE), 247
New Drug Application (NDA), 4, 174, 194
New drug entity (NDE), 170
New Drug Submission (NDS), 9, 15, 174
NIH-based National Clinical Assessment
        and Treatment Service, 101
Noncommunicable diseases (NCDs), 24
Nongovernmental funding models
    Angel investment, 76
    crowdfunding, 77
    private-angel investment, 76
    private-corporate investment, 77
    public-angel investment, 77
    pharmaceutical companies, 76
    public-venture philanthropy, 76
    venture capital, 76
Nonhuman primates
    animal models in development of
        biopharmaceuticals, 161
Nonprofit organizations, 77
No-observedadverse-effect-level (NOAEL),
        196
North American Free Trade Agreement
        (NAFTA), 17
Not-for-profit organization, 77

Not-for-profit research, 58
Novo Nordisk, 30
NRA. *See* National regulatory authority
    (NRA)
Nucleotide polymerase (NS5B) inhibitor, 44
Number of approvals of new molecular
    entities (NMEs), 32
  blockbuster era, 34

O

Office of Regulatory Affairs (ORA), 7
Olanzapine, 251
Omics technology, 93
One-size-fits-all paradigm, 41
Ontario Drug Benefit (ODB) plan, 263
Ontario government, 263
Open Investment Policy, 30
Optimal medication programs, 261
Oral bioavailability, 133
Oral drugs, 170
Orally ingested drug, *in vitro* screening
    assays, 136
Organization of Pharmaceutical Producers
    of India (OPPI), 275
Organs-on-a-chip, 163
Organ-specific cell, toxicity associated
    with, 136
Outsourcing, 21

P

Panitumumab, 234
Parallel artificial membrane permeation
    assay (PAMPA), 136
Parkinson's disease, 46
Patent Act in 1790, 16
Patent cliff, 34, 43
Patented Medicine Prices Review Board
    (PMPRB), 261
Patent protection, 43
Patents/exclusive marketing rights, 245
  defined, 245
  evergreening, 250–252
  global pharmaceutical market place,
    249–250
  Hatch–Waxman Act of 1984, 247–248
  product lifecycle, 248
  US Patent Law Amendments Act of
    1984, 246–247

Patient-Focused Drug Development
    program, 12
PD. *See* Pharmacodynamics (PD)
Personalized medicines, 51, 226
Pfizer, 35
Pgp–efflux pathway, 143
Pharmaceutical Advertising Advisory Board
    of Canada (PAAB), 274
Pharmaceutical Affairs Act (PAA) of Japan,
    5, 10, 11
Pharmaceutical Affairs Law (PAL), 10
Pharmaceutical Analytical Technology
    initiative, 173
Pharmaceutical and Medical Devices
    Agency (PMDA), 6
Pharmaceutical development, 169
  clinical trials materials, 175
    phase I clinical trial materials, 175
    phase II clinical trial materials, 176
    phase III clinical trial materials, 177
  concepts uses
    active pharmaceutical ingredient
      (API), 177
    chemical synthesis, 178
    critical impurity, 178
    critical process parameter (CPP), 178
    critical quality attribute (CQA), 178
    drug product, 178
    good manufacturing practice (GMP),
      178
    quality assurance, 178
    validation protocol, 178
  drug formulations/public health impact,
    175
    manufacturing quality problems, 175
  drug product specifications, 173
  drug shortages, 179
    Case II–crystal polymorphism, 181
    Case III: genotoxic impurity, 182
    Case I inconsistency in drug quality of
      metoprolol ER, 175
    categories by therapeutic class, 180
    genotoxic impurities, 182
    from January 2011 to June 2013, 184
    manufacturing problems, 180
      impurities, 180, 181
    repetitive cycle in drug manufacturing,
      183

Pharmaceutical development (*cont.*)
  sterility issues, 183
  strategies, 184–185
 formulation and manufacturing, 173
 formulation development, 174
 international conference on
      harmonisation (ICH) technical
      documents, 172
 manufacturing development, 174
 product formulation/manufacturing
      process, 171
 regulatory aspects of, 171
  overview, 171
 safety, efficacy and quality, 172
Pharmaceutical drug pricing, and
      ethics, 263
Pharmaceutical firms, 85
Pharmaceutical innovation, 30
 advances in technology, 36
 evolutionary trends in, 32
  global pharmaceutical discoveries, 32
   changing pharmaceutical
      productivity, 32
 factors contributing to setback, 38
  adverse drug reactions, challenge of, 39
  clinical development challenges, 43
  complex biological systems, 39
  economic strategies, 40
  patent protection, 43
  poor product strategies, 42
  regulatory burden, 45
  research and development (R&D)
      productivity, 38
  risk/return, Valley of Death, 41
 global pharmaceutical business (GPB),
      30, 31
Pharmaceutical market, 21
Pharmaceutical Price Regulation Scheme
      (PPRS), 259
Pharmaceutical product life cycle, 13
 labeling, 17
 modules for drug regulatory
      assessment, 13
  decision point I, 13
  decision point II, 15
  NRA/industry meetings, 15
 patents, 16
Pharmaceutical quality system (PQS), 5, 171

Pharmaceutical regulatory system, 5
 evolution of, 4–5
Pharmaceuticals and Medical Devices
      Agency (PMDA), 10
Pharmaceutical Shared-Risk programs, 69
Pharmaceutical value chain, firms
      involved, 66
 big pharmaceutical industries, 66
 biopharmaceutical industries, 66
 contract research organizations
      (CROs), 67
Pharmacodynamics (PD), 153
 effects, 194
 exposure/response (E/R) relationship of
      drugs, 230
 properties, 130
Pharmacoeconomics analysis, 198
Pharmacogenomics, 95, 98
 profiling, 233
Pharmacogenomics application, economic/
      social implications, 236
 economic considerations, 236
 national regulatory agencies, 237
 penetrance, 236
Pharmacogenomics, clinical
      implementation effectiveness, 230
 addressing adverse drug reactions, 232
 APOE4 gene, 236
 cancer drugs, 234
 in clinical practice, 231
 in clinical trials, 230
 human immunodeficiency virus
      (HIV), 233
 LRRTM3 in Alzheimer's disease, 235
 mental disorders, 235
 Vend, 234
Pharmacogenomics implementation,
      national regulatory agencies, 237
 personalized medicine program-
      University of Florida health, 238
Pharmacogenomics, in drug discovery
 biomarker, 226–227
 genetic and genomic strategies, 223
 genetic variations and implications, 227
  CYP2D6 isoform, 228
  cytochrome P450 (CYP)
      isoenzymes, 227
  pharmacodynamic outcomes, 230

pharmacokinetic outcomes, 229
population stratification, 228
one-size-fits-all approach, to clinical
practice, 226
overview, 222
personalized medicine, 226
pharmacogenetics, 224
polymorphism, 222
single nucleotide polymorphism
(SNP), 223
Pharmacokinetics (PK), 130, 153
Pharmacophore algorithm software
packages, 121
PharmGKB, 238
Phenotypic-centered approach, 90
Philanthropic seed funding, 77
Phosphoproteomics, 95
Physician-driven market, 262
PhysioLab model, 164
Physiologically-based pharmacokinetic
(PBPK) modeling, 153
Pipeline problem, 38
P450 isoform, 141
Placebo-controlled trials (PCTs), 204
Plavix, 35
PoC studies, 71
Point in time, 213
Polymorphism ADR, 224
Polypharmacological approaches, 39,
98–100, 102
Precautionary, 175
Preclinical development
animal models
of Alzheimer's disease, 159
of cancer, 159
of depressions, 159
development of
biopharmaceuticals, 161
insect models
fruit fly, 160
species selection and rationale, 158
Preclinical development, experimental
tools
Caco-2 cells, intestinal absorption studies
models, 137
cell culture systems, advances, 138
integrated microcell culture systems,
139

membrane-based multilayer
microfluidic devices, 139
microwell array technology–cell
function/toxicity assays, 138
three-dimensional cell patterning/
culturing, 139
metabolism/toxicology studies, *in vitro*
systems, 135–137
Preclinical disease models, predictability
of, 130
intracellular-level preclinical
evaluation, 131
trends in, 132
Pregnancy, 205
Prescription Drug User Fee Act
(PDUFA), 47
Prescription medicine advertising
codes, 276
governing the pharmaceutical
companies, 277
national codes of practice, 276
Prescription-only products, 272
Prices re-evaluation, 260
Private-angel investment, 76
Private-public sector groups, 78
Centre for Drug Research and
Development, 79
European Federation for Pharmaceutical
Sciences, 79
Innovative Medicines Initiative (IMI), 79
National Centre for Advancing
Translational Sciences (NCATS),
78
Progressive Licensing Model (PLM), 24
Project-portfolio management strategy, 63
Proof of concept (PoC), 59
Prospective Randomized Evaluation of
DNA Screening in a Clinical
Trial (PREDICT-1) study, 233
Pseudomonas aeruginosa, 45
PubChem, 36
Public health experts, 269
Public-venture philanthropy, 76

Q

Quality by Design (QbD), 172
Quantitative structure-activity relation
(QSAR) models, 118, 119

R

Ranbaxy, 35
Rapid Access Interventional Development
    (RAID), 73
R&D-based Pharmaceutical Association
    Committee (RDPAC), 276
REACH project, 135
Reductionist target-based approach, 92
Reference Member State, 9
Refinement, 165
Regulatory approval-benefit-risk
    assessment
    analytical framework, 11–13
Reproduction, 152
Respiratory symptoms, upper, 196
Return on investment (ROI), 76
Revenue-based ranking, 30
Rheumatoid arthritis, 37
    antibody, 49
Ritonavir, 181
RNA expression profiles, 93
Robotic liquid handlers, 110
Robust biological/biomedical research, 69
Rodents, 152

S

Safety pharmacology, 130, 150
Sanofi, 44
SBIR and Small Business Technology
    Transfer (STTR) program, 73
Schizophrenia, 46
Screening Center Network, 111
Screening tools, in drug discovery
    compound design, iterative process of, 124
    compound optimization, 123–125
    pathway, 125
    drug-like compounds into activity
        criteria, 117
    high throughput screening (HTS), 110
    bioassays, 112
    setbacks in application, 112
    in silico models, 114
    cheminformatics/bioinformatics
        technology, 122–123
    computer-aided drug design (CADD),
        116–118
    drug targeting, pharmacophore models
        of, 120

binding partner, protein recognize,
    121
pharmacophore approaches,
    limitations, 121
structure–activity relationships (SAR),
    118
limitations of, 120
virtual screening, 115–116
Seroquel, 35
Sickle-cell anemia, 85
Signaling proteins, 86
Single nucleotide polymorphism (SNP),
    140, 222
Small Business Innovative Research
    (SBIR), 73
Small molecule therapeutics (SMs), 161
Small-to-medium enterprises (SMEs), 74
SMART funds, 72
Socioeconomic status, 213
Staphylococcus aureus, 45
State Food and Drug Administration
    (SFDA), 21, 215
Sterilization processes, 172
Strange smell, 182
Stroke, 48
Structure–activity relationships (SAR), 118
Structure-based computer-aided drug
    design (SBCADD), 119
Sulfotransferase (SULT) enzymes, 136
Systems biology, 92
    approach, 100

T

Tafinlar, 51
Tailor-to-fit medicine, economic impact
    of, 236
Target-based drug discovery, 88
Target binding site, pharmacophore model
    of, 120
Target Drug Discovery (TD2), 88
Target identification, 88
Target-ligand cocrystal structures, 115
Target market profile (TMP), 267
Target product profile (TPP), 68
Taube-Koret Center (TKC) functions, 72, 77
Tax system, 74
The Technology Strategy Board and
    Technology Transfer Offices, 73

Therapeutic agent, cellular and molecular
       effects of, 150
Therapeutic confirmatory trials, 197
Therapeutic drug monitoring (TDM), 233
Therapeutic Products Directorate (TPD), 8
THxID BRAF mutation test, 51
Toprol XL, 175
Torcetrapib, 44
Toxicity, 151
   associated with organ-specific cell, 136
   profile, 129
Toxicology, 158
Trade Related Aspects of Intellectual
       Property Rights (TRIPS), 17
Trans-Atlantic Task Force on Antimicrobial
       Resistance, 24
Transcriptomics, 95
Translational Research Advisory
       Committee, 37
Tuberculosis, 46

U
UDP-glucuronosyltransferases (UGTs),
       136, 144
Uncertainty principle, 208
United States Code, 246
United States National Center for
       Biotechnology Information, 123
United States Pharmacopoeia (USP), 180
University of Florida (UF) Health
       Personalized Medicine Program,
       238
US Department of Health and Human
       Services, 257
US Food and Drug Administration (FDA),
       170
US National Venture Capital Association, 59

V
Valley of Death
   challenges, 60
      academic discovery/research
         limitations, 64–65
      biotech/small companies, vulnerability
         of, 61–62
      drug discovery, organization
         proportions and impact, 60

      lowest funding stage, key research
         activities, 62–63
      pharmaceutical innovation science,
         unpredictability of, 63
      target selection, 65
         Alzheimer's disease, 65
      contract research services, 67
      drug discovery and development
         progression, 59
      innovation failure, 67
      Path of Cash Flow, 64
      strategies for bridging, 67
         advancing corporate productivity, 69
         addressing investment limitations, 72
         big pharma/biotech company
            partnerships, 69–70
         biotechnology incubators,
            importance of, 72
         communication, 71–72
         industry–academic partnerships,
            70–71
         United Kingdom, 74
         United States, 73
      changing drug discovery landscape, 67
      investment, in discovery science, 69
      product forecasting, importance of, 68
Value-added indicator (VAI), 78
Vanderbilt University Medical Centre
       (VUMC), 232
Venture capital, 76
Verapamil, 143
Veterinary Medicinal Products (VICH), 18
Vioxx withdrawal, 32
Viracept®, 182
Virtual screening (VS), 115
Volume of distribution (VD), 132

W
Warfarin's target, 230
World Health Organization (WHO), 19, 268
World Trade Organization, 18
   TRIPS agreement, 249

Z
Zaltrap, 44
Zebrafish (Danio rerio), 144
   application of, 144

Printed in the United States
By Bookmasters